Video Contents

T0210225

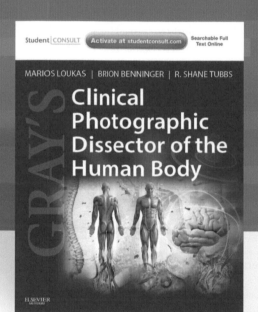

NETTER'S INTRODUCTION TO CLINICAL PROCEDURES

Marios Loukas, MD, PhD
Professor of Anatomical Sciences
Dean of Basic Sciences
School of Medicine
St. George's University
Grenada, West Indies

R. Shane Tubbs, MS, PA-C, PhD
Professor and Chief Scientific Officer
Seattle Science Foundation
Seattle, Washington;
Professor
Department of Anatomical Sciences
St. George's University
Grenada, West Indies

Joseph Feldman, MD, FACEP
Chairman, Emergency Services
Emergency & Trauma Center
Hackensack University Medical Center;
Volunteer Professor
Seton Hall-Hackensack-Meridian School of Medicine
Hackensack, New Jersey;
Professor of Emergency Medicine
St. George's University
Grenada, West Indies;
Clinical Associate Professor of Emergency Medicine
Rutgers School of Medicine
New Brunswick, New Jersey;
Adjunct Clinical Professor of Biomedical Engineering
Department of Chemistry, Chemical Biology, and Biomedical Engineering
Stevens Institute of Technology
Hoboken, New Jersey

Illustrations by **Frank H. Netter**

Contributing Illustrators
Carlos A.G. Machado, MD
Kristen Wienandt Marzejon, MS, MFA

ELSEVIER

ELSEVIER

1600 John F. Kennedy Blvd.
Ste 1800
Philadelphia, PA 19103-2899

NETTER'S INTRODUCTION TO CLINICAL PROCEDURES ISBN: 978-0-323-37055-4
Copyright © 2017 by Elsevier, Inc. All rights reserved.

Notices

Knowledge and best practice in this field are constantly changing. As new research and experience broaden our understanding, changes in research methods, professional practices, or medical treatment may become necessary.

Practitioners and researchers must always rely on their own experience and knowledge in evaluating and using any information, methods, compounds, or experiments described herein. In using such information or methods they should be mindful of their own safety and the safety of others, including parties for whom they have a professional responsibility.

With respect to any drug or pharmaceutical products identified, readers are advised to check the most current information provided (i) on procedures featured or (ii) by the manufacturer of each product to be administered, to verify the recommended dose or formula, the method and duration of administration, and contraindications. It is the responsibility of practitioners, relying on their own experience and knowledge of their patients, to make diagnoses, to determine dosages and the best treatment for each individual patient, and to take all appropriate safety precautions.

To the fullest extent of the law, neither the Publisher nor the authors, contributors, or editors, assume any liability for any injury and/or damage to persons or property as a matter of products liability, negligence or otherwise, or from any use or operation of any methods, products, instructions, or ideas contained in the material herein.

Library of Congress Cataloging-in-Publication Data

Names: Loukas, Marios, author. | Tubbs, R. Shane, author. | Feldman, Joseph,
    1955- , author. | Netter, Frank H. (Frank Henry), 1906-1991, illustrator.
    | Machado, Carlos A. G., illustrator. | Marzejon, Kristen Wienandt,
    illustrator.
Title: Netter's introduction to clinical procedures / Marios Loukas, R. Shane Tubbs, Joseph Feldman;
illustrations by Frank H. Netter ; contributing illustrators, Carlos A.G. Machado, Kristen Wienandt Marzejon.
Other titles: Introduction to clinical procedures
Description: Philadelphia, PA : Elsevier, [2017] | Includes bibliographical references and index.
Identifiers: LCCN 2016013126 | ISBN 9780323370554 (pbk. : alk. paper)
Subjects: | MESH: Clinical Medicine | Diagnostic Techniques and Procedures
Classification: LCC RC46 | NLM WB 102 | DDC 616--dc23
LC record available at http://lccn.loc.gov/2016013126

Executive Content Strategist: Elyse O'Grady
Senior Content Development Specialist: Marybeth Thiel
Publishing Services Manager: Patricia Tannian
Senior Project Manager: Carrie Stetz
Design Direction: Amy Buxton

Printed in Mexico

Last digit is the print number: 9 8 7 6 5 4 3

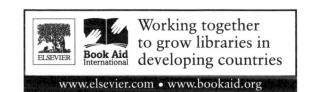

To my children, Nikol and Chris, for their kindness and endless support for my long hours of writing and research. I love you guys.

Marios Loukas

To Kaye and Ronald Raines; thank you for your understanding and support.

R. Shane Tubbs

To the teachers who have taught me and the students I have taught and will yet teach.

Joseph Feldman

About the Editors

Marios Loukas, MD, PhD, received his medical degree from Warsaw University School of Medicine, and a PhD from the Institute of Rheumatology at the Department of Pathology in Warsaw, Poland. He held a postdoctoral position at Ulm University Clinic in Germany and studied arteriogenesis.

Dr. Loukas began his academic career at Harvard Medical School, where he served as lecturer and laboratory instructor for the Human Body Course. In 2005, he joined St. George's University in Grenada and shortly after became Professor and Chair of the Department of Anatomical Sciences. Under his leadership, the Department of Anatomical Sciences developed a unique division of Ultrasound in Medical Education that instructs faculty members in how to teach the use and interpretation of ultrasound to medical students and residents and how to provide effective continuing medical education (CME) courses.

In 2012, Dr. Loukas was appointed Dean of Research for the School of Medicine at St. George's University. One of his main responsibilities is to develop a transdisciplinary research infrastructure to support translational research and to bridge basic science and clinical departments with the aim of enhancing student research.

Dr. Loukas' research has been continuously funded from St. George's University. He has been the recipient of numerous teaching and research awards, such as the 2007 Herbert M. Stauffer Award from the Association of University Radiologists and the Harvard Excellence in Tutoring Award from Harvard Medical School.

Dr. Loukas has published more than 600 papers in peer-reviewed journals, authored 12 books, including *Gray's Anatomy Review, Gray's Clinical Photographic Dissector of the Human Body, McMinn and Abrahams' Clinical Atlas of Human Anatomy, History of Anatomy,* and *Bergman's Comprehensive Textbook of Human Variation* and has authored 18 chapters in various medical and surgical textbooks, including *Gray's Anatomy.* He has also served as an editor and co-editor for 12 journals and reviewer for more than 50 journals. He is Co-Editor of the journal *Clinical Anatomy* and the Editor-in-Chief of the journal *Translational Research in Anatomy.* With this background, Dr. Loukas has been able to provide his medical knowledge in the anatomical sciences to a larger audience and in 2015 was elected President of the American Association of Clinical Anatomists. His scientific interests include surgical anatomy and techniques and cardiovascular pathology. Recently, his focus has been directed toward issues of integrated curriculum and faculty development in medical education with an emphasis on simulation and technology and effective teaching and testing. In February 2015, Dr. Loukas was named Dean of Basic Sciences at St. George's University School of Medicine.

R. Shane Tubbs, MS, PA-C, PhD, is a Professor of Anatomy and Chief Scientific Officer at the Seattle Science Foundation in Seattle, Washington. He has dedicated his career to the study and teaching of clinical anatomy. Dr. Tubbs has authored many books and papers in the anatomical sciences and is the Editor-in-Chief of the journal *Clinical Anatomy.* He is also an editor for works such as *Netter's Atlas of Anatomy,* fifth through seventh editions, *Gray's Anatomy,* 41st edition, and *Gray's Clinical Photographic Dissector of the Human Body.*

Joseph Feldman, MD, FACEP, has been with Hackensack-UMC since 1998, where he is an Attending Physician and Chairman of Emergency Medicine and Chairman of Emergency Medicine at HackensackUMC at Pascack Valley. Prior to coming to HackensackUMC, Dr. Feldman was the Assistant Director of Emergency Services at Columbia Presbyterian Medical Center. Dr. Feldman received two BS degrees from Stony Brook University prior to attending St. George University School of Medicine, where he obtained his medical degree. He completed his Emergency Medicine Residency at The Brooklyn Hospital Center and is board certified in Emergency Medicine. Dr. Feldman is a Fellow in the American College of Emergency Physicians.

Dr. Feldman holds academic appointments as Volunteer Professor at Seton Hall-Hackensack-Meridian School of Medicine, Professor of Emergency Medicine at St. George's University School of Medicine, Clinical Associate Professor of Emergency Medicine at the New Jersey Medical School at Rutgers University, and Adjunct Clinical Professor of Biomedical Engineering at Stevens Institute of Technology.

Dr. Feldman's scope of responsibility at HackensackUMC includes Emergency Medicine, Observational Services, Prehospital Care, and Disaster Preparedness, including the Mobile Satellite Emergency Department Program. He serves as the Medical Director of the Chest Pain Center, Director of Medical Education of the St. George's/HackensackUMC medical student program, Chairman of the ETC service line, and Chairman of the Forms and Order Set Committee, in addition to being a member of numerous other major hospital committees.

Dr. Feldman leads his department in quality and service excellence. The ETC has been the proud recipient of the Press Ganey Success Story, the Studer Group What is Right in Health Care Award, twice the recipient of the J.D. Powers Award for Outstanding Experience in Emergency Services, and also twice the recipient of the Health Grades Emergency Medicine Excellence Award. He has been a consultant of the Studer Organization on Physician Leadership and has served on the Press Ganey Physician Advisory Board. He was instrumental in creating the department's award-winning Take-a-Break Program and was honored by the Planetree Organization as the recipient of its Physician Champion Award for this program. He has also been the recipient of the Physician of the Year Award by the New Jersey State Society of Physician Assistants and received the Medal of Merit for his years of dedication and service to St. George's University School of Medicine.

Dr. Feldman has extensive research project management experience on a wide range of conditions and has made numerous contributions to the Emergency Medicine literature. He has administered executive oversight of a multi-million-dollar grant to develop a prototype of a rapidly deployable Mobile Satellite Emergency Department and several novel research projects for the Department of Defense. He has been the principal or sub-investigator for 25 research projects, has made numerous original contributions in referred journals, and has been invited to present both internationally and nationally over 60 times on various topics in health care. He has an extensive biography of speaking in the print, audio, and video media on a variety of medical topics.

Dr. Feldman is dedicated to developing educational programs that would benefit undergraduates interested in a career in medicine. To that end he is responsible for creating the HackensackUMC Careers in Medicine (CIM) program. CIM is a summer program that gives college students the ability to shadow health care providers. He also runs the National Alliance of Research Associates Program (NARAP), a program that allows college students to participate in clinical research year round. For undergraduate medical education, Dr. Feldman is director of St. George's/Hackensack School of Medicine for third- and fourth-year medical students. For graduate education, he has successfully implemented a 3-year ACGME for 12 residents per year at the Emergency Medicine Residency at HackensackUMC.

Dr. Feldman has made multiple contributions to the emergency medicine community at large for New Jersey in the way of disaster preparedness, education, and leadership. Through his leadership, the Mobile Satellite Emergency Department (MSED) has been successfully licensed in New Jersey as a Satellite Emergency Department and has been embedded as a Special Unit within the New Jersey EMS Task Force. He led five MSED deployments during Hurricane Sandy supporting efforts in northern and southern New Jersey, and an EMAC deployment to Long Beach Island, New York. Most recently the MSED was deployed prior to and during the Super Bowl.

Dr. Feldman lives in New York City with his wife, Julie; Jette, their playful German shepherd; and Sassy, their miniature poodle. In addition to his myriad contributions toward improving the practice of medicine for health care professionals, patients, and caregivers, in his free time Dr. Feldman participates in foundations that support higher education for New York City youth and organizations that promote global health initiatives.

About the Artists

Frank H. Netter, MD

Frank H. Netter was born in 1906 in New York City. He studied art at the Art Student's League and the National Academy of Design before entering medical school at New York University, where he received his MD degree in 1931. During his student years, Dr. Netter's notebook sketches attracted the attention of the medical faculty and other physicians, allowing him to augment his income by illustrating articles and textbooks. He continued illustrating as a sideline after establishing a surgical practice in 1933, but he ultimately opted to give up his practice in favor of a full-time commitment to art. After service in the United States Army during World War II, Dr. Netter began his long collaboration with the CIBA Pharmaceutical Company (now Novartis Pharmaceuticals). This 45-year partnership resulted in the production of the extraordinary collection of medical art so familiar to physicians and other medical professionals worldwide.

In 2005, Elsevier, Inc. purchased the Netter Collection and all publications from Icon Learning Systems. There are now over 50 publications featuring the art of Dr. Netter available through Elsevier, Inc. (in the US: www.us.elsevierhealth.com/Netter and outside the US: www.elsevierhealth.com).

Dr. Netter's works are among the finest examples of the use of illustration in the teaching of medical concepts. The 13-book *Netter Collection of Medical Illustrations*, which includes the greater part of the more than 20,000 paintings created by Dr. Netter, became and remains one of the most famous medical works ever published. *The Netter Atlas of Human Anatomy*, first published in 1989, presents the anatomical paintings from the Netter Collection. Now translated into 16 languages, it is the anatomy atlas of choice among medical and health professions students the world over.

The Netter illustrations are appreciated not only for their aesthetic qualities, but, more importantly, for their intellectual content. As Dr. Netter wrote in 1949, ". . . clarification of a subject is the aim and goal of illustration. No matter how beautifully painted, how delicately and subtly rendered a subject may be, it is of little value as a *medical illustration* if it does not serve to make clear some medical point." Dr. Netter's planning, conception, point of view, and approach are what inform his paintings and what make them so intellectually valuable.

Frank H. Netter, MD, physician and artist, died in 1991.

Learn more about the physician-artist whose work has inspired the Netter Reference collection: http://www.netterimages.com/artist/netter.htm.

Carlos Machado, MD

Carlos Machado was chosen by Novartis to be Dr. Netter's successor. He continues to be the main artist who contributes to the Netter collection of medical illustrations.

Self-taught in medical illustration, cardiologist Carlos Machado has contributed meticulous updates to some of Dr. Netter's original plates and has created many paintings of his own in the style of Netter as an extension of the Netter collection. Dr. Machado's photorealistic expertise and his keen insight into the physician-patient relationship inform his vivid and unforgettable visual style. His dedication to researching each topic and subject he paints places him among the premier medical illustrators at work today.

Learn more about his background and see more of his art at: http://www.netterimages.com/artist/machado.htm.

Kristen Wienandt Marzejon, MS, MFA

Kristen Wienandt Marzejon is a certified medical illustrator with a master's degree from the University of Illinois at Chicago's Biomedical Visualization graduate program. Her passion for both art and science from an early age makes her perfectly suited to this gratifying profession. She started her career as a staff illustrator at Rush University Medical Center in Chicago, then committed to self-employed status in 2001. She offers medical illustration and graphic design services to a variety of clients in the medical arena.

The work of Frank Netter has been a valuable part of Kristen's medical library throughout her 20-year career. She is honored to continue the Netter tradition by producing work authentic to his distinctive style.

Preface

Trainees in medicine and health-related professions are faced with learning a multitude of procedures, many of which can be invasive but are lifesaving. With a significant workload and the stressful environment that urgent situations hold, the intricate and multiple steps involved in many of these invasive procedures can be a challenge to master. The goal of this book is to provide the salient maneuvers of key clinical procedures in an easy, step-by-step format. The authors have gathered many of the most common clinical procedures that medical practitioners encounter in daily clinical scenarios or emergency settings.

This essential handbook combines clinical techniques with anatomical details illustrated with the dynamic imagery for which the Netter medical art legacy is known. It will certainly be a go-to reference for physicians, health care professionals, and students alike. Topics run the gamut from central venous catheterization to ingrown toenail removal. Other procedures covered in this text include thoracentesis, endotracheal intubation, reduction of dislocated joints, urinary bladder catheterization, skin abscess incision and drainage, digital nerve block, aspiration of joints, and nosebleed cauterization. In addition, each chapter contains several multiple-choice questions designed to facilitate student review in preparation for the USMLE and similar qualifying examinations.

Of note, certain procedures described in this book have been replaced in some parts of the world by newer procedures that are less risky and more sensitive and specific. However, these newer procedures require adjunct technologies and equipment (eg, ultrasound) that may not be available in all practice settings.

It is the hope of the authors that the reader will garner sufficient background and procedural information from each chapter to feel confident in performing these medical techniques safely and expeditiously after sufficient supervised training has occurred.

Editors and Contributors

EDITORS

Marios Loukas, MD, PhD
Professor of Anatomical Sciences
Dean of Basic Sciences
School of Medicine
St. George's University
Grenada, West Indies

R. Shane Tubbs, MS, PA-C, PhD
Professor and Chief Scientific Officer
Seattle Science Foundation
Seattle, Washington;
Professor
Department of Anatomical Sciences
St. George's University
Grenada, West Indies

Joseph Feldman, MD, FACEP
Chairman, Emergency Services
Emergency & Trauma Center
Hackensack University Medical Center
Hackensack, New Jersey

IMAGING AND VIDEO CONTRIBUTORS

Svetlana Zakharchenko, DO, RDMS
Director, Emergency Ultrasound
Hackensack University Medical Center
Hackensack, New Jersey
*Endotracheal Intubation, Thoracentesis, Expanded Focused
    Assessment With Sonography for Trauma (E-FAST)
    Examination, Central Venous Catheterization, Peripheral
    Intravenous Cannulation, Dislocated Shoulder Reduction,
    Abdominal Paracentesis, Elbow Joint Aspiration,
    Skin Abscess Incision and Drainage, Transurethral
    (Foley Catheter) and Suprapubic Urinary Bladder
    Catheterization; Videos 10.1 and 10.19*

Ellen J. Kurkowski, DO
Assistant Program Director
Emergency Medicine Residency
Associate Ultrasound Director
Emergency Trauma Department
Hackensack University Medical Center
Hackensack, New Jersey
*Videos 10.2, 10.3, 10.5, 10.6, 10.7, 10.9, 10.10, 10.11, 10.13,
    10.15, 10.17, and 10.19*

CONTRIBUTORS

Rebecca G. Andall, MD
Foundation Year 1 Doctor
NHS Tayside
Scotland, United Kingdom
Intercostal Nerve Block, Dental Nerve Blocks

Naomi R. Andall, MD
Foundation Year 1 Doctor
NHS Tayside
Scotland, United Kingdom
Cardiac Pacing, Digital Nerve Block

Weston G. Andrews, BS
Fourth Year Medical Student
Department of Anatomical Sciences
St. George's University School of Medicine
Grenada, West Indies
Tracheostomy, Tracheotomy, Cricothyroidotomy

Karan K. Arora
MD Candidate (2018)
Department of Anatomical Sciences
St. George's University School of Medicine
Grenada, West Indies
Ingrown Toenail Removal

Aparna Ashok, M.Eng
Medical Student Researcher (MSRI)
Department of Anatomical Sciences
St. George's University School of Medicine
Grenada, West Indies
Ingrown Toenail Removal, Thoracentesis

Jason C. Batey
MD Candidate (2017)
Department of Anatomical Sciences
St. George's University School of Medicine
Grenada, West Indies
*Intercostal Nerve Block, Abdominal Paracentesis, Nasogastric
    Tube Placement*

Claudine Brown, MD, MSPH
Pediatric Resident
Department of Pediatrics
Maimonides Medical Center
Brooklyn, New York
*Cerumen Removal, Burr Hole Craniotomy, Tracheostomy,
    Tracheotomy, Cricothyroidotomy*

Karolina Bukala
MD Candidate (2017)
Department of Anatomical Sciences
St. George's University School of Medicine
Grenada, West Indies
Intercostal Nerve Block

Alper Cesmebasi, MD, MSc
Intern
Division of Urology
St. Elizabeth's Medical Center
Brighton, Massachusetts
*Fasciotomy, Central Venous Catheterization, Thoracostomy,
    Expanded Focused Assessment With Sonography for
    Trauma (E-FAST) Examination, Lumbar Puncture,
    Peripheral Arterial Line Placement, Venous Cutdown,
    Transurethral (Foley Catheter) and Suprapubic Urinary
    Bladder Catheterization*

Daniel H. Chang, MS
MD Candidate
Medical Student III
St. George's University School of Medicine
Grenada, West Indies
Occipital Nerve block

Bradley Charran, MD
Department of Anatomical Sciences
St. George's University School of Medicine
Grenada, West Indies
Diagnostic Peritoneal Lavage, Venous Cutdown

Kaydeonne T. Ellis, MD
Intern
Internal Medicine
The General Hospital
Grenada, West Indies
*Skin Abscess Incision and Drainage, Dislocated Finger
    Reduction*

Jason A. Fisher, MS
MD Candidate
Department of Anatomical Sciences
St. George's University School of Medicine
Grenada, West Indies
Peripheral Intravenous Cannulation

Abigail Gabriel, MD
Department of Internal Medicine
Harlem Hospital
New York, New York
Intercostal Nerve Block

Sadia Ghani, MD
Psychiatry Resident
Department of Psychiatry
University of Arizona College of Medicine, South Campus
Tucson, Arizona
*Nasogastric Tube Placement, Transurethral (Foley Catheter)
    and Suprapubic Urinary Bladder Catheterization*

Rattandeep K. Ghotra, BS
Medical Student III
St. George's University School of Medicine
Grenada, West Indies
Endotracheal Intubation

Dylan J. Goodrich, BS
MD Candidate (2017)
Department of Anatomical Sciences
St. George's University School of Medicine
Grenada, West Indies
Burr Hole Craniotomy

Munawar Hayat, MD
Resident, Family Medicine
University of Texas Southwestern Medical Center
Dallas, Texas
*Dislocated Shoulder Joint Reduction, Tracheostomy,
    Tracheotomy, Cricothyroidotomy*

Taryn Elizabeth Hoffman, BS
MD Candidate (2017)
St. George's University
Grenada, West Indies
Nasogastric Tube Placement

Nikhil A. Jain
MD Candidate (2018)
Department of Anatomical Sciences
St. George's University School of Medicine
Grenada, West Indies
Ingrown Toenail Removal, Thoracentesis

Shamfa C. Joseph, MD
Department of Internal Medicine
Lincoln Medical and Mental Center
Bronx, New York
Abdominal Paracentesis

Aaron Kangas-Dick, MD
Fourth Year Medical Student
Department of Anatomical Sciences
St. George's University School of Medicine
Grenada, West Indies
Peripheral Arterial Line Placement

Farah Z. Kassamali
MD Candidate (2017)
St. George's University School of Medicine
Grenada, West Indies
Dislocated Shoulder Reduction

Akbar Khan, MD
Department of Pediatrics
SUNY Downstate Medical Center
Brooklyn, New York
*Ear and Nose Foreign Body Removal, Endotracheal
    Intubation*

Sung Deuk Kim, MD
Teaching Fellow
Department of Anatomical Sciences
St. George's University School of Medicine
Grenada, West Indies
*Auricular Hematoma Drainage, Peripheral Arterial Line
    Placement*

Vijay Krishna, MD, MSc
Resident Physician
Department of Family Medicine
MidMichigan Medical Center, Midland
University of Michigan Health System
Midland, Michigan
*Thoracostomy, Elbow Joint Aspiration, Dislocated Knee
    Reduction, Knee Joint Aspiration*

Precious Macauley, MD
Resident Physician
Department of Internal Medicine
Maimonides Medical Center
Brooklyn, New York
Cardioversion and Defibrillation, Abdominal Paracentesis

Adenieki Mornan, MD, MPH
Resident Physician
Department of Women's Medicine, Obstetrics and
    Gynecology
Atlantic Health System
Morristown, New Jersey
Introduction, Dislocated Shoulder Joint Reduction

Julie-Vanessa Munoz, MD
Instructor
Office of the Dean of Basic Sciences
St. George's University School of Medicine
Grenada, West Indies
Digital Nerve Block, Paronychia Incision and Drainage

Sonya Palathumpat, MD
Department of Pediatrics
University of Nevada School of Medicine
Las Vegas, Nevada
Dislocated Shoulder Joint Reduction

Dipen Patel, MD
Department of Anatomical Sciences
St. George's University School of Medicine
Grenada, West Indies
Nosebleed Cauterization, Lumbar Puncture

Jay V. Patel, MD
Critical Care Fellow
Division of Critical Care Medicine
Montefiore Medical Center/Albert Einstein College of
    Medicine
Bronx, New York
*Cardiac Pacing, Cardioversion and Defibrillation,
    Pericardiocentesis*

Kush Patel, MD
Department of Anatomical Sciences
St. George's University School of Medicine
Grenada, West Indies
*Expanded Focused Assessment With Sonography for Trauma
    (E-FAST) Examination, Dislocated Hip Reduction*

Sanjay Patel, MD, MSc
Resident Physician
Department of Medicine
University of Pittsburgh Medical Center
Mercy Hospital
Pittsburgh, Pennsylvania
*Fasciotomy, Central Venous Catheterization, Peripheral
    Intravenous Cannulation, Paronychia Incision and
    Drainage, Thoracentesis*

Swetal Dilip Patel, MD
Department of Internal Medicine
University of Nevada School of Medicine
Las Vegas, Nevada
*Cardiac Pacing, Cardioversion and Defibrillation,
    Pericardiocentesis*

Varun P. Patel, MD
Associate Chief Resident
New York Medical College
St. Michael's Medical Center
Newark, New Jersey
Cardiac Pacing, Cardioversion, and Defibrillation

Malika V. Rawal, MD
Teaching Fellow
Department of Anatomical Sciences
St. George's University School of Medicine
Grenada, West Indies
Occipital Nerve Block, Mask Ventilation

Azizul Rehman, MD
Internal Medicine Resident Physician
Maimonides Medical Center
Brooklyn, New York
Pericardiocentesis

Philip A. Ribeiro, MD
Internal Medicine Resident
Department of Internal Medicine
University of Nevada School of Medicine
Las Vegas, Nevada
Burr Hole Craniotomy

Mahmoud Sabha, MD
Resident Physician
Department of Family Medicine
University of Texas Southwestern Medical Center
Dallas, Texas
Pericardiocentesis, Shoulder Joint Aspiration

Sarah Uddin, MD
Resident Physician
Rutgers Robert Wood-Johnson
Centrastate Family Medicine Residency Program
Freehold, New Jersey
Nosebleed Cauterization

Reviewers

Hamed Abdolghafoorian
Bilawal Ahmed
Shehzad Amlani
Karina Angouw
Adinda K. Apriliani
Deren Aygin
Shreya Badhrinarayanan
Christopher B. Baker
Emalina Balasoglu
Joener B. Bangero
Carlos E. Barba
Tyler S. Beveridge
Usman Bhatti
Kaitlyn Marie Blackburn
Brandon Bodie
Gonçalo Borges
Michael Brisson
Dewey Brooke
Zhen Cahilog
Rhonda Carney
Bekim A. Cela
Alex J. Charboneau
YS Chen
Laura Cicani
Ryan Clark
Sam Cochran
Natasha Daniels
Taylor Davies
Nafi Mehmet Dilaver
Repetchi Dionisie
Darcelle DuBois
Larry L. Duenk
Faustine Dufka
Erin Duralde
Alexander Panayotou Ennes
Gregory M. Erb
Muhammed Said Erdem
Adam Fambiatos
Lisa Ferrando
Francis Fortin

Helene Fourie
Jameelah Franklin
Dariimaa Ganbat
Jose Angel Valdez Garcia
José Manuel Zúñiga García
Martha Luisa Figueroa
   Garcia
Lauren Garth
Andrew R. Ghaly
Alexandra Gol-Chambers
Joseph Gomes
Patricia Téllez González
Natalie Greco
Mr. Michalis Hadjiandreou
Emily Hagar
Randolph D. Haire
Guy P. Hamilton
Sara Seife Hassen
Stephanie Hawks
Georgina Highton
Sherri A. Hinchey
Stephanie Anne Hinds
Adriane Hines
P. Barrett Honeycutt
Craig Hricz
Warren Huang
Moudi Hubeishy
Cameron M. Ingram
Aaron Inouye
Courtney Jaket
Tolbert Dewayne Jefferies
Benjamen Jones
Hayden R. Jones
Viktorija Kaminskaite
Alan Klee
Matthew Krinock
Matthew Krzywicki
Gemma Therese Law
Caitlin M. Lawes
Natalia Soriano Lorié

Melodie M. Lowe
Zachary Lyon
Kamil M.
Precious Macauley
Ankita Mahajan
Hugh J. Malligan
Yobanny Kafruni Marcano
Livingston Martin
Maria Eduarda P.F. Martins
Amber McClure
Ramona Mittal
Eunice Monge
Sean Moran
Catherine Motosko
Nandita Natasha Naidu
Gemma Napaul
Nishchey Nayar
Ory S. Newman
Ann Margareth Wagner
   Nitsch
Eberechukwu G. Njoku
Caryl Joy C. Obaña
Abimbola Ogunseyila
Alain Garcia Olea
Philip Ong
Boingeanu Otniel
Deborah Pacik
Hollie Parfitt
Erika Paschal
Emma Pearson
D. Alexander Phillips
Alexandra Pires-Ménard
Kristian Rainge-Campbell
Joshua G. Ramsay
Charles Randolph
Nazanin Rassa
Craig Stuart Richmond
Megan Rogahn
Aurielle E. Rowe
Seena Saberi-Movahed

Sarah Sabir
Julienne Rowelie A. Sanchez
Andrea Lizeth Tarazona
   Santos
Danielle N. Sarlo
Dhruv Sarwal
Jelmer Savelkoel
Matthew R. Shane
Leung, Ka Shing
Jordan Shively
Naama H. Sleiman
Jessica Zarathena Smeaton
Valerie Smith
Jehu Strange
Brandon Stretton
Louisa Sutton
Benjamin Switzer
Zachary Szablewski
Alexis Tchaconas
Stella Thambirajah
Jeffrey D. Tompson
Tuyet Hong Tran
Tae Kyu Uhm
Raymond VanHam
Blessy Varughese
Matthew Verheyden
Tobias Vinycomb
Marta Costoya Viqueira
Gloria Z. Wang
Ow Kok Weng
Christopher Wike
Brent Wilson
Alex Wisbeck
Jennifer Woodard
Loo Li Yang
Mohammad Zaidi
Chen Zhang
Andrew J. Zovath

Chapters by Anatomic Region

Contents

Introduction

Health care professionals, especially emergency physicians, are expected to perform a wide range of procedures with competence and confidence. This book serves as a general guide for the emergency physician by addressing many common emergency procedures in terms of indications, contraindications, procedural techniques, and complications. In other words, this book outlines the basic standards and conditions under which these procedures should be performed. In addition, the salient anatomy necessary for performing each of the described procedures is reviewed and illustrated in each chapter.

The emergency department represents one of the most complex paradigms in medical care because there are many medical conditions whose successful outcome relies on the emergency physician quickly assessing and rectifying the problem (Fig. I.1). Even considering the fast pace of this medical discipline, certain principles, such as informed consent, time-out procedures, aseptic techniques, personal protection, and avoidance of needlestick injury, need to be followed despite the emergent nature of the patient complaints and the time sensitivity of certain medical procedures.

INFORMED CONSENT

It is generally accepted that informed consent is waived in an emergent setting because the time spent on obtaining informed consent might lead to a detrimental outcome for the patient. There are many emergent conditions that fall into this category, such as patients presenting unconscious or with altered consciousness, patients with minor injuries requiring immediate medical attention, or patients in cardiopulmonary arrest. However, in cases that are urgent but not emergent, verbal explanation of the procedure and obtaining verbal consent when a written one is not practical is considered sufficient. In such cases, the emergency physician must provide sufficient information in a timely manner. It is in these situations that chart documentation is very important in order to describe what occurred and what was said and done during this critical period.

Before attempting a procedure, it is imperative that the emergency physician has sufficient background knowledge regarding the procedure and a familiarity with the equipment and that the equipment is checked and found to be in good working order.

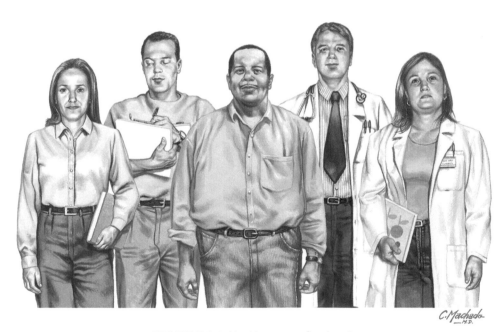

FIGURE I.1 Health care professionals

PERSONAL PROTECTION, UNIVERSAL PRECAUTIONS, NEEDLESTICK AVOIDANCE, ASEPTIC TECHNIQUES, TIME OUT

Even in emergent situations, donning of appropriate personal protective equipment, handwashing, and the use of aseptic techniques should always be followed. Good hand hygiene has been deemed the single most important preventive measure that directly correlates with the incidence of health care–associated infections.

Another vital consideration is the avoidance of needlestick or sharps injury. In many of the procedures discussed in this book, sharps are involved; hence there is a risk of injury. Following a proper technique is by far the best risk reduction strategy for avoiding a needlestick injury. When they do occur, the injured provider should promptly obtain postexposure prophylaxis.

Some general guidelines to prevent a needlestick injury include the following:

- Discard the needle and syringe as a single unit
- Do not resheathe needles
- Do not carry used sharps or give them to someone else to carry
- Do not overfill sharps containers

Time Out

A time out should always be performed prior to a procedure, including marking and identifying the site when applicable. A time out allows correct identification of the patient, verification of the procedure, and confirmation of the site where the procedure will be performed.

This text clearly describes emergency procedures, reviews their indications and contraindications, reviews the relevant anatomy and images, describes the equipment used, and outlines how to perform the procedure. The procedures outlined are the armamentarium an emergency physician needs to facilitate a positive outcome for a patient. These outlines are intended to improve patient care by promoting the performance of procedures with proficiency and timeliness.

Suggested Readings

Nutbeam T, Daniels R. *ABC of Practical Procedures*. Hoboken, NJ: Wiley-Blackwell; 2010.

Hartman KM, Liang BA. Exceptions to informed consent in emergency medicine. *Hosp Physician*. 1999:53–59.

Hazinski MF, Nolan JP, Billi JE, et al. 2010 International consensus on cardiopulmonary resuscitation and emergency cardiovascular care science with treatment recommendations. *Circulation*. 2010;122:S250–S275.

Endotracheal Intubation

INTRODUCTION

The emergency department requires quick thinking and immediate action. Clinical scenarios presented here are often a matter of life and death. One important skill that an emergency department physician should be an expert in executing is airway management. It is essential to secure the airway because without a functional airway, other efforts to save the patient will be futile.

Endotracheal intubation is the preferred procedure in the emergency department for stabilizing a patient with a compromised airway or an inability to adequately ventilate on his or her own. Rapid sequence intubation (RSI) utilizing a fiberoptic laryngoscope has become the gold standard method of intubation. Before implementing RSI, preoxygenation is necessary to ensure that the patient will not desaturate during the time it takes to perform intubation. Once the patient is preoxygenated, the medications used during RSI, such as neuromuscular blocking agents and sedatives, are simultaneously administered to facilitate intubation.

The medical provider should be able to determine both when it is appropriate to intubate and when it is not necessary. One must be able to identify a difficult airway and approach it in the most appropriate way possible. On occasion, a patient who is unconscious or apneic due to cardiac arrest may require a "crash intubation" to be performed without the use of RSI. There will also be clinical scenarios in which intubation is not possible, and the patient will need to be oxygenated and ventilated via bag-valve-mask (BVM) ventilation until airway intervention is no longer needed or a definitive airway can be established. Fiberoptic laryngoscopes have become standard equipment, especially in situations with a difficult airway. These fiberoptic scopes have dramatically improved the chances of success in establishing difficult airways on a "first-pass attempt." In addition, other ventilation methods, including continuous positive airway pressure (CPAP) and bilevel positive airway pressure (BiPAP), are now being utilized for patients who may traditionally have required intubation (eg, for congestive heart failure [CHF], chronic obstructive pulmonary disease [COPD], or asthma), thus avoiding an invasive procedure.

CLINICALLY RELEVANT ANATOMY

The trachea begins at the level of the cricoid cartilage and extends to the carina (Figs. 1.1 and 1.2). Its average length is 11.8 cm (range, 10–13 cm), which varies with the patient's height. It is composed of 18 to 22 cartilaginous rings that may be incomplete or bifid. On the body surface, the level of the carina of the trachea corresponds to the sternal angle or the fifth thoracic vertebra (T5).

Anatomically, the right main stem bronchus is more vertical compared with the left, which is more horizontal with respect to the trachea. The right main stem bronchus is therefore more prone to intubation if the endotracheal tube is inserted too far. In pediatric patients, the subcarinal angle between the bronchi is much wider, with the bronchi lying more transversely. The trachea generally has a larger diameter in males than in females, requiring a larger size endotracheal tube. Individuals who have a small physique or who are obese have a shorter trachea with a narrower diameter. In adults the airway is narrowest at the vocal cords, whereas in small children the narrowest point is at the cricoid cartilage.

To intubate an individual, the endotracheal tube must pass through the pharynx, a muscular tube situated immediately posterior to the nasal and oral cavities and ending superior to the esophagus. The pharynx can be divided into three parts: the nasopharynx, oropharynx, and laryngopharynx (or hypopharynx). The epiglottis, located at the base of the tongue, separates the larynx from the laryngopharynx. It prevents aspiration during swallowing by covering the opening of the larynx (glottis). The larynx, like the trachea, is composed of cartilage, but it also contains connecting ligaments and muscles, which delineate the upper airway from the lower airway. The glottis divides the larynx into a superior compartment, from the laryngeal outlet to the vocal cords, and an inferior compartment, from the vocal cords to the lower border of the cricoid cartilage. This will eventually lead into the trachea.

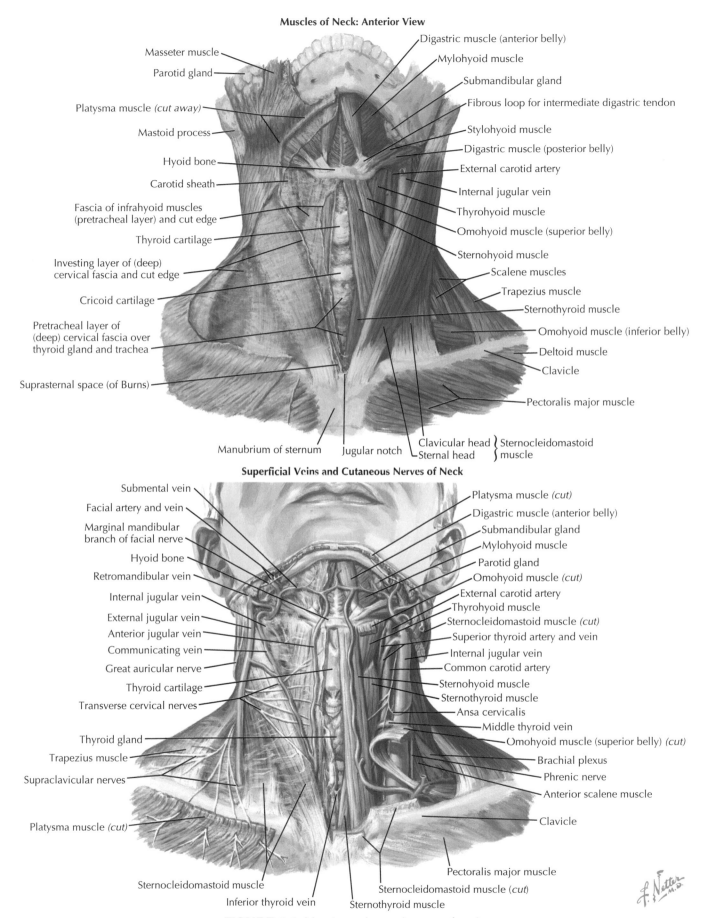

Muscles of Neck: Anterior View

Masseter muscle

Parotid gland

Platysma muscle *(cut away)*

Mastoid process

Hyoid bone

Carotid sheath

Fascia of infrahyoid muscles (pretracheal layer) and cut edge

Thyroid cartilage

Investing layer of (deep) cervical fascia and cut edge

Cricoid cartilage

Pretracheal layer of (deep) cervical fascia over thyroid gland and trachea

Suprasternal space (of Burns)

Digastric muscle (anterior belly)

Mylohyoid muscle

Submandibular gland

Fibrous loop for intermediate digastric tendon

Stylohyoid muscle

Digastric muscle (posterior belly)

External carotid artery

Internal jugular vein

Thyrohyoid muscle

Omohyoid muscle (superior belly)

Sternohyoid muscle

Scalene muscles

Trapezius muscle

Sternothyroid muscle

Omohyoid muscle (inferior belly)

Deltoid muscle

Clavicle

Pectoralis major muscle

Manubrium of sternum   Jugular notch   Clavicular head } Sternocleidomastoid
                                          Sternal head } muscle

Superficial Veins and Cutaneous Nerves of Neck

Submental vein

Facial artery and vein

Marginal mandibular branch of facial nerve

Hyoid bone

Retromandibular vein

Internal jugular vein

External jugular vein

Anterior jugular vein

Communicating vein

Great auricular nerve

Thyroid cartilage

Transverse cervical nerves

Thyroid gland

Trapezius muscle

Supraclavicular nerves

Platysma muscle *(cut)*

Sternocleidomastoid muscle

Inferior thyroid vein   Sternothyroid muscle

Platysma muscle *(cut)*

Digastric muscle (anterior belly)

Submandibular gland

Mylohyoid muscle

Parotid gland

Omohyoid muscle *(cut)*

External carotid artery

Thyrohyoid muscle

Sternocleidomastoid muscle *(cut)*

Superior thyroid artery and vein

Internal jugular vein

Common carotid artery

Sternohyoid muscle

Sternothyroid muscle

Ansa cervicalis

Middle thyroid vein

Omohyoid muscle (superior belly) *(cut)*

Brachial plexus

Phrenic nerve

Anterior scalene muscle

Clavicle

Pectoralis major muscle

Sternocleidomastoid muscle *(cut)*

FIGURE 1.1 Muscles, veins, and nerves of neck

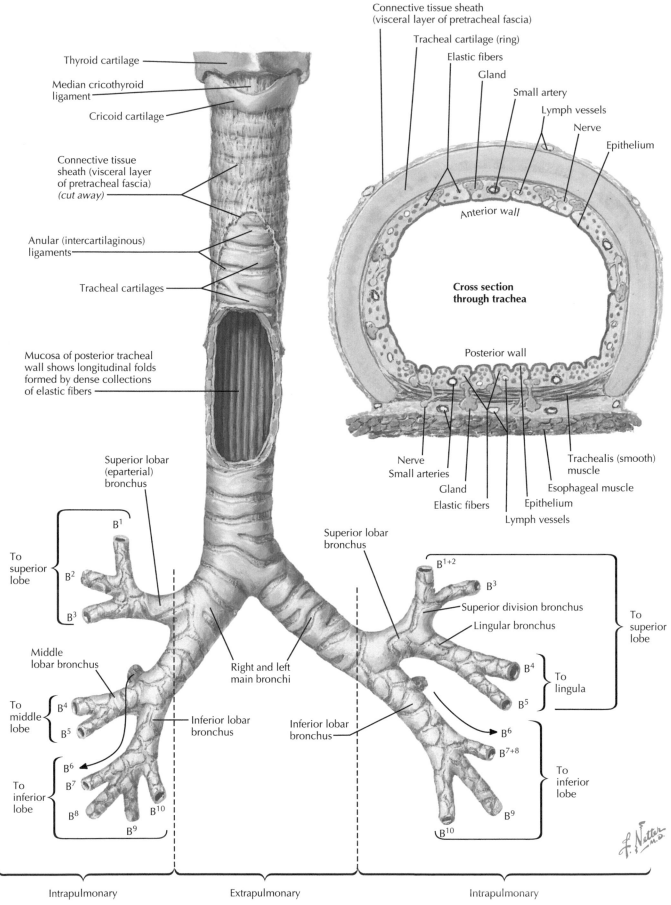

Thyroid cartilage

Median cricothyroid ligament

Cricoid cartilage

Connective tissue sheath (visceral layer of pretracheal fascia) *(cut away)*

Anular (intercartilaginous) ligaments

Tracheal cartilages

Mucosa of posterior tracheal wall shows longitudinal folds formed by dense collections of elastic fibers

Connective tissue sheath (visceral layer of pretracheal fascia)

Tracheal cartilage (ring)

Elastic fibers

Gland

Small artery

Lymph vessels

Nerve

Epithelium

Anterior wall

Cross section through trachea

Posterior wall

Nerve

Small arteries

Gland

Elastic fibers

Trachealis (smooth) muscle

Esophageal muscle

Epithelium

Lymph vessels

Superior lobar (eparterial) bronchus

To superior lobe

B^1

B^2

B^3

Middle lobar bronchus

To middle lobe

B^4

B^5

To inferior lobe

B^6

B^7

B^8

B^9

B^{10}

Right and left main bronchi

Inferior lobar bronchus

Superior lobar bronchus

B^{1+2}

B^3

Superior division bronchus

Lingular bronchus

To superior lobe

B^4

B^5

To lingula

Inferior lobar bronchus

B^6

B^{7+8}

B^9

B^{10}

To inferior lobe

Intrapulmonary

Extrapulmonary

Intrapulmonary

FIGURE 1.2 Trachea and major bronchi

INDICATIONS

The standard procedure for emergency airway management is endotracheal intubation using the RSI method. The decision to intubate should be determined by particular signs presented by the patient and careful assessment. Sometimes it is obvious, such as when a patient presents to the emergency department with severe injuries; at other times, it may not seem likely that intubation is needed because the patient seems to be responding well to treatment.

Indications for the insertion of an endotracheal tube in an emergency situation include cardiac arrest, acute respiratory insufficiency or failure, inability to protect the airway, and expected deterioration of the airway due to an evolving clinical situation (eg, inhalation burn, trauma with an expanding hematoma, and epiglottitis).

Respiratory failure can be indicated by the lack of airway patency, increased threat of aspiration, decreased ventilation, inability to oxygenate the blood, and the possibility of an acute injury eventually compromising the patency of the airway. Therefore, when assessing a patient before intubation, consider the following questions:

1. Is there failure of airway maintenance or protection?
   - If a patient can clearly speak and is alert and oriented, it signifies that the airway is patent and that the patient is ventilating well.
   - Inability to swallow or absence of a gag reflex suggests that the anatomical protective mechanisms are not intact, and thus intubation is required.
2. Is there failure of oxygenation or ventilation?
   - A restless and agitated patient is most likely hypoxic.
   - An obtunded, somnolent patient is most likely hypercapnic. Accumulation of CO_2 results in respiratory acidosis and affects the patient's mental status.
3. Is there an anticipated need for intubation?
   - Acutely injured patients may be awake and alert at first, but the progression of injuries could eventually hinder the airway. Consequently, early airway management can prevent a future crash airway (see below).

However, before taking any steps to stabilize the patient, be aware of his or her wishes, if possible, regarding resuscitation and extreme measures to save life.

CONTRAINDICATIONS

There are certain situations in which endotracheal intubation should be avoided. Endotracheal RSI can have absolute or relative contraindications. Absolute contraindications include when there is total upper airway obstruction or the loss of oropharyngeal landmarks, most commonly due to trauma or burns. When pathology exists at the glottis or supraglottis, endotracheal tube placement may be prohibited. Trauma by the laryngoscope blade could tear the trachea or create a false lumen. In all of these situations, an airway should be surgically established.

Difficult Airway

A difficult airway is present when intubation is unsuccessful due to facemask ventilation or problems with laryngoscopy or intubation, and it can be assessed using the LEMON rule. When dealing with a difficult airway, use a fiberoptic laryngoscope if available, which can greatly help overcome these anatomical or situational issues (eg, for a patient in a hard collar whose neck cannot be manipulated).

LEMON Rule

L: Look externally for abnormal anatomy/body habitus/facies.

E: Evaluate using the 3-3-2 rule.
   3: open mouth sufficiently to place three fingers between the incisors to determine the ease of access into the airway.
   3: place three fingers under the mandible to determine the degree of submandibular space.
   2: place two fingers in the superior laryngeal notch to locate the larynx in reference to the base of the tongue.

M: Mallampati classification: used to determine the ease with which intubation can take place on a scale of I to IV, with class I being relatively easy and class IV being difficult. This classification assesses the amount of oral/pharyngeal anatomy visible on inspection with the patient's mouth open.

O: Obstruction/obesity: intubation in patients with upper airway obstruction or who are obese tends to be difficult due to an obscured view of the glottis.

N: Neck mobility: an immobile cervical spine (eg, from cervical degenerative disease) prevents a proper view of the larynx, or the patient may be in a hard neck collar due to trauma and the neck must not be manipulated.

EQUIPMENT

Stylets

Laryngoscope (fiberoptic if available). Blade size and type are based on the body structure and size of the patient's jaw.

Endotracheal tube. Tube size is based on age, sex, and body structure. For pediatric patients, there are formulas to help to determine tube size.

Suction source and Yankauer suction catheter

Syringe, 10 mL

CO_2 detector

Ambu bag and mask

Pulse oximeter

Cricoid pressure assistant (optional)

Ventilator

Oxygen source

Nasal cannula

Nonrebreather mask

Lubricant

Tape or attachment device for the endotracheal tube

PROCEDURE

Obtain patient consent and perform a time out. See Fig. 1.3 and Video 1.1.

Rapid Sequence Intubation

Before the procedure is started, make sure all equipment is present and in good working order. This includes having the patient on a monitor with a pulse oximeter in place, and ensuring that the light source is working in the laryngoscope, there is an oxygen and suction source with a Yankauer suction catheter, the balloon in the endotracheal tube inflates, and a ventilator is available.

1. Preoxygenate with 100% oxygen via a nonrebreather mask or BVM ventilation (if the patient's ability to ventilate is compromised) for 2 to 3 minutes. Apneic oxygenation is a new method for delivering even more oxygen to the patient by administering 6 L of oxygen via a nasal cannula, in addition to using a nonrebreather mask. This creates a supersaturated oxygenation status, which allows more time to medicate and intubate before the patient will desaturate.
2. Premedicate the patient.
   - Etomidate is used as a short-acting anesthetic and sedative agent.
   - Succinylcholine is a short-acting paralytic.
   - Propofol should be started after intubation is completed as a long-term sedative agent.
3. Apply cricoid pressure (Sellick's maneuver) after the onset of deep sedation to occlude the esophagus and prevent passive regurgitation. Begin bag-valve-mask (BVM) ventilation (optional since this maneuver is falling out of favor).
4. Prepare the patient by removing dental appliances such as dentures and assess for loose teeth.
5. Elevate the patient's head by approximately 5 to 7 cm. Flex the neck (if the clinical situation allows it and if not using a fiberoptic laryngoscope) and extend the head to align the oral, pharyngeal, and laryngeal axes.
6. Open the patient's mouth with the right hand and hold the laryngoscope in the left hand. Insert the blade in the right side of the mouth, displacing the tongue to the left. (If using a fiberoptic scope, the procedure will differ depending on the type and brand of equipment used.)
7. Move the blade in a sweeping fashion toward the midline, and advance it to the base of the tongue.
8. Simultaneously move the lower lip away from the blade with the index finger. Be gentle and avoid applying pressure on the lips and teeth.

9. If using a curved blade, advance the tip into the vallecula. If using a straight blade, insert the tip under the epiglottis.
10. Expose the glottis opening by exerting upward traction on the handle. Point and firmly lift the end of the handle at an angle of 30 to 45 degrees above and toward the patient's feet. This creates a "sniffing" position. DO NOT use a prying motion, and do not use the upper teeth as a fulcrum.
11. Keep the vocal cords under direct vision and advance the lubricated tube from the right side of the mouth through the cords.
12. Continue inserting the tube until the cuff appears and completely passes through the cords.
13. Advance the tube approximately 1.25 to 2.5 cm into the trachea, corresponding to the 19- to 23-cm depth markings on the tube.
14. Remove the stylet if used.
15. Inflate the cuff with air, approximately 10 to 20 mL.
16. Confirm tube placement with a combination of physical examination (visualization of chest rising and 5-point auscultation to see if there are equal breath sounds), esophageal detector device, capnometry, and chest radiography.
17. Secure the tube with tape or a commercial tube holder. Frequently monitor the position of the tube.

Crash Airway Intubation for Cardiorespiratory Arrest

The term "crash airway" describes the airway in patients who are unresponsive, with no airway protective reflexes and without effective respiration or circulation. The steps of endotracheal intubation are part of the secondary survey. Patients with crash airways require chest compressions and positive-pressure ventilation before and after endotracheal intubation. When endotracheal intubation is performed for the crash airway, some intubation steps are modified based on the clinical situation.

ANATOMICAL PITFALLS

The trachea and esophagus share a common upper chamber, the pharynx. Because of this close anatomical relationship, there is a possibility of intubating the esophagus. However, as the esophagus is posterior to the trachea and is a muscular tube, anterior cricoid cartilage pressure can seal off the entrance to the esophagus and thus aid in the correct positioning of the endotracheal tube into the trachea. The right main stem bronchus is often intubated if the tube is advanced too far, owing to anatomical alignment with the trachea.

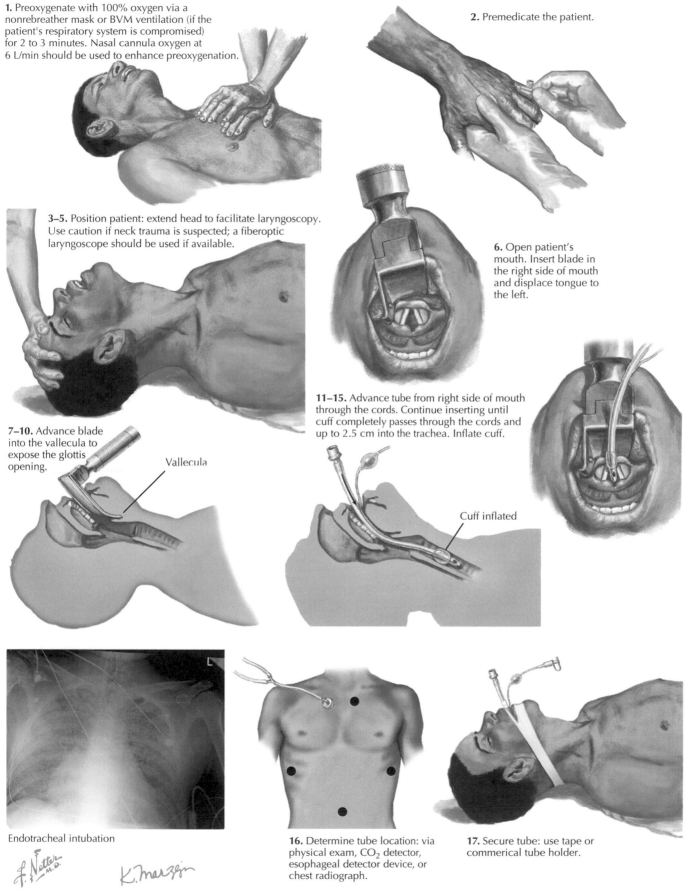

1. Preoxygenate with 100% oxygen via a nonrebreather mask or BVM ventilation (if the patient's respiratory system is compromised) for 2 to 3 minutes. Nasal cannula oxygen at 6 L/min should be used to enhance preoxygenation.

2. Premedicate the patient.

3–5. Position patient: extend head to facilitate laryngoscopy. Use caution if neck trauma is suspected; a fiberoptic laryngoscope should be used if available.

6. Open patient's mouth. Insert blade in the right side of mouth and displace tongue to the left.

7–10. Advance blade into the vallecula to expose the glottis opening.

Vallecula

11–15. Advance tube from right side of mouth through the cords. Continue inserting until cuff completely passes through the cords and up to 2.5 cm into the trachea. Inflate cuff.

Cuff inflated

Endotracheal intubation

16. Determine tube location: via physical exam, CO_2 detector, esophageal detector device, or chest radiograph.

17. Secure tube: use tape or commerical tube holder.

FIGURE 1.3 Endotracheal intubation: crash airway intubation for cardiorespiratory arrest

COMPLICATIONS

Endotracheal intubation usually takes places during high-risk situations. Training and a comprehensive understanding of the procedure will almost always lead to a successful intubation. However, there are instances in which a successful intubation is not achieved within the initial attempts.

The most common complication of endotracheal intubation is right main stem bronchial intubation, which simply requires an adjustment of the tube, usually by withdrawing it 2 to 3 cm. There have been many documented cases of esophageal intubation resulting in aspiration of gastric contents, requiring reintubation.

Laryngeal injuries can occur if there is trauma to the trachea during intubation. The use of a large endotracheal tube, aspiration of gastric contents, or not using muscle relaxant drugs can lead to injury, which may result in hoarseness, laryngeal edema, mucosal ulceration, vocal cord paralysis, swallowing impairment, sinusitis, and even respiratory failure upon extubation. Other complications such as pneumothorax, dental and soft tissue trauma, esophageal perforation, postintubation pneumonia, hypotension or hypertension, and aspiration can also occur as a result of intubation. In addition, laryngospasm or bronchospasm has been documented in many patients with asthma, COPD, or respiratory infection.

CONCLUSION

Endotracheal intubation is a complex procedure that requires training. It is used in a variety of emergent clinical situations. It is a life-saving procedure that creates a secure, definitive airway and allows for appropriate ventilation.

Suggested Readings

Field JM, Kudenchuk PJ, O'Connor R, VandenHoek T. *The Textbook of Emergency Cardiovascular Care and CPR*. Philadelphia: Lippincott Williams & Wilkins; 2012:273–294.

Gavel G, Walker W. Laryngospasm in anesthesia. *Contin Educ Anaesth Crit Care Pain*. 2013;14:47–51.

Grillo HC. *Surgery of the Trachea and Bronchi*. Ontario: BC Decker Inc; 2004:39–161.

Mosier JM, Whitmore SP, Bloom JW, et al. Video laryngoscopy improves intubation success and reduces esophageal intubations compared to direct laryngoscopy in the medical intensive care unit. *Crit Care*. 2013;17:R237.

Polansky M. Airway Management: The Basics Of Endotracheal Intubation. *Internet J Academic Physician Assist*. 1996;1:1–6.

Sellick BA. Cricoid pressure to control regurgitation of stomach contents during induction of anesthesia. *Lancet*. 1961;2:404–406.

REVIEW QUESTIONS

1. A 22-year-old man is admitted to the emergency department and is intubated. An endotracheal tube is passed through an opening between the vocal folds. What is the name of this opening?

   A. Piriform recess
   B. Vestibule
   C. Ventricle
   D. Vallecula
   E. Rima glottidis

2. If the endotracheal tube was advanced too far it would intubate the:

   A. Left main stem bronchus
   B. Esophagus
   C. Right main stem bronchus
   D. Right middle lobe of the lung
   E. Retropharyngeal space

3. All of the following are ways to check the placement of the endotracheal tube except:

   A. 2-point auscultation of the lung
   B. Capnometry
   C. Esophageal detector device
   D. Chest radiograph

Intercostal Nerve Block

INTRODUCTION

Analgesia of the chest and abdominal walls can be safely achieved through intercostal nerve blockade, a common technique first described by Braun in 1907. Intercostal nerve blocks (INBs) can be administered with a low incidence of infection, bleeding, or aspiration, little to no bladder and bowel dysfunction, and early mobilization. This is particularly useful for thoracic and abdominal surgical procedures, acute and chronic pain syndromes, and the treatment of traumatic chest wall injuries. Alternative methods, such as the use of oral analgesics, are of limited value because of the shorter duration of pain relief. A typical INB provides pain relief for 8 to 18 hours, especially if long-acting analgesics are used. Compared with general analgesia, regional nerve analgesia is associated with lower incidences of postoperative pneumonia, prolonged ventilatory support, and unplanned postoperative intubation, especially in surgical patients with chronic obstructive pulmonary disease.

The pain from rib fractures can cause respiratory compromise. Therefore INBs are indicated for patients with rib fractures or other chest wall trauma, as well as for those with preexisting respiratory disease, to minimize the complications of respiratory failure, atelectasis, and infection. Although ultrasound is not widely used for this purpose currently, improvements in INB administration have been achieved using ultrasound-guided techniques. The overlying rib casts an acoustic shadow, which prevents the direct visualization of the intercostal neurovascular structures. Despite this, ultrasound is useful for identifying the pleura–chest wall interface, which can minimize the incidence of pneumothorax and lung puncture.

CLINICALLY RELEVANT ANATOMY

The thoracic wall is made up of an osteocartilaginous cage that provides attachments for the intercostal muscles, which assist in active respiration and provide protection for the thoracic viscera (Fig. 2.1A). The head and neck of each rib articulate with the thoracic vertebrae posteriorly. The curved, flat body of the rib houses the intercostal neurovascular bundles in a groove along its inferior surface (Fig. 2.2). Intercostal nerves are derived from the ventral rami of the first 11 thoracic spinal nerves and travel within the plane between the internal and innermost intercostal muscles to give off cutaneous and muscular branches that innervate the thoracic and upper abdominal body walls (see Fig. 2.1B). In the bundle, the nerves lie inferiorly to the intercostal veins and arteries. Intercostal nerves arise from the somatic nervous system; therefore compression or irritation of these nerves due to chest wall trauma causes sharp, localized pain.

INDICATIONS

Major indications for INB include rib fractures, chest injuries, and flail chest as well as chronic pain syndromes (eg, postmastectomy, postthoracotomy, scar related), cancer pain, and postherpetic neuralgia.

CONTRAINDICATIONS

Contraindications to INB include hypersensitivity or allergy to anesthetic solutions, uncooperative patients (with confusion or altered mental state), bleeding or clotting disorders, anticoagulant therapy, and local or severe systemic infection.

EQUIPMENT

Ultrasound machine, if available
Sterile gloves, mask, and marking pen
Antiseptic solution
Sterile towels and gauze
20-mL sterile syringe and local anesthetic
38-mm, 22-gauge needle attached to extension tubing for intercostal local anesthetic injection
5- or 10-mL sterile syringe with 25- or 30-gauge needle for local anesthetic subcutaneous infiltration

A. Bony Framework of Thorax

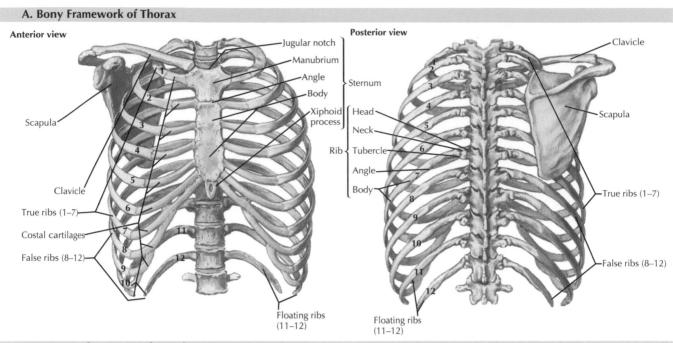

B. Intercostal Nerves and Arteries

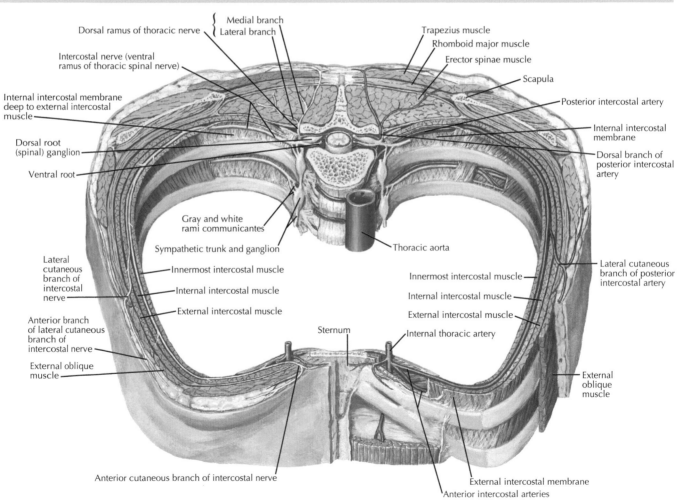

FIGURE 2.1 A, Bony framework of thorax. **B,** Intercostal nerves and arteries.

Spinal cord and ventral rami in situ

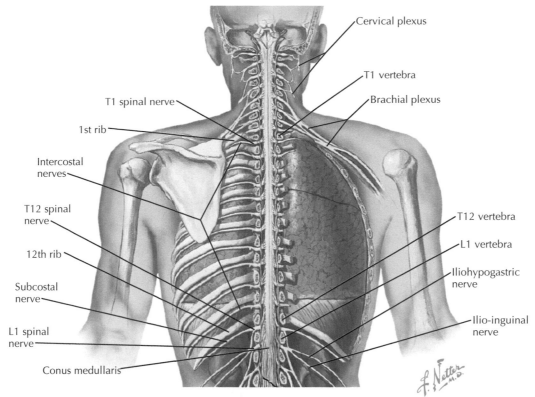

Cervical plexus

T1 vertebra

Brachial plexus

T1 spinal nerve

1st rib

Intercostal nerves

T12 spinal nerve

12th rib

Subcostal nerve

L1 spinal nerve

Conus medullaris

T12 vertebra

L1 vertebra

Iliohypogastric nerve

Ilio-inguinal nerve

Nerves of anterior abdominal wall

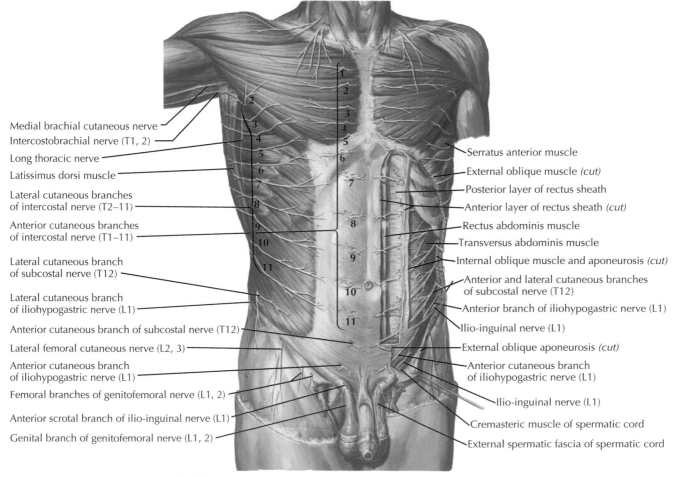

Medial brachial cutaneous nerve

Intercostobrachial nerve (T1, 2)

Long thoracic nerve

Latissimus dorsi muscle

Lateral cutaneous branches of intercostal nerve (T2–11)

Anterior cutaneous branches of intercostal nerve (T1–11)

Lateral cutaneous branch of subcostal nerve (T12)

Lateral cutaneous branch of iliohypogastric nerve (L1)

Anterior cutaneous branch of subcostal nerve (T12)

Lateral femoral cutaneous nerve (L2, 3)

Anterior cutaneous branch of iliohypogastric nerve (L1)

Femoral branches of genitofemoral nerve (L1, 2)

Anterior scrotal branch of ilio-inguinal nerve (L1)

Genital branch of genitofemoral nerve (L1, 2)

Serratus anterior muscle

External oblique muscle (cut)

Posterior layer of rectus sheath

Anterior layer of rectus sheath (cut)

Rectus abdominis muscle

Transversus abdominis muscle

Internal oblique muscle and aponeurosis (cut)

Anterior and lateral cutaneous branches of subcostal nerve (T12)

Anterior branch of iliohypogastric nerve (L1)

Ilio-inguinal nerve (L1)

External oblique aponeurosis (cut)

Anterior cutaneous branch of iliohypogastric nerve (L1)

Ilio-inguinal nerve (L1)

Cremasteric muscle of spermatic cord

External spermatic fascia of spermatic cord

FIGURE 2.2 Spinal cord and nerves of anterior abdominal wall

PROCEDURE

Obtain patient consent and perform a time out.

1. The patient is positioned in the seated, lateral decubitus, or prone position with the arms extended forward or hanging down the sides of the bed to rotate the scapula laterally out of the way (Fig. 2.3). If ultrasound is going to be used:
   - Use a linear (procedural) high-frequency probe. For patients with a body mass index of over 30 kg/m^2, use a curvilinear (abdominal) low-frequency probe.
   - To determine the proper intercostal space, place the probe perpendicular to the area that requires analgesia. Slide the probe caudad/cephalad and once again visualize the intercostal spaces. The shadow-free spaces represent the desired space. Continue by prepping the patient using sterile technique. The provider should wear appropriate personal protective equipment.
2. If ultrasound is not available for localization of the injection site, the inferior border of the appropriate rib is palpated and marked at the mid-posterior axillary line. An "X" is placed at the angle of the rib, denoting the injection site.
3. The area is sterilized with antiseptic solution, and 1 to 2 mL of local anesthetic is subcutaneously administered at the injection site.
4. An index finger is used to retract the skin over the rib.
5. A 38-mm, 22-gauge needle attached to a 10-mL syringe by extension tubing is inserted into the marked injection site at an 80-degree angle to the skin. The needle is advanced until the rib is met.
6. Retraction of the skin is discontinued, and the needle is then "walked off" the rib and advanced 3 mm below the inferior border.
7. Aspirate. If no blood, proceed.
8. If the aspirate is void of blood, other bodily fluid, or air, 2 to 5 mL of the local anesthetic agent is gradually injected.
9. If indicated, the procedure is repeated to achieve nerve blockade for other thoracic segments.
10. The patient should be observed for 20 to 30 minutes following the INB for any complications.

ANATOMICAL PITFALLS

An infraclavicular brachial plexus block may be required to supplement analgesia of the upper chest wall (Fig. 2.4). Achieving analgesia of the upper six thoracic levels is difficult

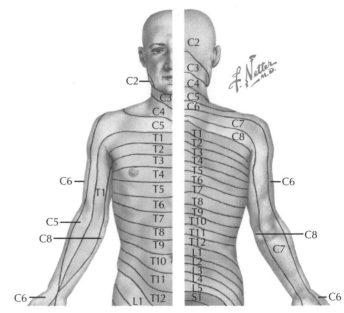

FIGURE 2.4 Dermatomes above the waist

because of the location of the scapula and the overlying muscles. Intercostal nerves do not typically innervate structures across the midline; thus bilateral blockade may be necessary. Furthermore, INB is challenging to administer to patients with a difficult anatomy (eg, morbid obesity or scoliosis).

Posteriorly, only a thin intercostal fascia separates the intercostal nerve from the parietal pleura and lungs; therefore administering INB in this position can result in pneumothorax or lung puncture. In addition, the intercostal nerve lies just inferior to the intercostal vein and artery, which explains the potential high plasma levels of local anesthetic caused by INBs, which can lead to anesthetic toxicity.

COMPLICATIONS

Complications of INB include pneumothorax, hemothorax, anesthetic toxicity, bleeding, subcapsular liver hematoma, nerve damage, infection, and abscess formation.

CONCLUSION

An INB is a highly effective and fairly simple procedure that is useful in minimizing the amount of general anesthesia required for thoracic and abdominal procedures and in managing postoperative rib fracture pain. Complications are few and can be minimized with an appropriate knowledge of the regional anatomy and the use of ultrasound guidance.

1. Place patient in chosen position.

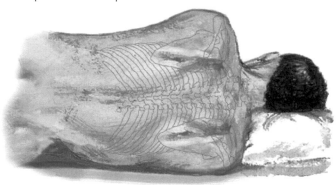

2. Palpate the inferior border of the appropriate rib and mark an X at the angle of the rib, the injection site.

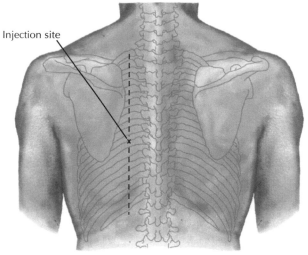

Injection site

3. Sterilize and anesthetize the area to be injected.

4. Retract skin over rib using index finger.

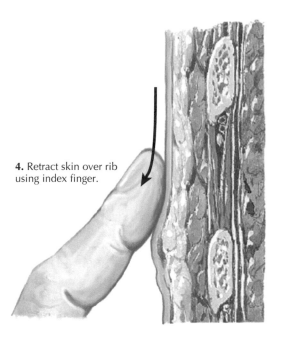

5. Insert needle at an 80° angle to the skin and advance until rib is met.

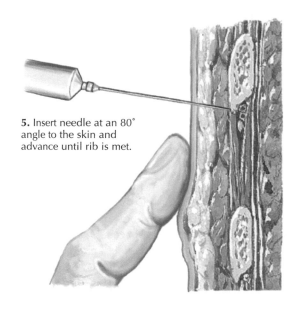

6–7. Discontinue retraction of the skin. The needle is "walked off" the rib and advanced 3 mm below the inferior border. Aspirate. If no blood, proceed.

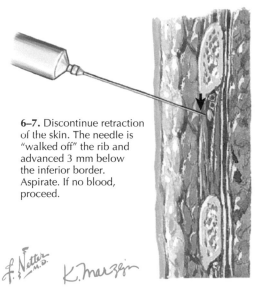

8. Gradually inject local anesthetic.

9–10. Repeat for other thoracic segments as needed. The patient should be observed for 20-30 min following the procedure for any complications.

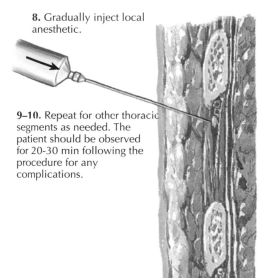

FIGURE 2.3 Intercostal nerve block

Suggested Readings

Abrahams MS, Horn JL, Noles LM, Aziz MF. Evidence-based medicine: ultrasound guidance for truncal blocks. *Reg Anesth Pain Med.* 2010;35:S36–S42.

Bhalla T, Sawardekar A, Dewhirst E, et al. Ultrasound-guided trunk and core blocks in infants and children. *J Anesth.* 2013;27:109–123.

Brascher AK, Blunk JA, Bauer K, et al. Comprehensive curriculum for phantom-based training of ultrasound-guided intercostal nerve and stellate ganglion blocks. *Pain Med.* 2014;15:1647–1656.

Clendenen NJ, Robards CB, Clendenen SR. A standardized method for 4d ultrasound-guided peripheral nerve blockade and catheter placement. *Biomed Res Int.* 2014;2014:920538.

Dillion DC, Gibbs MA. 2011. Local and regional anesthesia. In: Tintinalli JE, Stapczynski J, Ma O, et al., eds. *Tintinalli's emergency medicine: a comprehensive study guide.* 7th ed. New York: McGraw-Hill; 2011.

Hausman Jr MS, Jewell ES, Engoren M. Regional versus general anesthesia in surgical patients with chronic obstructive pulmonary disease: does avoiding general anesthesia reduce the risk of postoperative complications? *Anesth Analg.* 2015;120:1405–1412.

Karmakar MK, Ho AM. Acute pain management of patients with multiple fractured ribs. *J Trauma.* 2003;54:615–625.

Kilicaslan A, Topal A, Erol A, et al. Ultrasound-guided multiple peripheral nerve blocks in a superobese patient. *Case Rep Anesthesiol.* 2014;2014:896914.

Kolawole IK, Adesina MD, Olaoye IO. Intercostal nerves block for mastectomy in two patients with advanced breast malignancy. *J Natl Med Assoc.* 2006;98:450–453.

Moore DC. Intercostal nerve block: 1963. *Int Anesthesiol Clin.* 1998;36:29–41.

Naidu BV, Rajesh PB. Relevant surgical anatomy of the chest wall. *Thorac Surg Clin.* 2010;20:453–463.

Rathmell JP. Intercostal nerve block and neurolysis. In: Rathmell JP, ed. *Atlas of image-guided intervention in regional anesthesia and pain medicine.* 2nd ed. Philadelphia: Lippincott Williams & Wilkins; 2011:196–204.

REVIEW QUESTIONS

1. A 34-year-old man with a complaint of sharp, localized pain over the thoracic wall is diagnosed with pleural effusion. Through which intercostal space along the midaxillary line is it most appropriate to inject an anesthetic and insert a chest tube to drain the effusion?

   A. Fourth
   B. Sixth
   C. Eighth
   D. Tenth
   E. Twelfth

2. A 51-year-old man is admitted to the hospital with severe dyspnea. Radiographic examination reveals a tension pneumothorax. Adequate local anesthesia of the chest wall before the insertion of a chest tube is necessary for pain control. Of the following layers, which is the deepest that must be infiltrated with the local anesthetic to achieve adequate anesthesia?

   A. Endothoracic fascia
   B. Intercostal muscles
   C. Parietal pleura
   D. Subcutaneous fat
   E. Visceral pleura

3. A 34-year-old man with a complaint of sharp, localized pain over the thoracic wall is diagnosed with pleural effusion. A chest tube is inserted to drain the effusion through an intercostal space. At which of the following locations is the chest tube and the needle for the local anesthetic most likely to be inserted?

   A. Superior to the upper border of the rib
   B. Inferior to the lower border of the rib
   C. At the middle of the intercostal space
   D. Between the internal and external intercostal muscles
   E. Between the intercostal muscles and the posterior intercostal membrane

4. A 25-year-old man is brought to the emergency department because of a 1-week history of fever and cough productive of purulent sputum. His temperature is 38.9°C (102°F), pulse rate is 110 beats/min, respiratory rate is 24 breaths/min, and blood pressure is 110/70 mm Hg. Crackles, decreased breath sounds, and decreased fremitus are present in the right lower lobe. A chest radiograph shows pleural effusion over the lower third of the thorax on the right in the midscapular line. A thoracocentesis is scheduled. Which intercostal space in the midscapular line would be most appropriate for the insertion of the needle for the local anesthetic during this procedure?

   A. Fifth
   B. Seventh
   C. Ninth
   D. Eighth
   E. Eleventh

5. A 55-year-old man is admitted to the emergency department because of chills followed by a painful dry cough and fever for the past 3 days. The patient complains of painful breathing, and a pleural rub is heard on auscultation when the patient breathes. A radiograph shows signs of pleurisy. The physician decides to administer lidocaine to which of the following nerves?

   A. Intercostal nerves
   B. Phrenic nerve
   C. Vagus nerve
   D. Cardiopulmonary nerves
   E. Recurrent laryngeal nerve

6. A 57-year-old man is admitted to the emergency department after being hit by a truck while crossing a busy street. Radiographic examination reveals a flail chest. During physical examination, the patient complains of severe pain during inspiration and expiration. Which of the following nerves is most likely responsible for the sensation of pain during respiration?

   A. Phrenic nerve
   B. Vagus nerve
   C. Cardiopulmonary nerve
   D. Intercostal nerve
   E. Thoracic splanchnic nerve

Mask Ventilation

INTRODUCTION

Bag-valve-mask (BVM) ventilation, although difficult to master, is critical for basic airway management in scenarios where supportive intervention for inadequate ventilation is needed. Such scenarios may include airway obstruction, impaired respiratory effort, and cardiopulmonary resuscitation. This chapter summarizes airway management via basic BVM ventilation in adults.

CLINICALLY RELEVANT ANATOMY

BVM ventilation requires proper clinician technique as well as knowledge of the relevant anatomy of the airway. It is important to assess patients for factors that may impede proper administration of this procedure.

Anatomy of the Airway

The airway can be anatomically divided into upper and lower parts. The upper airway is made up of the structures superior to the vocal cords, including the nose, oral cavity, pharynx, and upper larynx (Figs. 3.1 and 3.2). The lower airway begins inferior to the vocal cords and consists of the lower larynx, trachea, bronchial tree, and lungs.

Assessment of the Patient's Anatomy

Before attempting the procedure, a careful examination of the patient should be performed, if possible, to evaluate for any obstacles to adequate mask ventilation. This should begin with an inspection of the patient's oral cavity to look for factors such as missing or loose teeth, capped teeth, a nonvisible uvula, enlarged tonsils, a small mouth opening, tumors, or dental appliances.

Measurement of the patient's thyromental distance (distance between the tip of the jaw and the thyroid cartilage [thyroid notch] on full neck extension with a closed mouth) should also be performed. An acceptable measurement is approximately 7 cm, with a shorter distance indicating possible difficulties with intubation. Other factors that may indicate limited airway mobility are if the patient has temporomandibular joint disease or is unable to open the mouth more than 4 cm. Additionally, patients should be evaluated for the ability to align their oral, pharyngeal, and laryngeal axes (neck mobility). If mechanical devices are needed to maintain the airway (ie, intubation), the procedure will be more difficult in a patient with limited neck mobility, temporomandibular joint disease, or a narrowed mouth opening.

In instances where intubation is required, the Mallampati airway classification can be used to determine the potential difficulty of the procedure. With the patient's mouth fully open and the head in neutral position, the posterior pharynx is visualized and the patient's airway is graded as class I to IV:

Class I (no difficulty): the soft palate, fauces, uvula, and pillars are visible
Class II (no difficulty): the soft palate, fauces, and a portion of the uvula are visible
Class III (moderate difficulty): the soft palate and base of the uvula are visible
Class IV (severe difficulty): only the hard palate is visible

INDICATIONS

Mask ventilation is indicated in any situation where there is evidence of insufficient ventilation, which may be due to altered respiratory effort or airway obstruction.

Respiratory Effort

The clinician must evaluate respiratory effort by the close observation of chest wall motion. Poor respiratory effort can result from intrinsic and extrinsic factors. Examples of intrinsic factors include pathological increases in intracranial pressure, seizures, cardiac arrest, and neuromuscular disease. Extrinsic factors include things such as drug overdose and carbon monoxide poisoning.

Airway Obstruction

Airway obstruction can result from soft tissue obstruction in a patient who has become unconscious. The tongue may occlude the posterior pharynx, or the muscle tone of the soft palate may be lost. The head-tilt, chin-lift maneuver or the jaw-thrust maneuver often resolves these problems. The clinician must also be alert for obstruction caused by foreign objects, tissue trauma, blood, and mucus secretions. Abnormal respiratory sounds facilitate the detection of airway obstruction. Partial obstruction of the upper airway by soft tissue or liquids may lead to grunting, gurgling, or sounds that resemble snoring. Complete airway obstruction may be associated with a complete absence of respiratory sounds along with abdominal retractions and accessory muscle use. In cases where a patient is making a respiratory effort but is not successfully ventilating due to obstruction, the clinician must determine the cause of the obstruction while simultaneously attempting to alleviate it. Chest thrusts, back blows, and abdominal thrusts have been shown to be effective. The 2015 American Heart Association Guidelines for Cardiopulmonary Resuscitation suggest it may take more than one technique to relieve an airway obstruction in the conscious patient and that

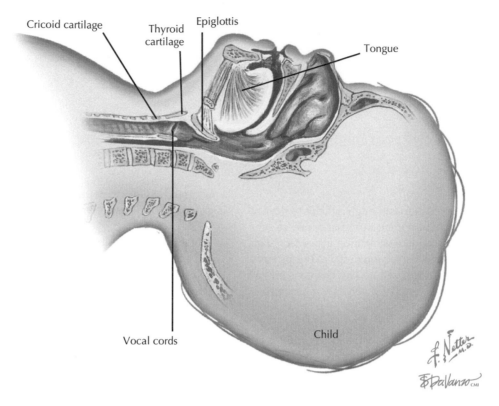

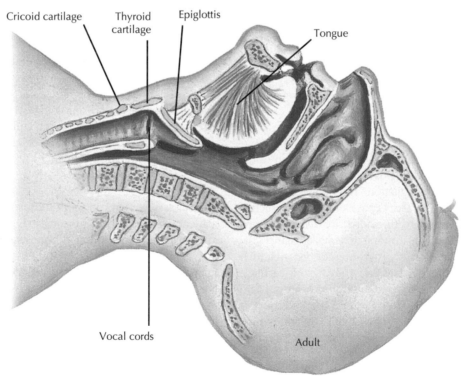

The pediatric airway is more anterior than an adult airway, requiring less manipulation to bring the oral, pharyngeal, and tracheal axes into alignment. The infant has a relatively large occiput, predisposing the neck to flexion and thus an increased propensity for airway obstruction when supine. Furthermore, extreme hyperextension may also result in airway obstruction in younger children as a result of the increased flexibility of the young airway. A child's airway is narrower and the tongue is relatively large compared to the jaw, increasing the risk of airway obstruction. The larynx is located more anteriorly and cephalad than the adult larynx, making the angle of entry into the trachea more acute.

FIGURE 3.1 Airway anatomy

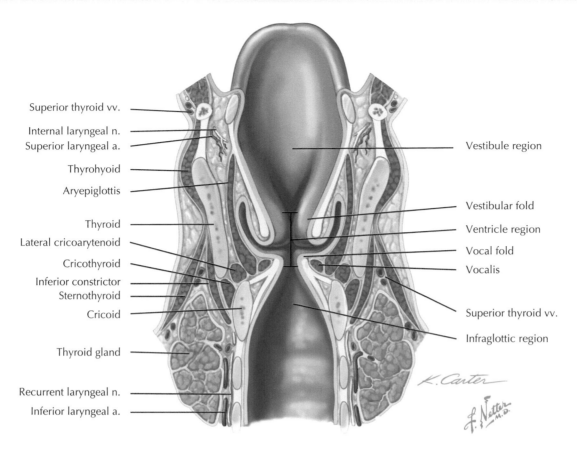

Superior thyroid vv.
Internal laryngeal n.
Superior laryngeal a.
Thyrohyoid
Aryepiglottis
Thyroid
Lateral cricoarytenoid
Cricothyroid
Inferior constrictor
Sternothyroid
Cricoid
Thyroid gland
Recurrent laryngeal n.
Inferior laryngeal a.

Vestibule region
Vestibular fold
Ventricle region
Vocal fold
Vocalis
Superior thyroid vv.
Infraglottic region

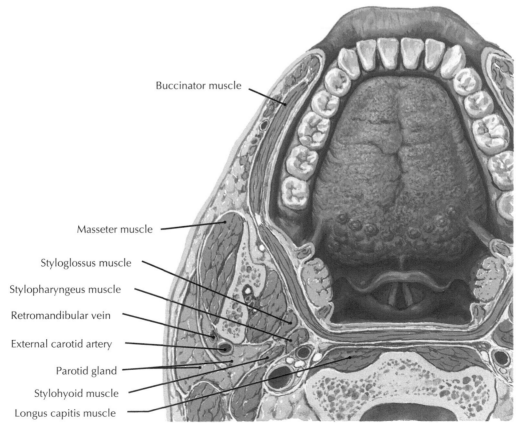

Buccinator muscle
Masseter muscle
Styloglossus muscle
Stylopharyngeus muscle
Retromandibular vein
External carotid artery
Parotid gland
Stylohyoid muscle
Longus capitis muscle

FIGURE 3.2 Larynx and tongue

abdominal thrusts, back blows, and chest thrusts are all effective. If the person's anatomy permits, one should start with a series of abdominal thrusts. This should be followed by chest thrusts if abdominal thrusts are not successful.

CONTRAINDICATIONS

Though safe in most patients, BVM ventilation should never be performed on patients with complete upper airway obstruction and should be performed with great caution in patients who are paralyzed or have undergone chemical paralysis and induction of anesthesia because there is an increased risk of aspiration.

EQUIPMENT

BVM device with cushioned rim
Tongue blade
Pulse oximeter (optional)
Oxygen source (if using flow-inflating bag)
Nasopharyngeal or oropharyngeal airways (optional)
Water-based lubricant (optional)
Gloves

PROCEDURE

Obtain patient consent if possible and perform a time out.

The clinician performing this technique must be certain to monitor his or her technique continuously. BVM ventilation is an interim procedure that provides oxygenation and ventilation of a patient requiring respiratory support and allows sufficient time for the clinician to plan definitive airway management such as endotracheal intubation. There are three elements required for effective BVM ventilation: a patent airway, an unbroken mask seal, and proper ventilation (volume and rate).

Opening the Airway

See Fig. 3.3.

1. An open airway is required prior to placement of the mask on a patient's face. An open airway can be obtained by using airway maneuvers (head-tilt, chin-lift; jaw-thrust; etc.) and airway adjuncts (nasopharyngeal airway or oropharyngeal airway).
2. Ensure that the mask is the proper size to allow for an adequate mask seal. A properly sized mask should encase the corners of the mouth and all airway openings.
3. After opening of the airway, the mask must be correctly placed on the patient's face. The bag should not be connected until the mask is properly placed.
4. Place the nasal portion of the mask (the apex of the triangle-shaped mask) on the bridge of the patient's nose.
5. The base of the mask must then be lowered to cover the nose and the mouth of the patient.
6. Patients with abnormal upper airway anatomy or excess soft tissue may require the use of a nasopharyngeal or oropharyngeal airway.

Sealing the Mask

The mask may be held in place by one of two methods: the single-hand (one hand, one person) or the two-hand (two hands, two persons) hold.

7A. Single-hand technique for BVM ventilation (one-rescuer method)
  a. The web space between the thumb and index finger is rested on the mask connector.
  b. The remaining three fingers are placed along the mandible and are used to pull the mandible up into the mask.
  c. A proper technique lifts the mandible up into the mask with the middle, ring, and little fingers and simultaneously holds the mask tightly against the patient's face using the thumb and index finger.
  d. Care should be taken to pull up on the mandible only, as pressure on the adjacent soft tissues may close the airway.

7B. Two-hand technique for BVM ventilation (two-rescuer method). Although the two-hand technique requires two people, it is the most effective way to open a patient's airway while providing ventilation and reducing provider fatigue.
  a. In this method, one rescuer has the sole responsibility of holding the mask against the patient's face and maintaining an adequate mask seal, as described above, or by placing both thenar eminences along the nasal aspect of the mask while using all remaining fingers to lift the mandible.
  b. The other rescuer is positioned to the side of the patient and has the sole responsibility of squeezing the bag to ventilate the patient.

8. Ventilation volume and rate. Connection of the bag to the mask is made and ventilation is begun. Ventilation errors that must be avoided are excessive tidal volume, forcing air too quickly, and excessive ventilation rate.
  • A tidal volume (up to 10 mL/kg) that causes the chest to rise is sufficient. The ventilation bag should be squeezed evenly over the course of 1 second at a rate of no more than 12 breaths/min.
  • Cricoid pressure (Sellick's maneuver) may be applied to avoid gastric insufflation if personnel are available. The role of cricoid pressure is controversial and is discussed elsewhere.

COMPLICATIONS

If BVM ventilation is performed incorrectly, complications, although rare, may occur. An improper ventilation rate may lead to either hypoventilation or hyperventilation. Failure to clear the oral cavity and upper airway of vomitus, blood, or foreign material as well as the process of BVM ventilation itself may lead to aspiration.

ANATOMICAL PITFALLS

Mask seal problems may be caused by facial hair. The seal can be improved by applying water or water-based lubricant. In patients who are edentulous, false teeth may be reinserted or gauze pads may be used to expand their cheeks. Other impediments to successful mask ventilation include obesity (body mass index >30), a history of obstructive apnea, and limited jaw protrusion.

Opening the Airway

1. Open the airway using airway maneuver: head-tilt, chin-lift; jaw-thrust; etc.

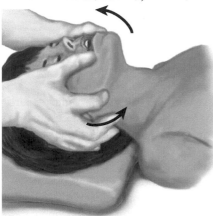

2. Ensure that mask is the proper size to allow for adequate seal. The mask should encase the corners of the mouth and all open airways.

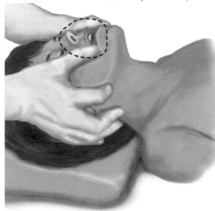

3. Place mask correctly on patient's face.

4. Place the nasal portion on the bridge of patient's nose.

5. Then lower to base to cover the nose and mouth.

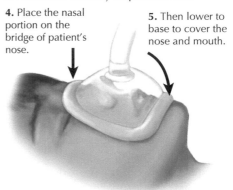

6. Use nasopharayngeal or oropharyngeal airway if patient has abnormal upper airway anatomy or excess soft tissue.

Sealing the Mask

7A. Single-hand technique

Rest web space between thumb and index finger on mask connector.

Place remaining three fingers along the mandible, pulling mandible up into the mask, but avoiding adjacent soft tissues so airway isn't inadvertently closed.

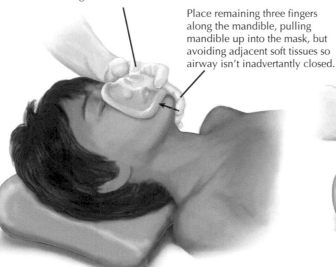

7B. Two-hand technique

One rescuer holds the mask on the patient's face by resting web space between thumb and index finger of both hands on mask connector.

The second rescuer is responsible for squeezing the bag to ventilate patient.

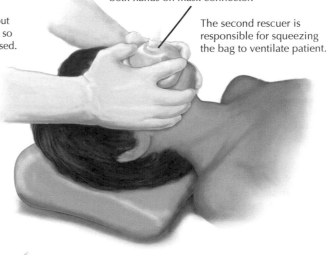

8. Connect the bag to the mask and squeeze to ventilate. Squeeze evenly over the course of 1 second, with no more than 12 breaths/min.

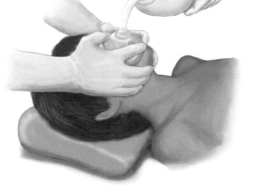

DRAGONFLY MEDIA GROUP

K. Marzin

FIGURE 3.3 Bag-valve-mask ventilation

CONCLUSION

Inadequate respiratory effort may be difficult to detect and requires close observation of chest wall motion. A common cause of airway obstruction is tongue prolapse into the posterior pharynx. This problem can be corrected by airway maneuvers such as the head-tilt, chin-lift or the jaw-thrust technique.

Oropharyngeal and nasopharyngeal airways are important ancillary devices for maintaining an open airway. An endotracheal tube, however, protects the trachea from secretions and gastric contents. It is critical that patients who are unable to protect their airways be intubated.

Adequate BVM ventilation depends on three elements: an open airway, a proper mask seal, and proper ventilation. Airway patency can be obtained through the use of maneuvers to open the airway and adjunct airway devices. Correct positioning and holding of the mask is critical to form a proper seal of the mask to the patient's face. If possible, a two-hand technique should be used. The thumb or the thenar eminences are pressed along the edge of the mask to securely hold it in place.

Common problems of BVM ventilation are poor mask seal, incorrect mask size, not using an adjunct airway when required, and improper airway maneuvers. Clinicians must avoid critical errors such as delivering excessive tidal volumes, squeezing the bag too forcefully, and ventilating at an excessive rate.

Suggested Readings

2005 International Consensus on Cardiopulmonary Resuscitation and Emergency Cardiovascular Care With Treatment Recommendations. *Circulation*. 2005;112(suppl I):III.

Aufderheide TP, Lurie KG. Death by hyperventilation: a common and life-threatening problem during cardiopulmonary resuscitation. *Crit Care Med*. 2004;32:S345.

Komatsu R, Kasuya Y, Yogo H, et al. Learning curves for bag-and-mask ventilation and orotracheal intubation: an application of the cumulative sum method. *Anesthesiology*. 2010;112:1525.

Mathru M, Esch O, Lang J, et al. Magnetic resonance imaging of the upper airway. Effects of propofol anesthesia and nasal continuous positive airway pressure in humans. *Anesthesiology*. 1996;84:273.

Travers AH, Rea TD, Bobrow BJ, et al. Part 4: CPR overview: 2010 American Heart Association Guidelines for Cardiopulmonary Resuscitation and Emergency Cardiovascular Care. *Circulation*. 2010;122:S676.

Wittels KA, Walls, RM, Grayzel J. Basic airway management in adults. Available at http://www.uptodate.com/contents/basic-airway-management-in-adults.

REVIEW QUESTIONS

1. A 45-year-old man is admitted to the emergency department with severe dyspnea. During physical examination, swelling in the floor of his mouth and pharynx is noticed and his airway is nearly totally occluded. In addition, there is a swelling in his lower jaw and upper neck. His physical history indicates that one of his lower molars was extracted a week ago and he had been feeling worse every day since that event. Which of the following conditions is the most likely diagnosis?

   A. Quinsy
   B. Torus palatinus
   C. Ankyloglossia
   D. Ranula
   E. Ludwig angina

2. A 54-year-old man is scheduled to undergo bilateral thyroidectomy. During this procedure, bilateral paralysis of the muscles that open the airway is possible. If a particular nerve is injured bilaterally, there is significant risk of asphyxiation postoperatively unless the patient is intubated or the airway is opened surgically. Which of the following muscle pairs opens the airway?

   A. Cricothyroids
   B. Posterior cricoarytenoids
   C. Arytenoids
   D. Thyroarytenoids
   E. Lateral cricoarytenoids

Thoracostomy

INTRODUCTION

Pneumothorax and pleural effusion are potentially life-threatening conditions that leave little room for error in diagnosis and management. In pneumothorax, the pleural cavity rapidly fills with air, whereas in pleural effusion, fluids such as blood, bile, or pus enter the pleural cavity. Chest tube thoracostomy is a procedure in which a tube is inserted into the pleural cavity to allow for the continuous drainage of large volumes of air or fluid. Without this intervention, patients are at great risk for morbidity and mortality.

When there is a significant amount of air or fluid in the thoracic cavity, the resulting rise in pressure greatly diminishes the capacity of the lung to fully expand. In turn, this restricts normal breathing and can result in hypoventilation and hypoxia. In pneumothorax, patients often present with the sudden onset of sharp chest pain, dyspnea with tachypnea, tachycardia, cough, fatigue, and cyanosis. In pleural effusion, the most commonly associated symptoms are pleuritic chest pain, progressive dyspnea, and cough.

In both these conditions, proper chest tube insertion allows for effective reexpansion of the lung. This optimizes ventilation/perfusion and minimizes mediastinal shift.

If available, ultrasonography should be utilized as an adjunctive guide in identifying the precise location for chest tube insertion, especially since ultrasound-guided chest tube thoracostomy is associated with lower complication rates. However, in many instances ultrasonography may not be readily available, and the procedure may need to be performed by standard blunt dissection. Therefore it is important to have a fundamental understanding of the relevant clinical anatomy encountered in performing thoracostomy.

CLINICALLY RELEVANT ANATOMY

The mediastinum is a space in the chest that is bounded by the lungs, sternum, and spine and contains the heart, esophagus, trachea, phrenic, vagus, and cardiac nerves, thoracic duct, thymus, and lymph nodes (Figs. 4.1 to 4.3). There are two pleural cavities in the chest. Each of these cavities is lined by a serous membrane called the pleural membrane (pleura). The pleura is composed of two continuous layers: the visceral pleura and parietal pleura. The visceral pleura covers the outer surface of the lung and adheres to all its surfaces. This layer is not sensitive to somatic pain. The parietal pleura lines the chest wall and extends over the diaphragm and mediastinum. Different portions of the parietal pleura are named according to their anatomic location. The cervical pleura rises into the neck and over the apex of the lung, the costal pleura covers the inner surface of the ribs and intercostal muscles, the diaphragmatic pleura lines the dome of the diaphragm, and the mediastinal pleura adheres to other thoracic viscera. Since the embryological derivative for the parietal pleura is the somatic mesoderm, it is highly sensitive to pain. In various portions of the parietal pleura, different nerve innervations are responsible for conveying pain: the phrenic nerve for the mediastinal and central region of the diaphragmatic portion and the intercostal nerves for the remaining lateral portions. The area between these two layers of pleura is known as the pleural space. Normally, there is only a small amount of fluid in the pleural space. The pleural fluid found within the pleural space allows both the visceral and parietal layers to effortlessly slide against each other during ventilation. This fluid also provides surface tension, allowing for greater inflation of the alveoli during inspiration.

Left lateral view

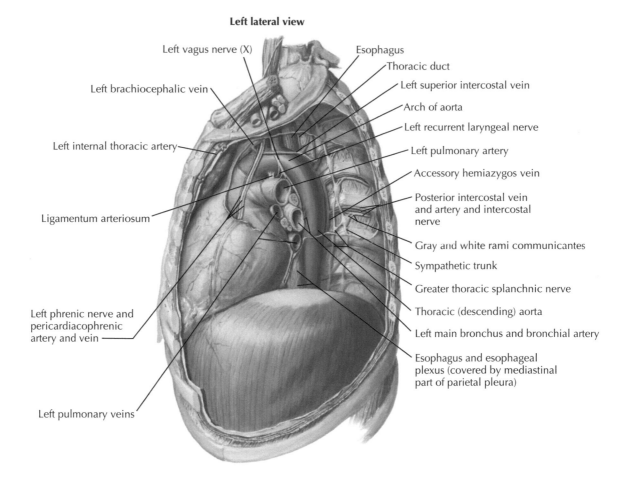

Left vagus nerve (X)

Esophagus

Thoracic duct

Left brachiocephalic vein

Left superior intercostal vein

Arch of aorta

Left recurrent laryngeal nerve

Left internal thoracic artery

Left pulmonary artery

Accessory hemiazygos vein

Posterior intercostal vein and artery and intercostal nerve

Ligamentum arteriosum

Gray and white rami communicantes

Sympathetic trunk

Greater thoracic splanchnic nerve

Thoracic (descending) aorta

Left phrenic nerve and pericardiacophrenic artery and vein

Left main bronchus and bronchial artery

Esophagus and esophageal plexus (covered by mediastinal part of parietal pleura)

Left pulmonary veins

Right lateral view

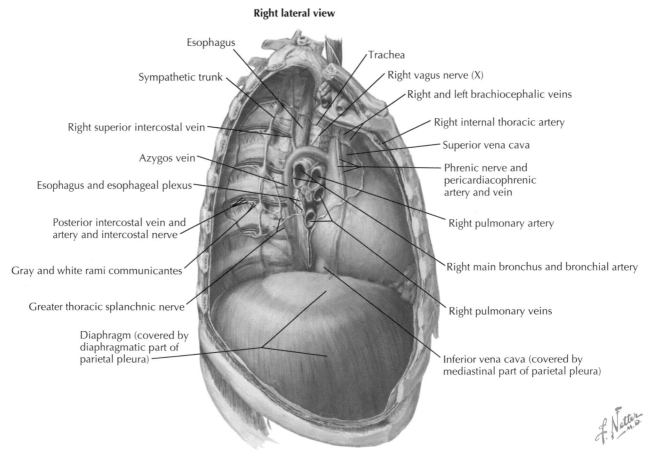

Esophagus

Trachea

Right vagus nerve (X)

Sympathetic trunk

Right and left brachiocephalic veins

Right superior intercostal vein

Right internal thoracic artery

Superior vena cava

Azygos vein

Phrenic nerve and pericardiacophrenic artery and vein

Esophagus and esophageal plexus

Right pulmonary artery

Posterior intercostal vein and artery and intercostal nerve

Gray and white rami communicantes

Right main bronchus and bronchial artery

Greater thoracic splanchnic nerve

Right pulmonary veins

Diaphragm (covered by diaphragmatic part of parietal pleura)

Inferior vena cava (covered by mediastinal part of parietal pleura)

FIGURE 4.1 Contents of the thorax: mediastinum

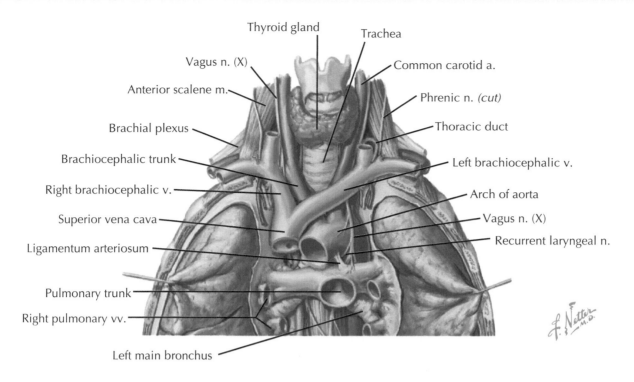

Thyroid gland

Trachea

Vagus n. (X)

Common carotid a.

Anterior scalene m.

Phrenic n. *(cut)*

Brachial plexus

Thoracic duct

Brachiocephalic trunk

Left brachiocephalic v.

Right brachiocephalic v.

Arch of aorta

Superior vena cava

Vagus n. (X)

Ligamentum arteriosum

Recurrent laryngeal n.

Pulmonary trunk

Right pulmonary vv.

Left main bronchus

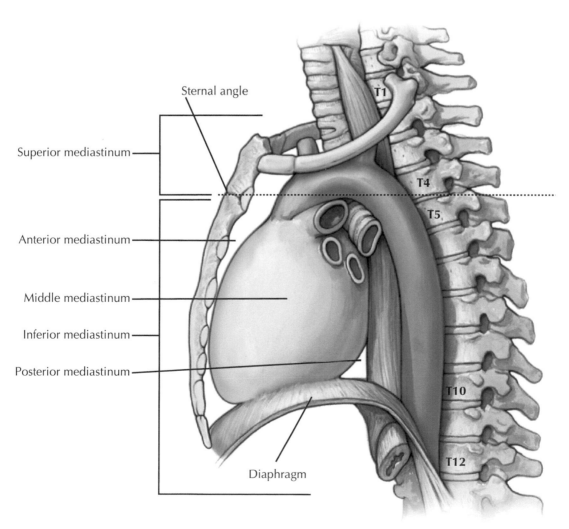

Sternal angle

T1

Superior mediastinum

T4

T5

Anterior mediastinum

Middle mediastinum

Inferior mediastinum

Posterior mediastinum

T10

T12

Diaphragm

FIGURE 4.2 Mediastinum

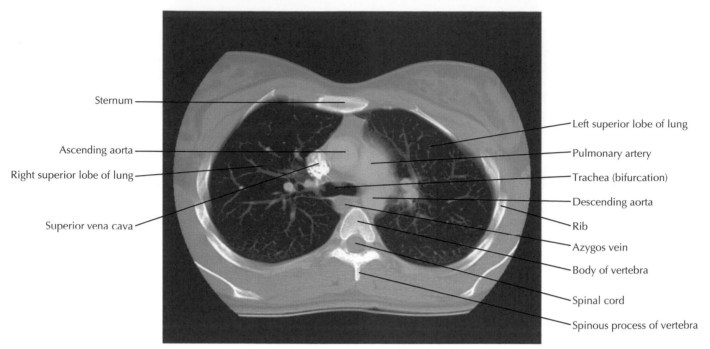

Sternum

Ascending aorta

Right superior lobe of lung

Superior vena cava

Left superior lobe of lung

Pulmonary artery

Trachea (bifurcation)

Descending aorta

Rib

Azygos vein

Body of vertebra

Spinal cord

Spinous process of vertebra

FIGURE 4.3 Imaging of mediastinum

Twelve pairs of ribs encircle the area from the spine to the sternum and protect the thoracic cavity. In between the ribs are the intercostal spaces, which contain three layers of muscles and the neurovascular bundle. The most superficial of the three muscles is the external intercostal, followed by the internal intercostal, and the deepest is the innermost internal intercostal. In between the internal intercostal and innermost intercostal muscles is the neurovascular bundle, a structure that is made up of the posterior intercostal vein superiorly and the posterior intercostal artery and intercostal nerve inferiorly. The neurovascular bundle travels along the inferior border of the rib. This anatomy has made it common practice to insert a chest tube just above the rib. However, if a chest tube is inserted as close as possible to the superior margin of the rib, laceration of the collateral intercostal arteries may occur. A recent study suggests that the optimal spot for chest tube insertion is between 50% and 70% down the intercostal space. The British Thoracic Society recommends using the "triangle of safety" when inserting a chest tube. This area corresponds to the anterior border of the latissimus dorsi, the lateral border of the pectoralis major, the apex of the axilla, and a line superior to the horizontal level of the nipple.

Several vital structures share a close anatomic relationship with the pleural cavities and lungs. The serratus anterior, long thoracic nerve, phrenic nerve, diaphragm, myocardium, liver, and other intrathoracic and intraabdominal organs are all at risk. Therefore it is important to be aware of this regional anatomy when performing chest tube thoracostomy.

INDICATIONS

Thoracostomy can be used for both diagnostic and therapeutic purposes.

Diagnostic Chest Tube Thoracostomy

Diagnostic thoracostomy is a nonemergent procedure that can be utilized to analyze pleural effusion, which can be either exudative or transudative. According to Light's criteria, fluid is exudative when one of the following is met:

- Effusion protein/serum protein ratio is more than 0.5
- Effusion lactate dehydrogenase (LDH)/serum LDH is more than 0.6
- Effusion LDH is more than two-thirds the upper limit of normal serum LDH

The fluid extracted can aid in diagnosing conditions that result in exudative or transudative effusion. Pathologies that produce exudative effusion are malignancy, infection, trauma, pulmonary infarction and embolism, autoimmune disorders, pancreatitis, ruptured esophagus, rheumatoid pleurisy, drug-induced lupus, and tuberculosis. Conditions that produce transudative effusions are congestive heart failure, liver cirrhosis, hypoproteinemia, nephrotic syndrome, acute atelectasis, myxedema, peritoneal dialysis, Meig syndrome, obstructive uropathy, and end-stage renal disease.

Therapeutic Chest Tube Thoracostomy

Therapeutic chest tube thoracostomy can be an emergent or nonemergent procedure. In nonemergent settings, a chest tube may be inserted as a palliative measure for chronic diseases or for prophylactic reasons. A chest tube may even be inserted to provide a vehicle for pharmacologic interventions, such as antibiotics for treating empyema, or for delivering sclerosing agents to prevent recurrent malignant effusions.

In emergent settings where patients are clinically unstable, a chest tube is indicated for pneumothorax, tension pneumothorax, hemopneumothorax, and esophageal rupture with gastric leakage into the pleural space. These indications are summarized in Table 4-1.

CONTRAINDICATIONS

There are few contraindications for chest tube placement. The only absolute contraindications are a lung adherent to the chest wall through the entire hemithorax or emergent situations (traumatic penetrating cardiac arrest) in which an open thoracotomy should be performed. Relative contraindications for this procedure include the use of anticoagulants, bleeding disorders, and an increased risk of infection at the chest tube insertion site.

EQUIPMENT

Sterile gloves and gown, mask, and cap
Sterile drapes
Adhesive tape
Sterile gauze squares
Petroleum-based gauze
Skin antiseptic (eg, chlorhexidine in alcohol)
Surgical marker
Razor
Syringes, 10 to 20 mL
Selection of syringe needles
Local anesthetic (eg, 1% to 2% lidocaine with epinephrine)
Scalpel with blade
Kelly clamps
Curved Mayo scissors
Straight suture scissors
Needle driver
Silk or nylon sutures, 1-0
Suction source and connecting tubing
Chest tube drainage device with water seal
Chest tube of appropriate size:
    Male: 28 to 32 Fr
    Female: 28 Fr
    Child: 12 to 28 Fr
    Infant: 12 to 16 Fr
    Neonate: 10 to 12 Fr
Ultrasound, if available

PROCEDURE

Obtain patient consent and perform a time out.

Ultrasound-Guided Blunt Dissection Technique

Ultrasonography is a tool that can be used to localize an area of fluid collection and to locate the precise site for chest tube placement. This mode of imaging also helps prevent the laceration of vital structures such as the serratus anterior, long thoracic nerve, phrenic nerve, diaphragm, myocardium, liver, and other intrathoracic and intraabdominal organs. The proposed site of chest tube insertion may first be confirmed by performing ultrasound-guided thoracocentesis. In emergency situations where ultrasound is not readily available, a traditional blind approach can still be used.

TABLE 4-1 Emergent Indications for Chest Tube Thoracostomy

Pneumothorax: spontaneous, tension, traumatic, iatrogenic, bronchopleural fistula
Hemothorax (postoperative): chest trauma (blunt or penetrating), thoracic or upper abdominal surgery
Pleural effusion: sterile effusion, empyema or parapneumonic effusion, malignant effusion, chylothorax
Pleurodesis

The following steps describe the most commonly used method for chest tube thoracostomy (Fig. 4.4 and Video 4.1):

1. Monitor the patient's vital signs.
2. Ensure the drainage system is properly connected to the suction source.
3. Position the patient in either a supine or a semirecumbent position. Abduct the patient's ipsilateral arm and flex the elbow to position the hand comfortably over the patient's head.
4. Use ultrasonography to examine the fourth and fifth intercostal spaces at the midaxillary or anterior axillary line for selecting a safe insertion site.
5. Locate the fourth and fifth intercostal spaces in the anterior axillary line at the horizontal level of the nipple. This area is one boundary of the "triangle of safety" and is the site of incision; the incision site is one intercostal space below the actual chest tube insertion site. Use a surgical marker to mark the spot for incision.
6. Prepare the skin around the area of insertion with antiseptic solution.
7. Drape the patient appropriately, exposing only the marked area.
8. Administer a local anesthetic (lidocaine 1% to 2%) to anesthetize a 2- to 3-cm area of skin and subcutaneous tissue at the site of incision.
9. Continue to anesthetize deeper subcutaneous tissues and intercostal muscles. Identify the rib inferior to the intercostal space where the tube will be inserted and anesthetize the periosteal surface. When anesthetizing the rib, identify the superior aspect of the rib and use this to help guide the needle at an angle on top of the rib.
10. Stop advancing the syringe needle when a flash of pleural fluid enters the syringe. This will confirm entry into the pleural space; in the case of pneumothorax, air will fill the syringe. Inject any remaining anesthetic to fully anesthetize the parietal pleura and completely withdraw the syringe.
11. Use a scalpel to make a 1- to 2-cm skin incision parallel to the rib.
12. Use a Kelly clamp to dissect a tract through the subcutaneous tissue and intercostal muscles by intermittently advancing the closed instrument and opening it.
13. Close the Kelly clamp and carefully pass through the intercostal muscles and parietal pleura, gently entering the pleural space.
14. Open the Kelly clamp while inside the pleural space and then withdraw it so that its jaws enlarge the dissected tract through all the layers of the chest wall.
15. Insert a finger into the pleural space and rotate it 360 degrees to feel for adhesions.
16. Use a Kelly clamp to grasp the fenestrated portion of the tube and introduce it through the incision and insertion sites. To advance the chest tube into the thoracic cavity, release the Kelly clamp. For the evacuation of air, aim the tube apically; for evacuation of fluid, aim the tube basally.
17. Use mattress or interrupted sutures on both sides of the incision to close the ends. Secure the chest tube to the chest wall using the suture's loose ends to wrap around the tube and tie them off.
18. Wrap petroleum-based gauze around the tube and cover it with several pieces of regular gauze. Secure the site with multiple layers of dressings, using adhesive tape to secure them to the chest.
19. Connect the chest tube to the drainage device.
20. Obtain an anteroposterior chest radiograph to confirm proper chest tube placement. A radiopaque line should be seen along the tube. If the drainage hole is outside the pleural space, drainage may be ineffective and leakage of air may result. If this occurs, remove the tube and insert a new chest tube.

Alternative Methods

Seldinger Technique

The Seldinger technique follows the same principles as the blunt dissection technique except that it utilizes a series of dilators over a guidewire to insert a small-bore chest tube; this is useful in draining air or fluid. This technique is typically performed with the aid of ultrasonography. One disadvantage, however, is the inability to assess the presence of pleural adhesions.

Trocar Method

The lesser-used trocar method requires a stabbing motion through skin, muscles, and parietal pleura. This technique is often difficult to control and can potentially damage the intrathoracic and intraabdominal organs. The trocar method is strongly advised against because it has historically been associated with higher complication rates.

ANATOMICAL PITFALLS

The clinically relevant anatomy must be considered in order to avoid vital structures. The neurovascular bundle runs parallel to the inferior edge of each corresponding superior rib. Furthermore, damage to intraabdominal organs may result if one enters at a lower intercostal space level.

Collateral Nerves and Vessels

The intercostal collateral nerve and vessels are usually located just superior to the rib. This neurovascular bundle may be higher within the intercostal space and can be damaged. In addition, the collateral intercostal vessels might run in a lace-like pattern around the anterior axillary line, resulting in abnormal bleeding during the procedure.

Long Thoracic Nerve

The long thoracic nerve runs close to the anterior axillary line and supplies the serratus anterior muscle. Injury to this nerve during blind chest tube insertion can result in scapular winging.

Relationship of the Intercostal Muscles to Lung Tissue

Approximately less than 1 cm of space is found between the intercostal muscles and lung. Thus care must be taken when performing blunt dissection through muscles to avoid injury to the lung.

1–3. Monitor patient's vital signs. Ensure drainage system is connected to suction source. Place patient in supine position. Abduct the patient's arm and flex elbow to position the hand over the patient's head.

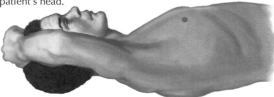

4–7. Use ultrasonography to locate the 4th and 5th intercostal spaces in the anterior axillary line at the level of the nipple. Mark this spot for incision. Cleanse the area with antiseptic and drape the patient.

— 4th rib

— 5th rib

— Anterior axillary line

8. Administer anesthetic to a 2- to 3-cm area of the skin and subcutaneous tissue at incision site (A). Continue to anesthetize deeper subcutaneous tissues and intercostal muscles (B).

A

B

C

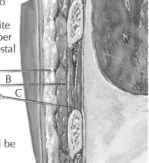

9. Identify the rib inferior to the intercostal space where tube will be inserted and anesthetize the periosteal surface (C).

10. Advance the needle until a flash of pleural fluid or air enters the syringe, confirming entry into the pleural space.

11. Use a scalpel to make a 1- to 2-cm incision parallel to the rib.

12–14. Dissect a tract through subcutaneous tissue and intercostal muscles by advancing a closed Kelly clamp and intermittently opening it. Close the clamp and gently enter the pleural space.

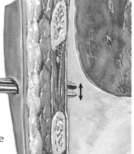

Open the clamp while inside the pleural space and then withdraw so that all layers of the dissected tract are enlarged.

15. Insert a finger into the pleural space and rotate 360 degress to feel for adhesions.

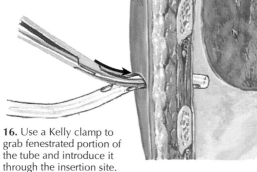
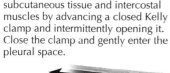
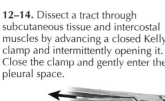
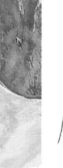
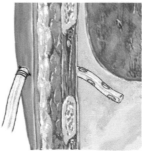

16. Use a Kelly clamp to grab fenestrated portion of the tube and introduce it through the insertion site.

17. Use sutures to close incision. Secure chest tube to chest wall using suture's lose ends to wrap around tube.

18–20. Wrap petroleum-based gauze around tube and cover with regular gauze. Secure the site with multiple dressings and adhesive tape to secure to chest. Connect chest tube to drainage device. Obtain a chest radiograph to confirm proper tube placement.

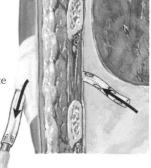

FIGURE 4.4 Thoracostomy

COMPLICATIONS

In emergent settings, chest tube thoracostomy is often blindly performed. However, this life-saving procedure is not without risk. Recent studies have shown that ultrasound-guided chest tube insertion significantly reduces complication rates. To further minimize complications, it is advised to keep to the "triangle of safety."

Complications can be grouped into two categories: technical or infectious. Technical complications include chest tube malposition and dislodgement, blocked chest tube, cardiac and vascular injuries, nerve injuries, esophageal injuries, reexpansion pulmonary edema, subcutaneous emphysema, residual/postextubation pneumothorax, fistulae, herniation through the insertion site, chylothorax, and cardiac dysrhythmias. Infectious complications include empyema, pneumonia, cellulitis, and necrotizing fasciitis.

The most common complication is chest tube malposition, which represents a form of penetrating trauma. Prior to the removal of a malpositioned chest tube, a second chest tube must first be successfully inserted into the pleural space. Premature chest tube removal could result in a tension pneumothorax. A clinician must be prepared to manage the bleeding and air leakage that may occur as a result of removing a malpositioned chest tube. The management of malpositioned chest tubes depends on where they are placed. If the tube is placed subcutaneously, the tube can be repositioned. If it is placed too far against the apical pleura, the tube can be gently retracted. However, the chest tube should be completely removed if it is accidentally placed in the abdominal cavity.

The most severe complication, which is extremely rare yet potentially fatal, is reexpansion pulmonary edema. This occurs after the rapid reexpansion of a large pneumothorax and in patients who have had large pleural effusions drained. Although the clinical presentation can be delayed up to 24 hours, patients typically present with cough, dyspnea, and hypoxemia soon after chest tube placement. Treatment is often supportive since this complication is usually self-limiting.

CONCLUSION

Chest tube thoracostomy can be a life-saving procedure. Through relieving pressure within the pleural cavity, patients can be stabilized through the insertion of a chest tube when presenting with life-threatening conditions. However, as no procedure is without risk, complications may arise due to inadequate knowledge of clinically relevant thoracic anatomy and deficiencies in training. Hence, a complete working knowledge of the clinically relevant anatomy can help minimize complications associated with this procedure.

Suggested Readings

Ball CG, Lord J, Laupland KB, et al. Chest tube complications: how well are we training our residents? *Can J Surg*. 2007;50:450–458.

Dev SP, Nascimiento B, Simone C, Chien V. Videos in clinical medicine: chest-tube insertion. *N Engl J Med*. 2007;357:15.

Doelken P. Placement and management of thoracostomy tubes. Available at http://www.uptodate.com/contents/placement-and-management-of-thoracostomy-tubes.

Gareeboo S, Singh S. Tube thoracostomy: how to insert a chest drain. *Br J Hosp Med*. 2006;67:M16–M18.

Havelock T, Teoh R, Laws D, Gleeson F. Pleural procedures and thoracic ultrasound: British Thoracic Society pleural disease guideline 2010. *Thorax*. 2010;65:i61–i76.

Hogg JR, Caccavale M, Gillen B, et al. Tube thoracostomy: a review for the interventional radiologist. *Semin Intervent Radiol*. 2011;28:39–47.

Irwin RS, Rippe JM. Chest tube insertion and care. In: Irwin RS, Rippe JM, eds. *Irwin and Rippe's Intensive Care Medicine*, ed 7. Philadelphia, PA: Lippincott Williams & Wilkins; 2011; 86–94.

Khandhar SJ, Johnson SB, Calhoon JH. Overview of thoracic trauma in the United States. *Thoracic Surg Clin*. 2007;17:1–9.

Ladwa M, Kaul S, Anderson J. An evaluation of ultrasound-guided chest drain insertion in intensive care. *Am J Respir Crit Care Med*. 2010;181:1662.

Laws D, Neville E, Duffy J. BTS guidelines for the insertion of a chest drain. *Thorax*. 2003;58:ii53–ii59.

Meredith JW, Hoth JJ. Thoracic trauma: when and how to intervene. *Surg Clin North Am*. 2007;87:95–118.

Wraight WM, Tweedie DJ, Parkin IG. Neurovascular anatomy and variation in the fourth, fifth, and sixth intercostal spaces in the mid-axillary line: a cadaveric study in respect of chest drain insertion. *Clin Anat*. 2005;18:346–349.

REVIEW QUESTIONS

1. A 34-year-old man with a complaint of sharp, localized pain over the thoracic wall is diagnosed with pleural effusion. Through which intercostal space along the midaxillary line is it most appropriate to insert a chest tube to drain the effusion fluid?

   A. Fourth
   B. Sixth
   C. Eighth
   D. Tenth
   E. Twelfth

2. A 51-year-old man is admitted to the hospital with severe dyspnea. Radiographic examination reveals a tension pneumothorax. Adequate local anesthesia of the chest wall prior to the insertion of a chest tube is necessary for pain control. Of the following layers, which is the deepest that must be infiltrated with a local anesthetic to achieve adequate anesthesia?

   A. Endothoracic fascia
   B. Intercostal muscles
   C. Parietal pleura
   D. Subcutaneous fat
   E. Visceral pleura

3. A 50-year-old man was involved in a motor vehicle crash and was rushed to the emergency department, where a chest tube was placed to drain fluid. Which of the following structures makes up the deepest layer of the thoracic wall?

   A. Internal intercostal muscle
   B. Skin
   C. Innermost intercostal muscle
   D. Parietal pleura
   E. External intercostal muscle
   F. Visceral pleura

Thoracentesis

INTRODUCTION

Pleural effusion is the excess accumulation of fluid between the lung and chest wall. The severity of the effusion depends on the underlying cause and degree of respiratory symptoms. Thoracocentesis is a procedure in which a needle is inserted to remove the excess fluid accumulated in the pleural space.

Pleural effusions occur as a result of many disease processes, including cancer, pneumonia, congestive heart failure, pulmonary embolism, and liver cirrhosis. Depending on the cause, the accumulated fluid can be classified as an exudate (protein rich) or transudate (watery). Furthermore, effusions can be distinguished by the specific type of fluid found in the pleural space: hemothorax (blood), empyema (pus), chylothorax (lymph), hydrothorax (serous fluid), and urinothorax (urine). Analysis of the fluid allows the diagnosis of the cause of the pleural effusion.

Many patients with pleural effusion are asymptomatic. The most common symptoms, regardless of the type of fluid, are dyspnea and chest pain. The accumulation of fluid makes it difficult for the lungs to fully expand, resulting in dyspnea. Clinical manifestations are predominantly indicative of and dependent on the underlying disease process. Pleural effusion may be diagnosed by chest radiography, chest computed tomography, chest ultrasound, and thoracentesis. The etiology of the pleural fluid can be confirmed by laboratory analysis.

CLINICALLY RELEVANT ANATOMY
Boundaries

The thoracic cage is bounded superiorly by the thoracic inlet and inferiorly by the thoracic outlet, and is surrounded by the rib cage. The thoracic inlet is defined by the body of the first thoracic vertebra, first pair of ribs and their costal cartilages, and jugular notch of the sternum. It communicates with the neck and the upper extremities (Fig. 5.1). The thoracic outlet is defined by the twelfth thoracic vertebra, eleventh and twelfth pairs of ribs, costal cartilages of ribs 7 to 10 (costal margin), and xiphisternal joint. This outlet is closed by the diaphragm, a musculotendinous partition that serves as a septum between the thoracic and abdominal cavities and functions as the major muscle of respiration.

Viscera

Within the framework of the thoracic cage are the lungs and pleural cavities and interposed mediastinum. Important structures within the mediastinum include the heart, great vessels, trachea, and esophagus.

Pleurae and Pleural Cavity

The pleura is a double-layer serous membrane made up of the visceral pleura that adheres to and covers the lung and the parietal pleura that covers the internal surface of the thoracic wall. The visceral pleura is insensitive to pain, whereas the parietal pleura is sensitive to pain and is innervated by the intercostal (costal and cervical pleura), phrenic (mediastinal and central diaphragmatic pleura), and lower fifth to sixth intercostal nerves (peripheral diaphragmatic pleura). Between the parietal and visceral pleurae is a potential space known as the pleural cavity. It normally contains a thin film of serous fluid but can accumulate fluid in pathological conditions.

Musculature

Extensive musculature covers the thoracic cage in order to aid with respiration, to effect movement of the upper limbs and back, and to maintain an upright posture. The muscles of the anterior thoracic wall can be divided into superficial and deep groups. The superficial muscles are the pectoralis major, pectoralis minor, subclavius, and serratus anterior. Below these are the superficial, middle, and deep layers of the deep group. External intercostal muscles and internal intercostal muscles constitute the superficial and middle layers, respectively, whereas the innermost intercostal muscles, the subcostal muscles, the transversus thoracis muscles, and the levatores costarum make up the deep layer. Similarly, the muscles of the back are classified as belonging to the superficial, intermediate, or deep groups. The trapezius, latissimus dorsi, levator scapulae, rhomboid major, and rhomboid minor form the superficial group. A thin layer of muscles, the serratus posterior superior and serratus posterior inferior, forms the intermediate group. Finally, the deep group includes the erector spinae muscle.

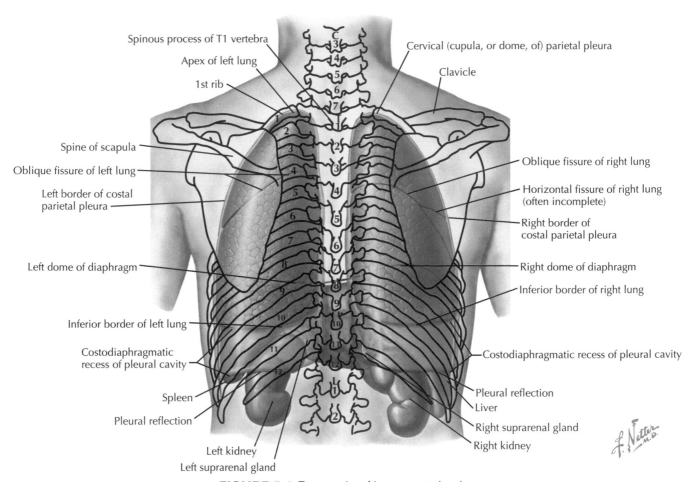

Spinous process of T1 vertebra

Apex of left lung

1st rib

Spine of scapula

Oblique fissure of left lung

Left border of costal parietal pleura

Left dome of diaphragm

Inferior border of left lung

Costodiaphragmatic recess of pleural cavity

Spleen

Pleural reflection

Left kidney

Left suprarenal gland

Cervical (cupula, or dome, of) parietal pleura

Clavicle

Oblique fissure of right lung

Horizontal fissure of right lung (often incomplete)

Right border of costal parietal pleura

Right dome of diaphragm

Inferior border of right lung

Costodiaphragmatic recess of pleural cavity

Pleural reflection

Liver

Right suprarenal gland

Right kidney

FIGURE 5.1 Topography of lungs: posterior view

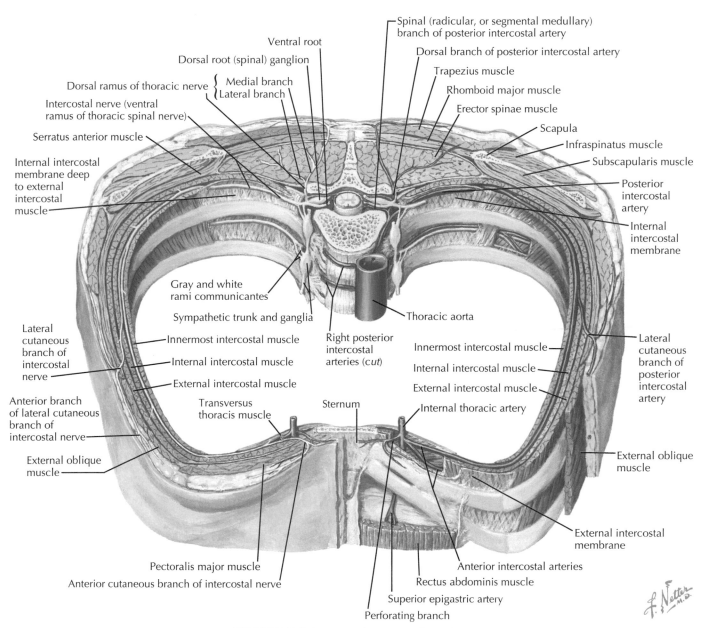

Spinal (radicular, or segmental medullary) branch of posterior intercostal artery

Dorsal branch of posterior intercostal artery

Trapezius muscle

Rhomboid major muscle

Erector spinae muscle

Scapula

Infraspinatus muscle

Subscapularis muscle

Posterior intercostal artery

Internal intercostal membrane

Ventral root

Dorsal root (spinal) ganglion

Dorsal ramus of thoracic nerve { Medial branch / Lateral branch

Intercostal nerve (ventral ramus of thoracic spinal nerve)

Serratus anterior muscle

Internal intercostal membrane deep to external intercostal muscle

Gray and white rami communicantes

Sympathetic trunk and ganglia

Thoracic aorta

Right posterior intercostal arteries (cut)

Lateral cutaneous branch of intercostal nerve

Innermost intercostal muscle

Internal intercostal muscle

External intercostal muscle

Innermost intercostal muscle

Internal intercostal muscle

External intercostal muscle

Internal thoracic artery

Lateral cutaneous branch of posterior intercostal artery

Anterior branch of lateral cutaneous branch of intercostal nerve

External oblique muscle

Transversus thoracis muscle

Sternum

External oblique muscle

External intercostal membrane

Pectoralis major muscle

Anterior cutaneous branch of intercostal nerve

Superior epigastric artery

Perforating branch

Anterior intercostal arteries

Rectus abdominis muscle

FIGURE 5.2 Intercostal nerves and arteries

Neurovascular Structures

In order to support these body wall structures, branches of nerves, arteries, and veins travel between the layers of muscles and along the costal margins. Neurovascular bundles (intercostal vein, artery, and nerve), running along the inferior borders of the ribs and between the internal and innermost intercostal muscles, supply the anterior and posterior thoracic walls. The intercostal arteries are branches of the anterior intercostal arteries, the internal thoracic artery that arises from the subclavian artery, and the posterior intercostal arteries that arise directly from the aorta (Fig. 5.2). The azygos venous system drains the intercostal veins that run along with the arteries and nerves. The intercostal nerves are the ventral primary rami of thoracic spinal nerves and branch into lateral and anterior cutaneous nerves. These nerves also provide segmental sensory and sympathetic innervation and have considerable overlap with the adjacent nerves. Apart from the nerves in the neurovascular bundle that are derived from the ventral primary rami, the thoracic spinal nerves give rise to dorsal primary rami that supply the deep muscles and skin of the back.

INDICATIONS

Thoracentesis is indicated for pleural effusions of unknown etiology and can provide both diagnostic and therapeutic benefits. Diagnostically, analysis of the fluid allows classification as an exudate or a transudate. Therapeutically, if a significant amount of fluid is present in the pleural space, thoracentesis is used to alleviate respiratory distress (eg, dyspnea). However, one must be cautious when removing large amounts of fluid.

The presence of transudates in the pleural space is due to an imbalance of hydrostatic and oncotic pressures, often caused by congestive heart failure, liver cirrhosis, or nephrotic syndrome. In contrast, exudates are due to increased capillary permeability or lymphatic obstruction resulting in fluid accumulation and stagnation in the pleural space. Exudative pleural effusions are commonly caused by pneumonia or cancer. Diagnostic thoracentesis can often be deferred if the patient shows overt signs of congestive heart failure without atypical features or if only a small amount of fluid is present in the pleural space.

Light's criteria are used to distinguish transudates from exudates. Transudates are characterized by a pleural fluid protein/serum protein ratio less than 0.5, pleural fluid lactate dehydrogenase (LDH)/serum LDH less than 0.6, or pleural fluid LDH less than two-thirds of the upper limit of normal. Exudates have pleural fluid protein/serum protein ratios more than 0.5, pleural fluid LDH/serum LDH more than 0.6, or pleural fluid LDH more than two-thirds of the upper limit of normal.

CONTRAINDICATIONS

There are no absolute contraindications to performing a thoracentesis. Relative contraindications include severe coagulopathies, thrombocytopenia, or current use of anticoagulant medications. Other relative contraindications include an inability of the patient to cooperate, mechanical ventilation (positive end-expiratory pressure), minimal fluid volume, altered chest wall anatomy, severe pulmonary disease, uncertain fluid location, and active cutaneous infection at the point of needle insertion.

EQUIPMENT

Sterile field preparation
  Skin cleaning antiseptic solution: chlorhexidine or povidone-iodine solution
  Sterile gauze
  Sterile gloves
  Sterile fenestrated drape (24 × 30 inches) with adhesive strip
Anesthesia
  Lidocaine (1% to 2%), 10-mL ampule
  Syringe, 10 mL
  22-gauge needle, 1.5 inches
  25-gauge needle, 1 inch
  Hemostat (optional)
Fluid collection
  Prepackaged thoracocentesis kit; if a kit is unavailable, the following components should be collected:
  • Over-the-needle catheter, 18 or 20 gauge
  • Syringe, 60 mL
  • Three-way stopcock
  • Drainage tubing
  • Large evacuated container
  Scalpel, No. 11 blade
  Specimen tubes
  Sterile occlusive dressing
  Adhesive dressing
Ultrasound (if available)

PROCEDURE

Obtain patient consent and perform a time out.

Prior to Procedure

Patient Positioning
• Upright, for stable patients:
  • Patient should be upright, sitting at the edge of the bed while leaning slightly forward and resting the arms on a raised table (eg, Mayo stand).
• Lateral recumbent position, for unstable patients or those who cannot sit up:
  • Patient should be lying supine on the bed with the ipsilateral hand placed behind the head.
  • Raise the contralateral shoulder with a towel or a pillow to facilitate a posterior axillary approach.

Ultrasonography
See Fig. 5.3.
• Goals
  • Locate the pleural effusion
  • Mark the size
  • Determine the site of needle insertion

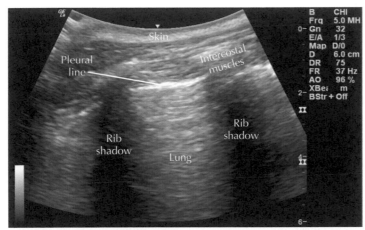

Left thoracocentesis with ribs

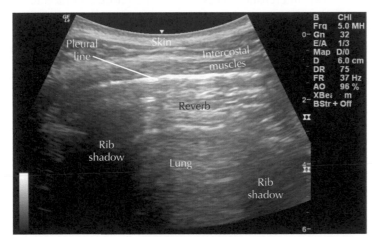

Left thoracocentesis

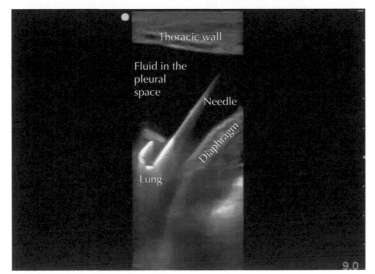

Thoracocentesis

FIGURE 5.3 Ultrasonography for thoracentesis

- Equipment
  - Curvilinear transducer (5 to 2 MHz) or high-frequency linear transducer (7.5 to 1 MHz)
- Landmarks
  - Identify the hyperechoic diaphragm
  - Fluid from the pleural effusion will appear dark
  - In motion mode (M-mode), the lung can be visualized as a sinusoidal wave pattern due to respiratory movement
- Using bedside ultrasonography with the patient upright, the upper extent of the effusion in the pleural cavity can be observed.

Site Verification

- Confirm the level of pleural effusion on the posterior chest wall by the following:
  - Auscultation: Listen for decreased or absent breath sounds
  - Percussion: dullness to percussion
  - Fremitus: diminished or absent vibrations
- Mark the site of needle insertion two intercostal spaces below the upper border of the effusion, 5 to 10 cm lateral to the spine at the midscapular line.
  - Puncture site should be at the superior border of the lower rib of the chosen intercostal space to minimize injury to the neurovascular bundle at the inferior border of the rib.
  - Note that the needle should not be inserted below the ninth rib to avoid injury to the diaphragm or abdominal organs.

Procedural Steps

See Fig. 5.4 and Video 5.1.

1. Create a sterile field by cleaning the skin with antiseptic (povidone-iodine or chlorhexidine solution) in concentric circles starting from the marked incision site outwards.
   a. Once dry, drape the area with a fenestrated sterile drape.
   b. Extend the field with another larger drape.
2. Using a 25-gauge needle, inject a subcutaneous wheal of anesthetic (lidocaine) at the incision site above the superior border of the rib below the selected intercostal space.
3. Using a 22-gauge needle, anesthetize the deeper subcutaneous tissues up to the parietal pleura.
   a. Be careful to avoid the inferior border of the upper rib where the neurovascular bundle lies.
   b. "Walk" or serially inject lidocaine along superior border of the rib.
   c. Aspirate every 2 to 3 mm to:
      i. Ensure that no lidocaine is intravascularly injected (ie, blood returns) and
      ii. Determine the depth of the intrapleural space (ie, fluid returns).
         A. Mark the depth with a hemostat on the needle.
         B. Slightly withdraw the needle and inject lidocaine to provide anesthesia to the parietal pleura.

4. Assemble the thoracentesis device by attaching a syringe to an 18-gauge over-the-needle catheter.
5. Slowly insert the needle at the superior border of the rib up to the predetermined depth while pulling back on the plunger until fluid is aspirated.
   a. Once fluid is aspirated, immediately stop advancing the needle.
6. Guide the plastic catheter over the needle and insert until firmly anchored in the skin.
   a. A small nick may be made with the scalpel if the catheter is difficult to insert.
   b. When the catheter is fully inserted, remove the needle as the patient exhales or hums.
   c. The exposed port of the catheter should be immediately covered to prevent the entry of air into the pleural space.
7. Attach the large syringe (35 to 60 mL) to the catheter hub with a three-way stopcock.
8. Diagnostic thoracentesis:
   a. With the stopcock in the open position, aspirate fluid until the syringe is full (50 to 60 mL).
   b. When the syringe is full, turn the stopcock to the closed/off position.
   c. The stopcock should only be open when fluid is being aspirated.
9. Therapeutic thoracentesis:
   a. If additional fluid needs to be drained, attach one end of the sterile drainage tubing to the second port on the stopcock and the other end of the tubing to the evacuated container.
   b. Open the stopcock and allow the evacuated container to fill.
   c. Do not remove more than 1500 mL of pleural fluid. Removing too much fluid may result in postexpansion pulmonary edema.
10. When fluid collection is complete, close the stopcock.
11. Rapidly remove the catheter as the patient holds the breath in end expiration (Valsalva maneuver) and immediately cover the incision site with sterile gauze and an occlusive dressing to prevent the entry of air.

Postprocedure

Fluid Analysis

The fluid can be sent for laboratory analysis to determine the underlying etiology of the pleural effusion. In general, evaluation includes cell count, protein levels, LDH, pH, glucose, amylase, bacterial culture, and cytology.

ANATOMICAL PITFALLS

The primary structures at risk during thoracentesis are those contained in the intercostal neurovascular bundle. As described previously, the intercostal vein, artery, and nerve in the bundle travel along the inferior border of each rib. Any incisions made in the intercostal spaces must be positioned above the superior borders of ribs to avoid damaging any of

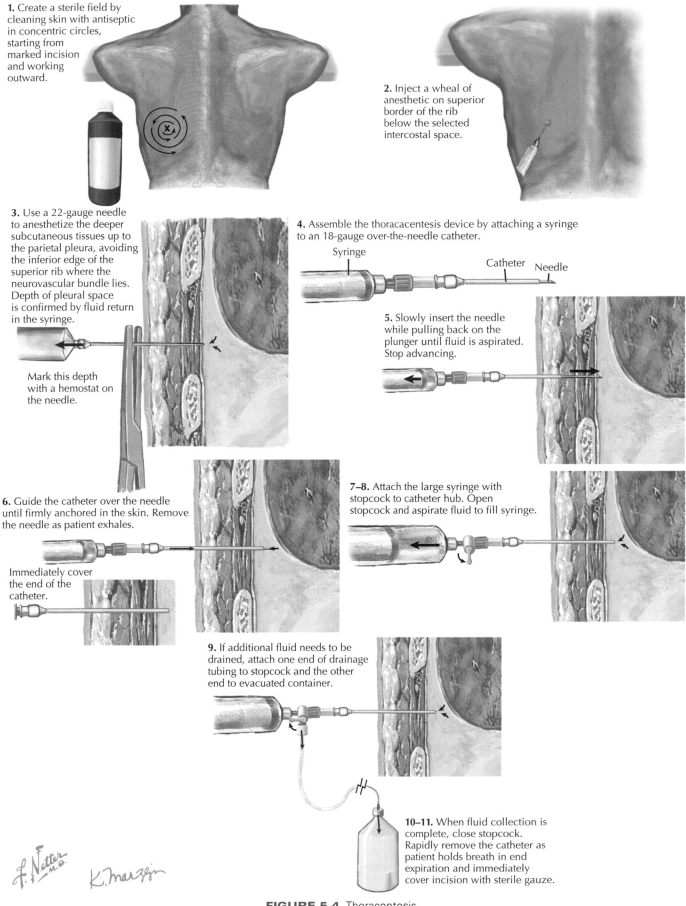

1. Create a sterile field by cleaning skin with antiseptic in concentric circles, starting from marked incision and working outward.

2. Inject a wheal of anesthetic on superior border of the rib below the selected intercostal space.

3. Use a 22-gauge needle to anesthetize the deeper subcutaneous tissues up to the parietal pleura, avoiding the inferior edge of the superior rib where the neurovascular bundle lies. Depth of pleural space is confirmed by fluid return in the syringe.

Mark this depth with a hemostat on the needle.

4. Assemble the thoracacentesis device by attaching a syringe to an 18-gauge over-the-needle catheter.

Syringe
Catheter Needle

5. Slowly insert the needle while pulling back on the plunger until fluid is aspirated. Stop advancing.

6. Guide the catheter over the needle until firmly anchored in the skin. Remove the needle as patient exhales.

Immediately cover the end of the catheter.

7–8. Attach the large syringe with stopcock to catheter hub. Open stopcock and aspirate fluid to fill syringe.

9. If additional fluid needs to be drained, attach one end of drainage tubing to stopcock and the other end to evacuated container.

10–11. When fluid collection is complete, close stopcock. Rapidly remove the catheter as patient holds breath in end expiration and immediately cover incision with sterile gauze.

FIGURE 5.4 Thoracentesis

these structures. In addition, the incision should be made 5 to 10 cm lateral to the spine to avoid damage to the posterior intercostal arteries and veins or nerve branches that emerge immediately lateral to the spine. The needle should not be inserted below the ninth rib to avoid injury to the diaphragm or the abdominal viscera.

COMPLICATIONS

The most common clinically significant complication of thoracentesis is pneumothorax, an abnormal collection of air and gas in the pleural space causing the lung to collapse. Pneumothorax is suspected after thoracentesis if patients are symptomatic (eg, chest pain, dyspnea, and hypoxemia) or if air is aspirated during the procedure. Although the pneumothorax may resolve spontaneously, the patient may require chest tube thoracostomy. Use of ultrasound guidance lowers the risk of pneumothorax, as does greater operator experience.

Hemothorax is due to bleeding caused by iatrogenic injury to the intercostal arteries. The neurovascular bundle (intercostal vein, artery, and nerve) is found at the inferior border of the ribs. When performing a thoracentesis, injury to these structures can be avoided by inserting the needle superior to the rib.

Potential complications of thoracentesis also include pain at the puncture site, bleeding, liver or spleen puncture, empyema, reexpansion pulmonary edema, vasovagal events, and infection. Immediately after the procedure, chest radiography and other imaging can be used to rule out many of the potential complications of thoracentesis.

CONCLUSION

Thoracentesis is a minimal-risk diagnostic and/or therapeutic intervention for patients with pleural effusion of unknown cause. Laboratory analysis of the pleural fluid allows classification as a transudate or exudate, which is suggestive of the underlying pathophysiology. For patients with respiratory distress, thoracentesis is used to remove fluid to alleviate symptoms caused by the pleural effusion. Ultrasonography is performed to confirm the presence and location of the effusion and can effectively minimize complications of the procedure. Complications of thoracentesis are often the result of inadequate knowledge of the relevant clinical anatomy and/or lack of training and experience. Although no procedure is without risks, careful understanding and application of the proper technique and procedure can improve patient outcomes.

Suggested Readings

Binder D, Goldsmith G. Thoracentesis. Available at https://www.youtube.com/watch?v=UBY3cQiQ6Ko; 2011.
Brauner M, Bailey R. Thoracentesis. Available at http://emedicine.medscape.com/article/80640-overview; 2013.
Cleveland Clinic. Pleural effusion. Heart & Vascular Institute Overview. Available at http://my.clevelandclinic.org/health/diseases_conditions/pleural-effusion; 2013.
Gordon C, Feller-Kopman D, Balk E, Smetana G. pneumothorax following thoracentesis: a systematic review and meta-analysis. *Arch Intern Med.* 2010;170(4):332–339.
Heffner J. Diagnostic thoracentesis. Available at http://www.uptodate.com/contents/diagnostic-thoracentesis; 2015.
Johns Hopkins Medicine. Thoracocentesis. Available at http://www.hopkinsmedicine.org/healthlibrary/test_procedures/pulmonary/thoracentesis_92, p07761.
Lechtzin N. Thoracentesis. Available at http://www.merckmanuals.com/professional/pulmonary-disorders/diagnostic-pulmonary-procedures/thoracentesis; 2013.
Light R. Pleural effusion. *N Engl J Med.* 2002;346(25):1971–1977.
Light R. Pleural effusion. Available at http://www.merckmanuals.com/professional/pulmonary-disorders/mediastinal-and-pleural-disorders/pleural-effusion; 2014.
National Heart, Lung, and Blood Institute. What is thoracocentesis? Available at http://www.nhlbi.nih.gov/health/health-topics/topics/thor; 2012.
Thomsen T, DeLaPena J, Setnik G. Thoracocentesis. *N Engl. J Med.* 2006;355(16). Available at http://www.nejm.org/doi/full/10.1056/NEJMvcm053812.
Yu H. Management of pleural effusion, empyema, and lung abscess. *Semin Intervent Radiol.* 2011;28(1):075–086.

REVIEW QUESTIONS

1. A 21-year-old female gymnast is admitted to the hospital with severe dyspnea after a fall from the uneven parallel bars. Radiographic examination reveals that her right lung is collapsed and the left lung is compressed by a great volume of air in her right pleural cavity. On physical examination, she has no signs of external injuries. The patient suddenly becomes tachycardic with a systolic blood pressure of 90 mm Hg. Which of the following conditions most likely describes this case?

   A. Flail chest with paradoxical respiration
   B. Emphysema
   C. Hemothorax
   D. Chylothorax
   E. Tension pneumothorax

2. A 34-year-old man with a complaint of sharp, localized pain over the thoracic wall is diagnosed with pleural effusion. A chest tube is inserted to drain the effusion through an intercostal space. At which of the following locations is the chest tube most likely to be inserted?

   A. Superior to the upper border of the rib
   B. Inferior to the lower border of the rib
   C. At the middle of the intercostal space
   D. Between the internal and external intercostal muscles
   E. Between the intercostal muscles and the posterior intercostal membrane

Tracheostomy, Tracheotomy, Cricothyroidotomy

INTRODUCTION

Tracheotomy and cricothyroidotomy are two surgical procedures used to gain access to an otherwise compromised airway in both emergency and routine situations. Tracheostomy is the term given to the stoma created by the tracheotomy procedure in which access to the airway is gained through the anterior wall of the trachea. Tracheotomy is considered a more complicated yet more permanent procedure compared with cricothyroidotomy, which is an emergency procedure. Commonly used techniques include percutaneous tracheotomy and cricothyroidotomy, open tracheotomy, and surgical cricothyroidotomy. These are the general procedures described in this chapter, but some procedures may vary depending on available kits and instrumentation, the patient's anatomy, and institutional practices.

CLINICALLY RELEVANT ANATOMY

The key surface landmark is the cricoid cartilage (Fig. 6.1), which is usually found by using the suprasternal notch below and the thyroid cartilage above as reference points. The cricothyroid membrane, which spans the anterior aspect of the thyroid and cricoid cartilages, can be identified by palpating a slight indentation in the skin inferior to the thyroid notch.

Along the superior aspect of this membrane, a pair of cricothyroid arteries runs horizontally and anastomoses in the midline (Fig. 6.2). On the anterior surface of the cricoid cartilage, the cricothyroid muscles arise and extend superiorly and posteriorly to attach to the lateral surfaces of the thyroid cartilage. The brachiocephalic artery transverses from left to right anterior to the trachea at the superior thoracic inlet and deep to the suprasternal notch.

The thyroid gland lies anterior to the trachea and is made up of two lateral lobes and an isthmus that crosses anteriorly at the level of the second to fourth tracheal rings (see Fig. 6.2). The recurrent laryngeal nerves travel in the tracheoesophageal grooves and are outside the surgical field unless dissection strays significantly. The inferior thyroid veins ascend near the midline to the inferior poles of the thyroid gland and are superficial to the trachea. The great vessels are lateral to the dissection area and should always be avoided.

INDICATIONS

The indications for performing tracheotomy include the provision of a safe airway and/or the prevention of aspiration in patients with neurological disease or trauma when endotracheal intubation is not suitable. In the intensive care unit (ICU), the need for prolonged mechanical ventilation is the most common reason for tracheotomy. The risk of oral and upper airway damage, including tracheal stenosis and vocal cord paresis, increases during extended endotracheal intubation. By replacing an endotracheal tube with a tracheostomy tube, dependence on sedatives can be reduced, giving the patient more mobility, social interaction, and the possibility of earlier weaning. In the emergency department, tracheotomy may be required to manage acute airway obstruction, which can occur due to edema from an infection, allergic reaction, or direct trauma to the trachea. A tracheotomy can be performed in such cases as a preventative measure. A well-trained physician may perform one as an emergency procedure, although emergent airway obstruction is most often managed by performing a cricothyroidotomy with subsequent conversion to a tracheotomy if required for ongoing care.

Cricothyroidotomies are performed only in emergency situations where endotracheal intubation ventilation has failed—hence the phrase "can't intubate, can't ventilate." It is considered a last-resort procedure when the patient's life is at risk. Anticipation of the potential for sudden airway obstruction coupled with the widespread use of fiberoptic laryngoscopes has seen a reduction of the need for surgical airways. However, there will be occasions when the only option is surgical establishment of an airway in order to ventilate the patient.

CONTRAINDICATIONS
Tracheotomy

There is no absolute contraindication for tracheotomy except for when the patient requires an emergency airway. The relative contraindications are as follows:
- Children younger than 12 years
- Palpable pulses over the tracheotomy site
- Active infection over the tracheotomy site
- Anatomic abnormalities of the trachea, including tracheomalacia
- Thyroid mass or goiter over the tracheotomy site
- Obese neck or nonpalpable laryngotracheal landmarks
- Thrombocytopenia
- Positive end-expiratory pressure more than 15 cm H_2O
- Coagulopathy

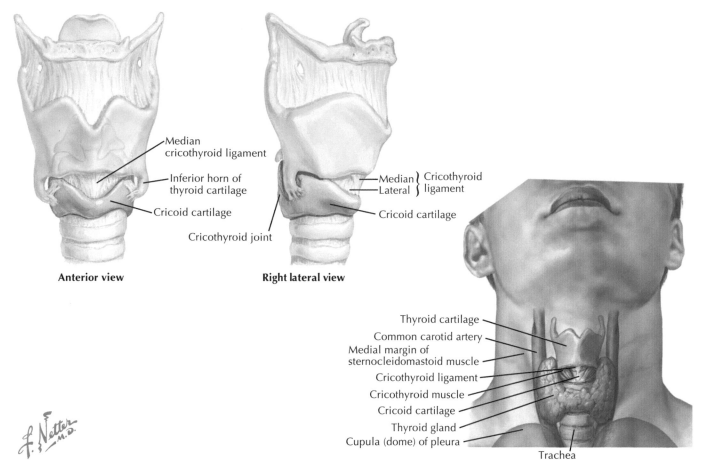

Median cricothyroid ligament

Inferior horn of thyroid cartilage

Cricoid cartilage

Cricothyroid joint

Anterior view

Median } Cricothyroid
Lateral } ligament

Cricoid cartilage

Right lateral view

Thyroid cartilage
Common carotid artery
Medial margin of sternocleidomastoid muscle
Cricothyroid ligament
Cricothyroid muscle
Cricoid cartilage
Thyroid gland
Cupula (dome) of pleura

Trachea

FIGURE 6.1 Cricoid cartilage

- History of difficult intubation
- Limited ability to extend the neck, especially with an unstable spine

There are few absolute contraindications for either the traditional cricothyroidotomy or percutaneous cricothyroidotomy, as both are emergency procedures of last resort. They may be contraindicated when there is complete or partial transection of the airway, significant injury to the cricoid cartilage, or a severely fractured larynx.

EQUIPMENT
Tracheotomy

Skin marker
No. 15 scalpel blade
Cricoid hook
Kitner sponge
Tracheostomy tube
Bag-valve-mask device
Oxygen source

Cricothyroidotomy

Bag-valve-mask device
Oxygen source
No. 15 scalpel blade
Hemostats
Tracheal hook

Scissors
Trousseau dilator
Tracheostomy tube

PROCEDURE

Tracheotomy can be performed via an open surgical approach or a percutaneous approach called a percutaneous dilation tracheotomy. Cricothyroidotomy can also be completed percutaneously (needle cricothyroidotomy) or surgically.

As with all procedures, the provider should explain the procedure and indications for it to the patient and the family. Consent should always be obtained if the clinical situation allows. In addition, all providers should wear appropriate personal protective equipment, and a time out should be performed before beginning the procedure.

Cricothyroidotomy

This procedure, similar to tracheotomy, can be completed by two methods: needle cricothyroidotomy and surgical cricothyroidotomy.

Needle Cricothyroidotomy

1. Position the patient supine with the neck hyperextended to expose the laryngotracheal complex, as in standard open tracheotomy, and palpate the cricothyroid membrane

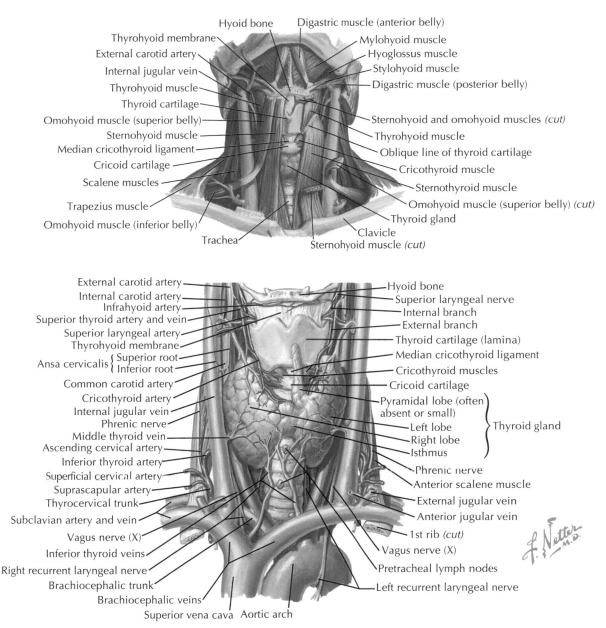

Hyoid bone — Digastric muscle (anterior belly)

Thyrohyoid membrane — Mylohyoid muscle
External carotid artery — Hyoglossus muscle
Internal jugular vein — Stylohyoid muscle
Thyrohyoid muscle — Digastric muscle (posterior belly)
Thyroid cartilage —
Omohyoid muscle (superior belly) — Sternohyoid and omohyoid muscles (cut)
Sternohyoid muscle — Thyrohyoid muscle
Median cricothyroid ligament — Oblique line of thyroid cartilage
Cricoid cartilage — Cricothyroid muscle
Scalene muscles — Sternothyroid muscle
Trapezius muscle — Omohyoid muscle (superior belly) (cut)
Omohyoid muscle (inferior belly) — Thyroid gland
Trachea — Clavicle
Sternohyoid muscle (cut)

External carotid artery — Hyoid bone
Internal carotid artery — Superior laryngeal nerve
Infrahyoid artery — Internal branch
Superior thyroid artery and vein — External branch
Superior laryngeal artery — Thyroid cartilage (lamina)
Thyrohyoid membrane — Median cricothyroid ligament
Ansa cervicalis { Superior root / Inferior root } — Cricothyroid muscles
Common carotid artery — Cricoid cartilage
Cricothyroid artery — Pyramidal lobe (often absent or small)
Internal jugular vein —
Phrenic nerve — Left lobe
Middle thyroid vein — Right lobe } Thyroid gland
Ascending cervical artery — Isthmus
Inferior thyroid artery — Phrenic nerve
Superficial cervical artery — Anterior scalene muscle
Suprascapular artery — External jugular vein
Thyrocervical trunk — Anterior jugular vein
Subclavian artery and vein — 1st rib (cut)
Vagus nerve (X) — Vagus nerve (X)
Inferior thyroid veins — Pretracheal lymph nodes
Right recurrent laryngeal nerve — Left recurrent laryngeal nerve
Brachiocephalic trunk —
Brachiocephalic veins —
Superior vena cava   Aortic arch

FIGURE 6.2 Thyroid gland and suprahyoid and infrahyoid muscles

located 1.5 to 2 cm in width and 2 to 3 cm below the laryngeal prominence. Prepare skin with Betadine.
2. Inject lidocaine (usually 1%) into the skin and subcutaneous tissue where the needle will be placed.
3. Standing at the head of the patient and, using the nondominant hand, insert a 12- or 14- gauge needle attached to a 5- or 10-mL syringe containing 2 to 3 mL of normal saline at a 30- to 45-degree angle caudally towards the suprasternal notch.
4. Aspirate the syringe while advancing through the cricothyroid membrane, paying close attention for bubbles seen in the syringe to indicate entry into the trachea.
5. Hold the needle in place and advance the catheter to the hub.
6. Withdraw the needle when the catheter is in place.

7. Confirm proper placement by withdrawing approximately 10 mL of air into the catheter and expel it into the airway. If resistance is felt, the catheter is likely too far advanced into the posterior trachea. If the catheter is located subcutaneously, the air will expand the skin. Adjust the catheter accordingly.
8. Remove the syringe and secure the catheter. Connect it to a jet ventilation apparatus, which consists of a flow regulator connected to an oxygen source.

Surgical Cricothyroidotomy

1. Position the patient and identify the cricothyroid membrane as described for the needle cricothyroidotomy.
2. Inject lidocaine (usually 1%) into the skin and subcutaneous tissue where the incision will be placed.

3. Prepare the neck and upper chest with povidone-iodine solution and drape the surgical site.
4. Standing at the head of the patient, stabilize the larynx with the nondominant hand.
5. Use the No. 15 scalpel to make a single 3- to 5-cm vertical incision through the skin and subcutaneous tissue in the midline over the thyroid cartilage, extending to below the inferior border of the cricoid cartilage.
6. Expose the cricothyroid membrane. Use the scalpel to make a horizontal incision perforating the membrane in its inferior half, nearer to the cricoid cartilage. This reduces the chance of damage to the vocal cords and cricothyroid vessels.
7. Use a Trousseau dilator to penetrate and widen the membrane entry site. A Kelly clamp, curved hemostat, right angle instrument, or the handle of the scalpel may be used as an alternative to the dilator.
8. Insert a tracheostomy or endotracheal tube and connect to a bag-valve-mask device for ventilation. If an endotracheal tube is used, the end should be placed no more than 2 to 3 cm into the trachea to avoid placement into the right main stem bronchus.
9. Confirm that bilateral breath sounds are present.
10. Secure the tube in place with a tracheal tie, suture, or adhesive tape.

If the airway is needed for more than 48 hours, the surgical cricothyroidotomy should be converted to a tracheostomy. If a needle cricothyroidotomy was performed, the patient should have a formal tracheostomy as soon as possible because ventilation through the catheter is suboptimal and there is a risk of catheter dislodgment.

Percutaneous Dilation Tracheotomy

Percutaneous dilation tracheotomy has become a commonly used bedside procedure, especially in ICU and trauma units. This minimally invasive procedure involves the placement of a tracheostomy tube without direct visualization of the trachea. It therefore should only be performed on patients with an endotracheal tube in place. It can be performed using bronchoscopic guidance at the bedside. This procedure should be performed by clinicians who are well trained in the technique and are prepared to convert to an open tracheotomy if needed.

1. Drape and position the patient as mentioned previously in the standard open tracheotomy procedure.
2. Palpate the skin to locate the laryngotracheal framework and make an incision in the skin. Using blunt dissection, clear the pretracheal tissue.
3. Withdraw the endotracheal tube until the cuff is just at the level of the glottis. The tip of the bronchoscope can be placed in the tube so that the light from the tip is visible through the surgical incision, highlighting the target area.
4. Enter the tracheal lumen below the second tracheal ring with a needle introducer and insert the guide wire through the needle.
5. Using a series of dilators, dilate the tract from the skin to the tracheal lumen using the guide wire as a guide.
6. Insert the tracheostomy tube (#8 for males and #6 for females) under direct bronchoscopic visualization over the dilator.
7. Confirm tube placement by viewing the tracheobronchial tree through the tracheostomy tube. Remove the dilator and endotracheal tube. Secure the tracheostomy tube as mentioned above in standard open tracheotomy.

Open Tracheotomy

This surgical procedure can be performed in the operating room, trauma bay, or at the bedside in a monitored setting such as the ICU. It is traditionally performed under general anesthesia in a previously intubated patient (Fig. 6.3, Video 6.1). In emergency situations when a patient presents in acute distress, this procedure can be performed under local anesthesia while the patient breathes spontaneously.

1. Place the patient supine with a bolster underneath the shoulders to extend the neck and expose the laryngotracheal landmarks. (This maneuver is contraindicated in patients with cervical spine injuries or atlantoaxial instability because of the risk of spinal cord compression.)
2. Palpate the major landmarks of the neck, including the thyroid cartilage, cricoid cartilage, and suprasternal notch. Use a skin marker or pen to indicate the position of each landmark.
3. Inject lidocaine (usually 1%) into the skin and subcutaneous tissue where the incision will be placed.
4. Prepare the neck and upper chest with povidone-iodine solution and drape the surgical site.
5. Make a 2- to 3-cm incision in the vertical or horizontal plane. A horizontal incision yields a more cosmetically pleasing postoperative scar, as it will follow the relaxed skin tension lines. In the case of emergency tracheotomy, a vertical incision should be used to avoid bleeding from the anterior jugular venous system.
6. Incisions
   a. A vertical incision starts just below the cricoid cartilage.
   b. A horizontal incision is placed approximately two finger breadths below the cricoid cartilage or halfway between the cricoid cartilage and the suprasternal notch, corresponding to the second or third tracheal ring.
7. Divide the subcutaneous tissue using either a No. 15 blade or electrical cautery to the level of the strap muscles. Avoid damage to the anterior jugular vein. When identified, it should be ligated or lateralized to avoid bleeding.
8. Identify the strap muscles and dissect them laterally through the midline raphe, separating right and left sides, until the thyroid isthmus is exposed.
9. Retract the thyroid isthmus either superiorly or inferiorly or divide and ligate it to expose the second and third tracheal rings, allowing for creation of a tracheal window.

1. Place patient on table with a bolster underneath shoulders to extend the neck and expose laryngotracheal landmarks.

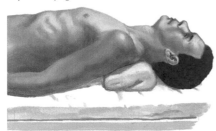

2–3. Palpate major landmarks of the neck. Inject lidocaine into the skin and subcutaneous tissue where incision will be made.

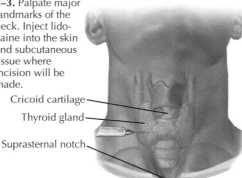

Cricoid cartilage

Thyroid gland

Suprasternal notch

4–6. Prepare neck and upper chest with Betadine solution. Make a 2- to 3-cm incision midway between the cricoid cartilage and the suprasternal notch.

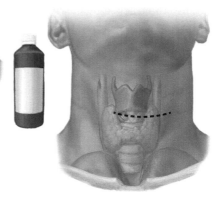

7–9. Divide the subcutaneous tissue to the level of the strap muscles. Divide strap muscles vertically along midline raphe until thyroid isthmus is exposed. Retract isthmus to expose 2nd and 3rd tracheal rings.

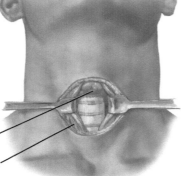

Thyroid isthmus

Strap muscles

10–11. Using a cricoid hook, move cricoid into superior and superficial position to allow easier access to trachea. Using a Kitner sponge, dissect pretracheal fascia off proximal trachea.

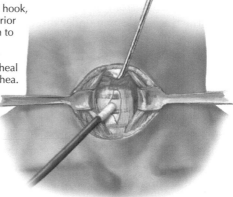

12–13. Enter the trachea by making a tracheal window. Insert a tracheal dilator to make the lumen larger, without causing excessive trauma to cartilaginous framework.

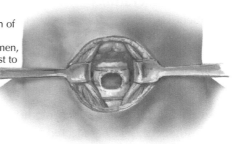

14. Upon visualization of the endotracheal tube within the tracheal lumen, ask the anesthesiologist to withdraw tube until posterior trachea is observed.

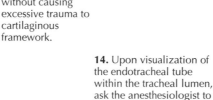

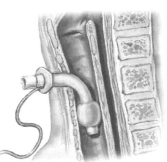

15–16. Place the tracheostomy tube into the tracheal lumen. Confirm proper placement by connecting tracheostomy tube to the ventilator, inflating the cuff, and observing end-tidal CO_2.

17–18. Close the fascia and the skin and suture tracheostomy tube collar in place through the flanges of the tube. Place ties around patient's neck. Perform a post-tracheotomy chest radiograph to assess tube positioning and survey for pneumothorax or pneumomediastinum.

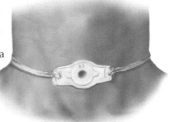

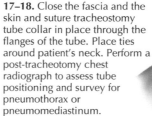

FIGURE 6.3 Open tracheotomy

10. With a cricoid hook, place traction on the cricoid cartilage to move it superiorly and superficially to allow easier access into the trachea.
11. With a Kitner sponge, dissect the pretracheal fascia off the proximal trachea.
12. Enter the trachea by making a window by using one of the following techniques:
    a. Single horizontal intercartilaginous incision
    b. H-type incision
    c. Removing 1-cm-wide portion of the anterior aspect of the second or third tracheal ring with a scalpel, Metzenbaum scissors, or a tracheal punch
13. After entering the trachea, use a tracheotomy dilator to open the tracheal lumen further, taking care to prevent excessive trauma to the cartilaginous framework. Stay sutures can be placed superiorly and inferiorly to the stoma.
14. Upon visualization of the endotracheal tube within the tracheal lumen, ask the anesthesiologist to withdraw the tube until the posterior tracheal wall is visualized.
15. Place the tracheostomy tube (#8 for men or #6 for women) into the tracheal lumen under direct visualization.
16. Confirm proper placement by connecting the tube to the ventilator, inflating the cuff, and observing end-tidal CO_2. Once placement is established and chest auscultation reveals bilateral breath sounds, remove the cricoid hook.
17. Close the fascia and skin and suture the tracheostomy tube collar in place using nonabsorbable sutures placed through the flanges of the tube. Place the tracheostomy ties around the patient's neck.
18. Perform a posttracheostomy chest radiograph to assess tube positioning and to look for pneumothorax or pneumomediastinum.

Surgical Considerations

If the patient is unable to tolerate either lying supine or having the neck extended due to significant kyphoscoliosis, cervical osteoarthritis, or other conditions, tracheotomy should be performed with the patient in a sitting position without neck extension.

Procedure Under Local Anesthesia

Local anesthetic should be injected into the pretracheal tissues prior to opening the trachea to provide proper analgesia. In addition, 2% lidocaine solution can be applied inside the trachea to provide topical endoluminal anesthesia.

Flap Construction

A Bjork flap can be made to facilitate reinsertion of the tracheostomy tube in cases of accidental decannulation, which occurs frequently in obese patients or those with difficult anatomy. A horizontal incision is made between the second and third tracheal rings and down the lateral aspects of the third tracheal ring. The flap is then pulled down and sutured to the skin with nonabsorbable sutures.

ANATOMICAL PITFALLS IN CHILDREN

It should be noted that the laryngotracheal landmarks used in adult tracheotomy are located relatively more superiorly within the neck in pediatric patients. As the pleural apices lie within the cervical compartment, particular attention should be paid to avoid straying laterally, which might result in pleural puncture leading to pneumothorax.

Tracheal incisions are generally made vertically through two or three tracheal rings, usually between the second and the fifth rings. These incisions need to be long enough to allow easy passage of the tracheostomy tube to prevent damage to the cartilaginous framework. Incisions that are too small or intercartilaginous horizontal incisions may lead to collapse of the suprastomal tracheal ring as the curved tube exerts a backward pressure on the ring above the incision.

During the procedure, nylon sutures are placed on both sides of the trachea before the incision is made to allow traction on the tracheal ring during cannulation. After the tracheostomy tube is placed and secured in a fashion similar to that used in adults, the traction sutures are tied loosely and taped to the skin of the anterior chest wall. Tape is used to clearly mark the right and left sutures so they are not reversed when used to recannulate the trachea.

Tube position can be confirmed by passing a pediatric flexible endoscope through the tube or by obtaining a postoperative chest radiograph. The tip of the tube should be 5 to 20 mm away from the carina and should not be so short that the lumen faces posteriorly or is at risk for exiting the tracheal window.

Of note, obese children or those with metabolic storage diseases may have excessively long tracts between the skin and trachea, requiring a custom tracheostomy tube with extra-long proximal, extratracheal portions.

COMPLICATIONS

These procedures, while fairly routine, do not come without possible complications. These are mostly self-limited but can include cardiovascular compromise and death. Complications can occur intraoperatively and postoperatively. Bleeding is the most frequent intraoperative complication. Laceration of the anterior jugular vein can cause profuse bleeding immediately after the initial incision. Damage to the thyroid gland vessels will result in extensive bleeding as well. A second frequent complication involves damage to or perforation of the posterior wall of the trachea due to blind needle puncture. There is also an increased risk of esophageal perforations since the esophagus lies directly posterior to the trachea. Performing tracheotomy with bronchoscopy and having sufficient training can reduce these complications. Awareness of the position of the recurrent laryngeal nerve reduces the risk of laceration and subsequent vocal damage. Fractures of both the cricoid and thyroid cartilage can occur. The tube may be misplaced either anterior or lateral to the trachea. Absence of bilateral breath sounds or lack of end-tidal CO_2 indicates improper placement.

Postoperative decannulation and/or displacement is a frequent complication. Pneumothoraxes and pneumomediastinum can occur from routine tracheotomies but typically follow difficult procedures. Tracheostomies bypass a large part of the airway that is crucial for humidifying air. The dry air increases the viscosity of bronchial secretions and may contribute to lung infections, impaired gas diffusion, and atelectasis. A dry cough due to tracheitis has also been associated with dry air, so the use of properly humidified air and nebulizers is encouraged. Routine cleaning and changing of the tracheostomy tube can reduce infection at the stoma site. Improperly sized tracheostomy tubes can lead to irritation, tracheomalacia, tracheal stenosis, trachea–innominate artery fistula, and tracheoesophageal fistula, so regular inspection and cleaning of the inner cannula is recommended. Introduction of a tracheostomy tube also predisposes patients to aspiration due to compression of the esophagus.

CONCLUSION

The four procedures described above have had a profound impact on airway management for critically ill patients. A compromised airway is one of the most dangerous and life-threatening occurrences seen in hospitals. Proper training and knowledge of head and neck anatomy allow physicians to treat patients efficiently and safely in both emergency and routine situations.

Suggested Readings

Apfelbaum JL, Hagberg CA, Caplan RA, et al. Practice guidelines for management of the difficult airway: an updated report by the American Society of Anesthesiologists Task Force on Management of the Difficult Airway. *Anesthesiology*. 2013;118(2):251–270.

Ben-Nun A, Altman E, Best LA. Emergency percutaneous tracheostomy in trauma patients: an early experience. *Ann Thorac Surg*. 2003;77(3):1045–1047.

Bhatti NI, Mohyuddin A, Reaven N, et al. Cost analysis of intubation-related tracheal injury using a national database. *Otolaryngol Head Neck Surg*. 2010;143:31–36.

Blankenship DR, Kulbersh BD, Gourin CG, et al. High-risk tracheostomy: exploring the limits of the percutaneous tracheostomy. *Laryngoscope*. 2005;115(6):987–989.

Chan TC, Vilke GM, Bramwell KJ, Davis DP, Hamilton RS, Rosen P. Comparison of wire-guided cricothyrotomy versus standard surgical cricothyrotomy technique. *J Emerg Med*. 1999;17:957.

Dierks EJ. Tracheotomy: elective and emergent. *Oral Maxillofacial Surg Clin North Am*. 2008;20:513–520.

Epstein SK. Late complications of tracheostomy. *Respir Care*. 2005;50:542–549.

Griffiths J, Barber VS, Morgan L, Young JD. Systematic review and meta-analysis of studies of the timing of tracheostomy in adult patients undergoing artificial ventilation. *Br Med J*. 2005;330:1243.

Grillo HC. Development of tracheal surgery: A historical review. Part 1: techniques of the tracheal surgery. *Ann Thorac Surg*. 2003;75:610–619.

Hart KL, Thompson SH. Emergency cricothryotomy. *Atlas Oral Maxillofac Surg Clin North Am*. 2010;18:29–38.

Heard AM, Green RJ, Eakins P. The formulation and introduction of a "can't intubate, can't ventilate" algorithm into clinical practice. *Anaesthesia*. 2009;64:601–608.

Helm M, Hossfeld B, Jost C, Lampl L, Bockers T. Emergency cricothyroidotomy performed by inexperienced clinicians: surgical technique versus indicator-guided puncture technique. *Emerg Med J*. 2013;30:646–649.

Langvad S, Hyldmo PK, Nakstad AR, Vist GE, Sandberg M. Emergency cricothyrotomy: a systematic review. *Scand J Trauma Resuscitation Emerg Med*. 2013;21:43.

Malata CM, Foo IT, Simpson KH, Batchelor AG. An audit of Bjork flad tracheostomies in head and neck plastic surgery. *Br J Oral Maxillofac Surg*. 1996;34(1):42–46.

Morris LL, Afifi MS. *Tracheostomies: The Complete Guide*. New York: Springer; 2010:17–38.

Nekhendzy V, Guta C, Champeau MW. *Tracheotomy/Tracheostomy and Cricothyroidotomy: Anesthetic Consideration. Anesthesiologist's Manual of Surgical Procedures*. Philadelphia: Lippincott Williams & Wilkins; 2009:187–189, 277–299.

Kost KM. Endoscopic percutaneous dilatational tracheotomy: a prospective evaluation of 500 consecutive cases. *Laryngoscope*. 2005;115(10 Pt 2):1–30.

Tabaee A, Geng E, Lin J, et al. Impact of neck length on the safety of percutaneous and surgical tracheotomy: a prospective, randomized study. *Laryngoscope*. 2005;115(9):1685–1690.

REVIEW QUESTIONS

1. A 35-year-old woman is admitted to the emergency department after a violent automobile crash. The patient's upper airway is obstructed with blood and mucus, and a midline tracheotomy inferior to the thyroid isthmus is performed. Which of the following vessels are most likely to be present at the site of incision and will need to be cauterized?

    A. Middle thyroid vein and inferior thyroid artery
    B. Inferior thyroid artery and inferior thyroid vein
    C. Inferior thyroid vein and thyroidea ima artery
    D. Cricothyroid artery and inferior thyroid vein
    E. Left brachiocephalic vein and inferior thyroid artery

2. A 22-year-old woman is admitted to the emergency department unconscious after falling over the handlebars of her bicycle. An emergency tracheotomy is performed to insert a tracheostomy tube. What is the most common tracheal cartilage level at which a tracheotomy incision is performed?

    A. First to second
    B. Second to third
    C. Third to fourth
    D. Fourth to fifth
    E. Fifth to sixth

3. A 32-year-old man is admitted to the emergency department unconscious after a severe car crash. During an emergency cricothyroidotomy, an artery is accidentally injured. Two days later the patient shows signs of aspiration pneumonia. Which of the following arteries was most likely injured?

    A. Superior thyroid
    B. Inferior thyroid
    C. Cricothyroid
    D. Superior laryngeal
    E. Suprahyoid

4. A 34-year-old woman bursts through the doors of the emergency department. She is straining to take a breath but can only mouth, "I can't breathe" before collapsing. She is placed on a stretcher. Her tongue is swollen and protruding from her mouth. The patient has only minimal air movement with bag-valve-mask ventilation. Oxygen saturation is approximately 80%. Attempts at oral intubation are unsuccessful due to massive soft tissue edema of her pharynx. A decision is made to perform a cricothyrotomy. After palpating the neck to identify the appropriate landmarks, an incision should most likely be made at which of the following locations?

A. The cricothyroid membrane, which is located at the junction of the clavicle and the sternum

B. The cricothyroid membrane, which is located between the thyroid cartilage and the cricoid cartilage below

C. The thyrohyoid membrane, which is located between the thyroid cartilage and the hyoid bone above

D. The suprasternal notch, which is located at the medial junction of the clavicle and the sternum

E. The trachea, which is located below the cricoid cartilage

Cardiac Pacing

INTRODUCTION

Cardiac pacing introduces electrical impulses into the heart to induce cardiac depolarization and contraction. Since the advent of external electric stimulation in 1952 by Zoll and associates, the role of cardiac pacing has been constantly evolving. Currently, there are many different methods of pacing, and given its wide acceptance, it is important to have a strong clinical understanding of the anatomy of the surrounding structures and the uses and management of cardiac pacing. Pacing can be performed pharmacologically, transcutaneously, or transvenously on an emergency basis.

CLINICALLY RELEVANT ANATOMY FOR TRANSVENOUS PLACEMENT

The subclavian vein courses medially as a continuation of the axillary vein, starting from its emergence out of the axilla at the first rib (Figs. 7.1 to 7.3). The subclavian vein travels under the clavicle anterior to the subclavian artery, where it joins with the internal jugular vein, creating the brachiocephalic vein. The internal jugular vein begins in the jugular foramen at the base of the skull and traverses inferiorly through the anterior triangle of the neck, where it lies lateral to the carotid artery in the carotid sheath and joins with the innominate vein. The superior vena cava (SVC) is valveless and is formed by the union of the two brachiocephalic veins at the level of the sternal angle; the left brachiocephalic vein is longer than its right-sided counterpart. The SVC empties into the superior right atrium, which creates the superior right border of the heart.

ELECTROCARDIOGRAPHY

Electrocardiographic (ECG) tracing is determined by the net vector of electrical currents in relation to the sensing electrode, with vectors pointing toward the electrode causing a positive deflection and those pointing away from the electrode causing a negative deflection. In the human heart, electrical current travels from the sinoatrial (SA) node (the primary intrinsic pacemaker of the heart) at the junction of the right atrium and SVC to the atrioventricular (AV) node, which lies at the inferior portion of the interatrial septum, depolarizing the atria along its course (represented by the P wave). From there, the current travels to the bundle of His in the interventricular septum and subsequently splits into the left and right fascicles. The current then courses the length of the interventricular septum until reaching the apex of the heart, where it is transmitted to the Purkinje fibers and then

to the ventricular myocytes (represented by the QRS complex; Fig. 7.4).

When placing a transvenous pacemaker using the internal jugular or subclavian approach, the sensing electrode is initially advanced to the level of the high right atrium. ECG tracing changes as the sensing electrode travels from the right atrium to the right ventricle. At this point, the net vector of electrical conduction is traveling *away* from the sensing electrode, resulting in a negative P wave and QRS complex, with the P wave becoming larger as the electrode nears the SA node. Once in the mid-right atrium, the current initially travels toward the electrode for the first half of atrial depolarization and then continues away from the electrode to the AV node, resulting in a biphasic P wave. As the electrode approaches the ventricles, the QRS complex gains in amplitude. Once at the level of the tricuspid valve, the P wave is positive. As the sensing electrode passes into the right ventricle, the P wave begins to diminish in size, whereas the QRS complex increases.

When the catheter makes contact with the right ventricular wall, ST segment elevation will be seen (ideal placement). If the electrode is passed through the right ventricular outflow tract into the pulmonary artery, it will lie above the sinus node, resulting in atrial depolarization traveling away from the electrode, a negative P wave, and the shrinking of QRS amplitude. If the electrode enters the inferior vena cava, the QRS amplitude will shrink further. However, since the electrode is below the AV node, the atrial depolarization will be *toward* it, and the P wave will still be positive.

INDICATIONS

The indications for cardiac pacing are bradycardia with hemodynamic compromise, ventricular tachyarrhythmias secondary to bradyarrhythmias, second-degree AV block type II or third-degree AV block with hemodynamic compromise, overdrive pacing, complicated myocardial infarction, and cardiac surgeries that may promote bradycardia.

In life-threatening bradyarrhythmias, initial resuscitation measures (ie, basic life support and advanced cardiac life support) should take priority, with attempts at pharmacologic and then transcutaneous methods of pacing. If this fails or if the patient is successfully resuscitated and needs permanent pacing, transvenous pacing can be used as a bridge to a permanent implantable pacemaker. In cases of tachycardia caused by a reentrant circuit, pacing can safely be used to overdrive the circuit by pacing at a faster rate than the

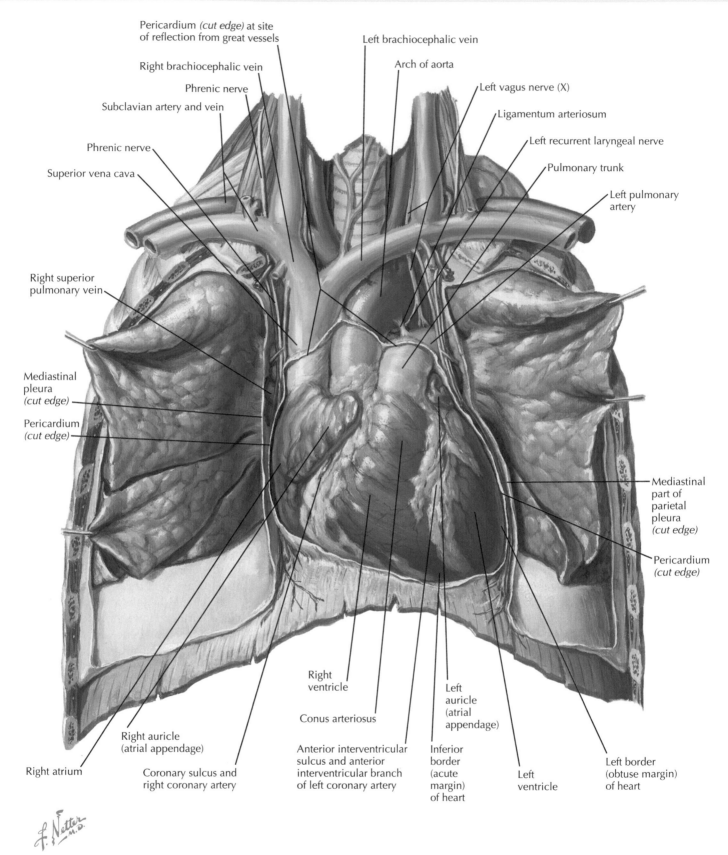

FIGURE 7.1 Heart: anterior exposure

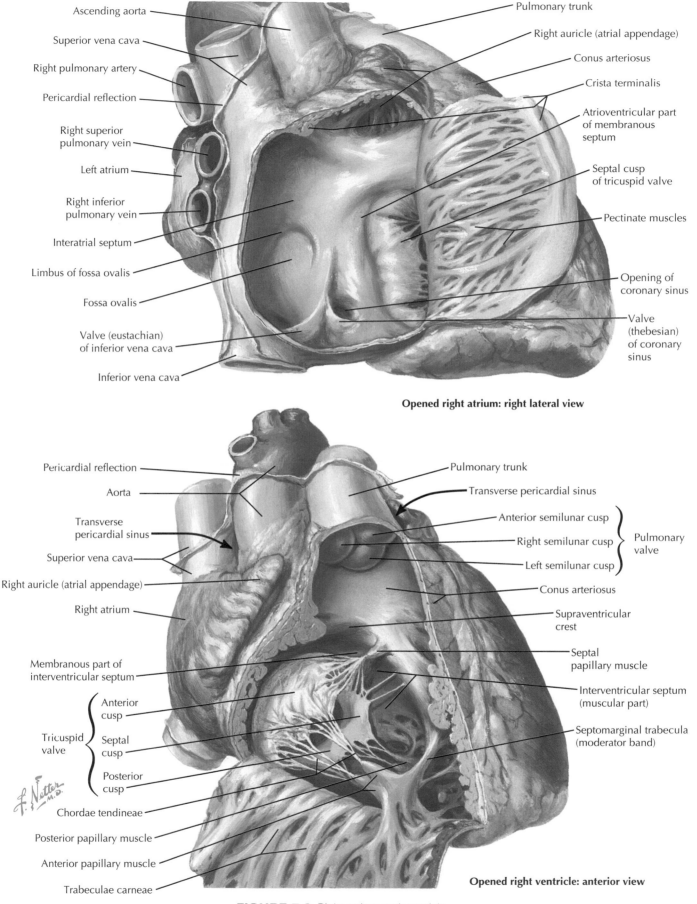

Ascending aorta

Superior vena cava

Right pulmonary artery

Pericardial reflection

Right superior
pulmonary vein

Left atrium

Right inferior
pulmonary vein

Interatrial septum

Limbus of fossa ovalis

Fossa ovalis

Valve (eustachian)
of inferior vena cava

Inferior vena cava

Pulmonary trunk

Right auricle (atrial appendage)

Conus arteriosus

Crista terminalis

Atrioventricular part
of membranous
septum

Septal cusp
of tricuspid valve

Pectinate muscles

Opening of
coronary sinus

Valve
(thebesian)
of coronary
sinus

Opened right atrium: right lateral view

Pericardial reflection

Aorta

Transverse
pericardial sinus

Superior vena cava

Right auricle (atrial appendage)

Right atrium

Membranous part of
interventricular septum

Anterior
cusp

Tricuspid
valve

Septal
cusp

Posterior
cusp

Chordae tendineae

Posterior papillary muscle

Anterior papillary muscle

Trabeculae carneae

Pulmonary trunk

Transverse pericardial sinus

Anterior semilunar cusp

Right semilunar cusp

Pulmonary
valve

Left semilunar cusp

Conus arteriosus

Supraventricular
crest

Septal
papillary muscle

Interventricular septum
(muscular part)

Septomarginal trabecula
(moderator band)

Opened right ventricle: anterior view

FIGURE 7.2 Right atrium and ventricle

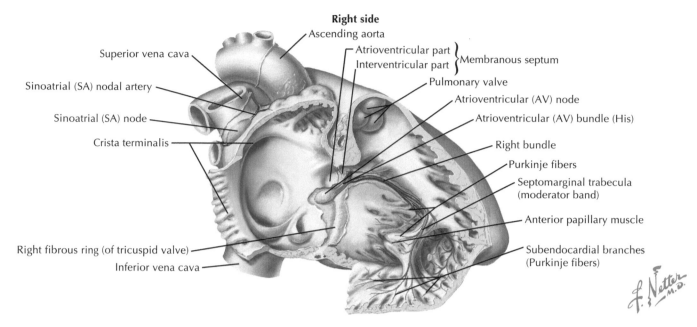

Right side
Ascending aorta
Atrioventricular part
Interventricular part } Membranous septum
Superior vena cava
Pulmonary valve
Sinoatrial (SA) nodal artery
Atrioventricular (AV) node
Sinoatrial (SA) node
Atrioventricular (AV) bundle (His)
Crista terminalis
Right bundle
Purkinje fibers
Septomarginal trabecula (moderator band)
Anterior papillary muscle
Right fibrous ring (of tricuspid valve)
Subendocardial branches (Purkinje fibers)
Inferior vena cava

FIGURE 7.3 Conducting system of the heart

intrinsic rhythm. This method can also be used to pace bradycardia in order to prevent the R-on-T phenomenon, which predisposes to torsades de pointes. Asystole is no longer an indication for pacing.

CONTRAINDICATIONS

There are no absolute contraindications to pacing. Hypothermia predisposes the patient to pacing-induced ventricular fibrillation, and pacing in this clinical situation is usually deferred until the patient's core temperature has risen. Pacing in the presence of a prosthetic tricuspid valve also presents challenges because of the altered anatomy. Reversible causes, such as drug-induced arrhythmias, may also interfere with attempts at pacing.

PHARMACOLOGIC PACING

In the emergency setting, the pharmacologic approach to pacing is generally the first choice because medication can be administered quickly and easily. Atropine (muscarinic antagonist) is the first-line drug for bradycardia. Because of the AV nodal mechanism of action, many cases of high-degree AV block will not respond to atropine or may worsen. In these situations, isoproterenol (β_1 and β_2 agonist) may be a better option.

TRANSCUTANEOUS PACING

Transcutaneous pacing is accomplished by sending generator-induced electrical impulses through pads that are attached to the skin. It is well established as a safe, timely, and efficient means of temporary pacing and has the added benefit of being readily available.

1. Clean and dry the skin. Trimming or shaving the hair at the site may be required before applying the pads.
2. Place the patient on a continuous ECG monitor.

3. Place the electrode pads according to the manufacturer's instructions. One method is to place one pad posteriorly between the left scapula and the spine and the other between the xiphoid process and the left nipple. Alternatively, a pad can be placed on the right upper chest and another at the apex of the heart.
4. Configure the rate of pacing (initially 60 to 90 beats/min) and set the pacing output to minimal; it can be increased until the QRS complex and T waves are appropriately established.
5. Check the ECG to confirm electrical capture (QRS complexes identified after the pacing spike), and check the patient's pulse to ensure that adequate ventricular contractions are occurring.

TRANSVENOUS PACING

Transvenous pacing is a more definitive means of temporary emergency pacing. It is more tolerable than transcutaneous pacing, although the pacemaker is more difficult to place and the procedure takes approximately 30 minutes to perform. It is usually prudent to pace transcutaneously initially while a transvenous pacemaker is prepared. The procedure involves gaining central venous access and then placing a wire in contact with the right ventricular wall.

EQUIPMENT

Sterile drapes
Sterile gown, gloves, mask, and hat
Chlorhexidine swabs
1% to 2% lidocaine solution (with or without epinephrine)
25-gauge needle
18- to 21-gauge needle
3- to 5-mL Luer-Lok syringes

Repolarization

When heart is fully depolarized, there is no electrical activity for brief period (ST segment). Then repolarization begins from epicardium to endocardium, producing electrical vector directed downward and to left, causing upward (positive) deflection in both leads I and aVF (T waves). A period of no electrical activity follows, with tracing at baseline until next impulse originates at SA node.

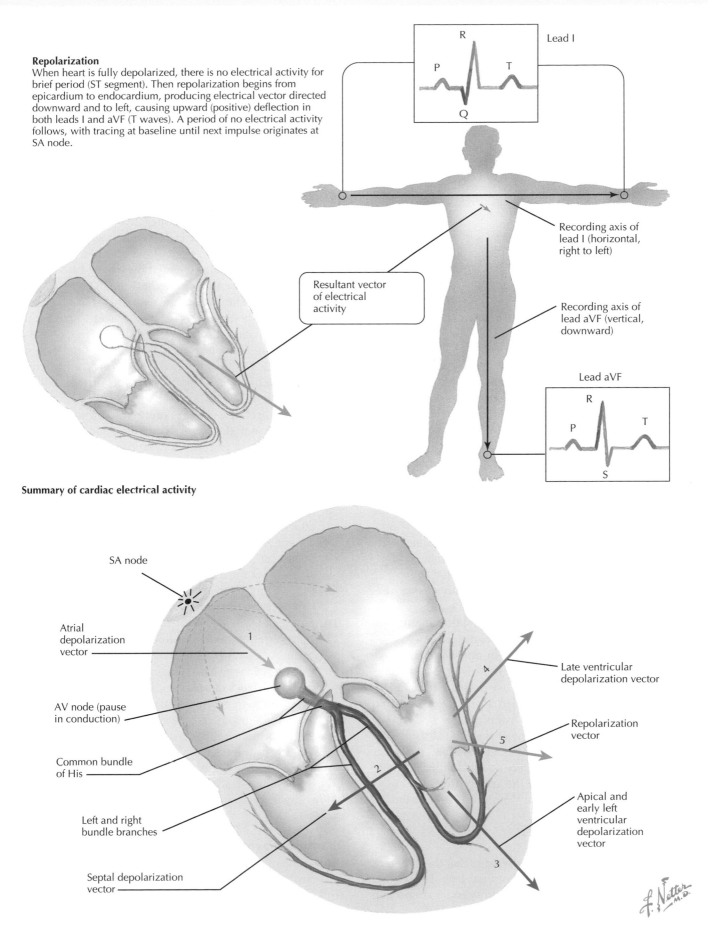

Lead I

Resultant vector of electrical activity

Recording axis of lead I (horizontal, right to left)

Recording axis of lead aVF (vertical, downward)

Lead aVF

Summary of cardiac electrical activity

SA node

Atrial depolarization vector

AV node (pause in conduction)

Common bundle of His

Left and right bundle branches

Septal depolarization vector

Late ventricular depolarization vector

Repolarization vector

Apical and early left ventricular depolarization vector

FIGURE 7.4 Cardiac depolarization and repolarization

10-mL non–Luer-Lok syringe
Guide wire with J tip
Dilator
Sutures (0 or 1-0 nonabsorbable)
Needle driver
Scalpel
4 × 4 gauze pads
Introducer sheath
Sterile sleeve
Transvenous pacing catheter
Adapter pins
Pacing generator with connector cable
Pacing pads
ECG machine
Ultrasound machine (preferably with cardiac and vascular probes)

PROCEDURE

Obtain patient consent, and perform a time out.

Central Venous Access

1. Identify the venous access point, which can be the right or left internal jugular, subclavian, femoral, or brachial vein, by a cutdown. The right internal jugular and left subclavian vein approaches are preferred because of easier anatomical access to the right side of the heart and fewer adverse effects. Ultrasound with a vascular probe should be used for visualization if available.
2. Place the patient in the Trendelenburg position if using these approaches to increase central venous pressure, which increases lumen diameter, and to decrease the chance of an air embolus to the brain.
3. Thoroughly clean the area with a chlorhexidine swab. Wash your hands with a chlorhexidine scrub.
4. Gown and glove following sterile technique.
5. Place a sterile drape over the patient, with adequate exposure of the access point.
6. Anesthetize the area generously with lidocaine, using a 25-gauge needle and a 3- to 5-mL syringe.
7. Gain central venous access with an 18- to 21-gauge needle attached to a 10-mL non–Luer-Lok syringe, making sure to maintain negative pressure throughout.
8. Remove the syringe and thread a J-tip guide wire into the vein using the Seldinger technique.
9. Nick the subcutaneous tissue at the edge of the needle with a scalpel to allow for adequate dilation.
10. Remove the needle and insert the dilator, making sure throughout not to let go of the guide wire.

Also see Chapter 14, "Central Venous Catheterization."

Transvenous Pacemaker Placement

See Fig. 7.5.

1. Before starting the procedure, ensure that the catheter's balloon tip is inflatable and does not leak. Ensure that the generator has a functional battery and that a backup battery is ready and charged.

2. Remove the dilator and insert the introducer sheath, making sure not to release the guide wire. Once the sheath is in an adequate position, the guide wire may be removed.
3. Attach the sterile sleeve to the introducer sheath. The combination of the sleeve and sheath allows for seamless positioning of the long pacing catheter while maintaining sterile technique.
4. The pacing catheter has a one-pronged end consisting of the electrode and a three-pronged end consisting of a proximal or positive end, a distal or negative end, and a port for a syringe to inflate or deflate the balloon. Attach an adapter pin to the negative terminal and connect it to a continuous ECG monitor, which should be positioned directly in front of the operator.
5. Insert the one-pronged end of the pacing catheter into the sterile sleeve and advance it through the introducer sheath until the SVC is reached. This is usually about 15 cm for the right internal jugular and 17 cm for the left subclavian approach.
6. Inflate the balloon using a 3- to 5-mL Luer-Lok syringe filled with air. Leave the syringe attached to confirm balloon inflation and for further balloon manipulation.
7. While observing changes on the ECG monitor, carefully advance the pacing catheter. Proper right ventricular apex placement will correlate with small positive P waves and large QRS complexes with marked ST segment elevation. Once this is achieved, deflate the balloon and leave the syringe attached.
8. Remove the negative lead from the ECG machine and attach both positive and negative leads to the pacing generator using the connector cable.
9. Set the rate at 10 to 20 beats/min higher than the intrinsic rate. Set the output to greater than 4 mA. Observe the ECG for electrical capture. Check the pulse for the confirmation of mechanical capture.
10. Suture in place.
11. Immediately confirm placement by checking the pulse again. A 12-lead ECG reading should then be obtained. Correct right ventricular placement should show left bundle branch block morphology with left axis deviation.
12. Chest radiographs (posteroanterior and lateral views preferred) should also be obtained to confirm placement and rule out postcatheterization complications. The tip of the catheter should be visible at the apex of the heart. Two-dimensional ultrasound using a cardiac probe can also help verify placement and rule out complications.

Additional Pacing Techniques

Transesophageal Pacing

Placement of a lead in the esophagus or stomach allows for cardiac pacing through the left atrium and ventricle. This method has proved to be effective and safe for atrial pacing. However, given the distance of the left ventricle from the esophagus, ventricular pacing is

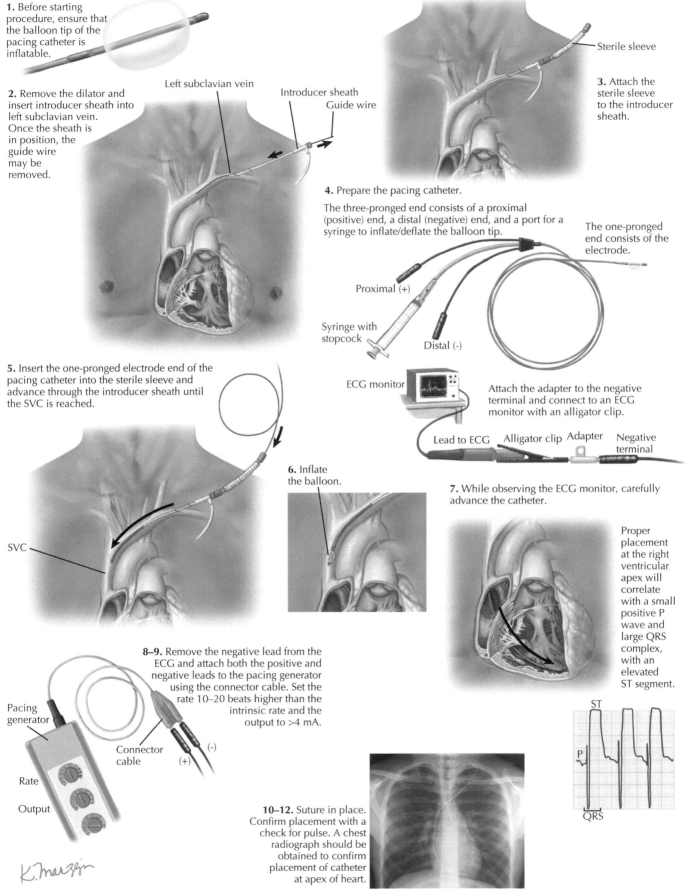

1. Before starting procedure, ensure that the balloon tip of the pacing catheter is inflatable.

2. Remove the dilator and insert introducer sheath into left subclavian vein. Once the sheath is in position, the guide wire may be removed.

Left subclavian vein

Introducer sheath
Guide wire

3. Attach the sterile sleeve to the introducer sheath.

Sterile sleeve

4. Prepare the pacing catheter.

The three-pronged end consists of a proximal (positive) end, a distal (negative) end, and a port for a syringe to inflate/deflate the balloon tip.

The one-pronged end consists of the electrode.

Proximal (+)

Syringe with stopcock

Distal (-)

ECG monitor

Attach the adapter to the negative terminal and connect to an ECG monitor with an alligator clip.

Lead to ECG   Alligator clip   Adapter   Negative terminal

5. Insert the one-pronged electrode end of the pacing catheter into the sterile sleeve and advance through the introducer sheath until the SVC is reached.

SVC

6. Inflate the balloon.

7. While observing the ECG monitor, carefully advance the catheter.

Proper placement at the right ventricular apex will correlate with a small positive P wave and large QRS complex, with an elevated ST segment.

8–9. Remove the negative lead from the ECG and attach both the positive and negative leads to the pacing generator using the connector cable. Set the rate 10–20 beats higher than the intrinsic rate and the output to >4 mA.

Pacing generator

Connector cable

(-)
(+)

Rate

Output

ST
P
QRS

10–12. Suture in place. Confirm placement with a check for pulse. A chest radiograph should be obtained to confirm placement of catheter at apex of heart.

K. marzejon

FIGURE 7.5 Transvenous pacemaker placement

difficult, making AV block difficult to treat. Because of the mobility of the gastrointestinal tract itself and the intolerability of the procedure for conscious patients, transesophageal pacing has not gained much favor in the emergency setting.

Epicardial Pacing

In the postcardiac surgery period, particularly after cardiopulmonary bypass, the patient is vulnerable to AV block, usually warranting the placement of a temporary epicardial pacemaker intraoperatively with removal soon thereafter. The leads are placed directly into the epicardium during open-heart surgery. Pediatric patients also benefit from epicardial pacing because anatomical anomalies may make transvenous access unfeasible.

ANATOMICAL PITFALLS

Cardiac pacing via the transvenous approach involves guiding a catheter from venous access to the heart. While aiming for the vein, an artery may be inadvertently punctured. Because of the anatomical relationships, the lead can be misplaced in many other locations, including the left ventricle, left atrium, coronary sinus, and pulmonary artery. Misplacement may also cause a pneumothorax. Confirmation of lead misplacement may be demonstrated by the lack of backflow of blood, seeing the needle in the internal jugular vein on ultrasound, connecting the line to an arterial line transducer to confirm the absence of arterial waves, analyzing a venous blood gas, and obtaining a chest radiograph to check for pneumothorax. In hypotensive patients, low-flow states can mimic "venous" characteristics even when the line is intraarterial.

COMPLICATIONS

Transcutaneous Pacing

The complications for transcutaneous pacing are few and less severe than for transvenous pacing. An added benefit is the lack of complications associated with mechanical manipulation of the endocardium. However, transcutaneous pacing is generally limited by patient discomfort and associated soft tissue injury, inconsistent capture, and ECG disturbances, which can lead to the masking of underlying malignant arrhythmias.

Transvenous Pacing

Complications may arise with venous access, catheter placement, and lead malfunction. The risks of venous access include infection and thromboembolism.

Mechanical irritation of the ventricular endocardium during right heart catheterization can lead to serious ventricular dysrhythmias at rates of 1.5% to 2.3%. If this occurs, the catheter tip may simply be repositioned to a less arrhythmogenic location in the right ventricle. The most common complication of transvenous catheter placement is a friction rub audible on physical examination. Although mostly benign, this may also indicate right

ventricular perforation and tamponade, which has been reported at a rate of 0.14%.

Lead malfunction can result in pacing failure. Lead fracture or dislodgment and inflammation or fibrosis around the catheter site can also lead to failure. A sign of this is a change from baseline in the amplitude of pacing spikes on the surface ECG and in the pacing threshold. In this situation, check the connections and the battery and increase the threshold; if capture still does not occur, the pacing lead will need to be replaced.

CONCLUSION

Cardiac pacing provides an emergency corrective measure for restoring the innate electrical activity of the heart and is usually performed when pharmacologic management is inadequate. Several types of cardiac pacing approaches can be used based on clinical appropriateness, as determined by the clinician, and can be administered with minimal adverse effects.

Suggested Readings

Bannon MP, Heller SF, Rivera M. Anatomic considerations for central venous cannulation. *Risk Manag Health Policy*. 2011;4:27–39.

Khorsandi M, Muhammad I, Shaikhrezai K, Pessotto R. Is it worth placing ventricular pacing wires in all patients post-coronary artery bypass grafting? *Interact Cardiovasc Thorac Surg*. 2012;15:489–493.

Kim WY, Lee CW, Sohn CH, et al. Optimal insertion depth of central venous catheters: is a formula required? A prospective cohort study. *Injury*. 2012;43:38–41.

Neumar RW, Otto CW, Link MS, et al. Adult advanced cardiovascular life support. Part 8. 2010 American Heart Association Guidelines for Cardiopulmonary Resuscitation and Emergency Cardiovascular Care. *Circulation*. 2010;122:S729–S767.

Steele R, Irvin CB. Central line mechanical complication rate in emergency medicine patients. *Acad Emerg Med*. 2001;8:204–207.

REVIEW QUESTIONS

1. A 62-year-old female accountant is admitted to the emergency department with severe chest pains that radiate to her left arm. An ECG reveals that the patient has had an acute myocardial infarction. Coronary angiography is performed, and a stent is placed at the proximal portion of the left anterior descending artery. Because of the low ejection fraction of the right and left ventricles, a cardiac pacemaker is also placed in the heart. The function of which of the following structures is essentially replaced by the insertion of a pacemaker?

   A. AV node
   B. SA node
   C. Purkinje fibers
   D. Bundle of His
   E. Bundle of Kent

2. A 62-year-old male internist is admitted to the emergency department with a complaint of severe chest pain. Physical examination reveals acute myocardial infarction. After the patient is stabilized, angiography is performed and the ejection fraction of the left ventricle is reduced to

30% of normal. A cardiac pacemaker is placed to prevent fatal arrhythmias. What is the location of the tip of the pacemaker?

A. Right atrium
B. Left atrium
C. Right ventricle
D. Left ventricle
E. Superior vena cava

3. In the same patient as question 2, the ECG recording shows positive P waves. What is the location of the tip of the pacemaker?

A. Right atrium
B. Tricuspid valve
C. Right ventricle
D. SA node
E. Superior vena cava

Cardioversion and Defibrillation

INTRODUCTION

Providing immediate cardiopulmonary resuscitation (CPR) for patients with sudden cardiac arrest (SCA) delays the onset of asystole and extends the window for defibrillation to occur. Early defibrillation is associated with an increased likelihood of survival, which decreases by 5% with every minute after collapse.

Cardioversion and defibrillation are common procedures that are used to terminate potentially lethal cardiac arrhythmias. *Cardioversion* is the synchronized delivery of current during the R wave of the QRS complex, avoiding the delivery of a shock during the relative refractory period of the cardiac cycle, which could degenerate into ventricular fibrillation (Fig. 8.1). Cardioversion is used for "stable rhythms."

In contrast, *defibrillation* is the unsynchronized delivery of current at any time during the cardiac cycle, which is important in rhythms that are too rapid or disorganized to quickly locate a QRS complex. Defibrillation is used with the two "unstable rhythms," ventricular fibrillation and ventricular tachycardia without a pulse. These two rhythms are too disorganized and rapid for synchronization to be successful in locating the R wave. Because most deaths outside the hospital in witnessed SCA are from ventricular fibrillation, the need to learn and understand the application of defibrillation is crucial to preventing death. This is especially true for the lay public with access to automated external defibrillators (AEDs).

Cardiac arrhythmias have many causes, including coronary artery disease, electrolyte imbalance, hypovolemia, hypoxia, hypothermia, drug intoxication, cardiac tamponade, tension pneumothorax, pulmonary embolism, and trauma. Patients may present in a variety of ways, depending on the underlying cause of the arrhythmia; however, those with some of the stable arrhythmias may be completely asymptomatic. When patients become hemodynamically unstable, cardioversion or defibrillation may help stabilize them by converting the cardiac rhythm back to normal sinus rhythm.

Since the inception of basic life support and advanced cardiac life support, the machines used for cardioversion or defibrillation have evolved and become more portable. AEDs are now present in most public locations. Many individuals are being trained to use AEDs for minimizing the downtime after SCA.

CLINICALLY RELEVANT ANATOMY AND PATHOPHYSIOLOGY

In order to understand how the procedure works, it is important to have a strong understanding of the various arrhythmias and their origins. Electrical impulses in the heart begin in the sinu-atrial (SA) node, which is located in the right atrium near the entrance of the superior vena cava (Fig. 8.2). The SA node generates impulses that send a signal down the electrical pathway to the atrioventricular (AV) node. The AV node, which is located in the posteroinferior aspect of the interatrial septum near the coronary sinus opening, normally has an approximate 0.12-second delay of impulse before sending the signal to the bundle of His. This delay allows time for the atria to eject the blood into the ventricles before ventricular contraction. Once the signal passes through the AV node and down the bundle of His, it spreads throughout the Purkinje fibers to allow for a synchronous ventricular contraction. When impulses follow this normal, synchronized pattern, it is called "normal sinus rhythm."

When electrical activity becomes disorganized, there is electrical dyssynchrony, with cardiac cells in different stages of depolarization and repolarization. This results in an arrhythmia, which may be atrial, junctional, or ventricular in origin. Arrhythmias interrupt the sequential contraction of the myocardium, which results in blood being inadequately ejected from the ventricles, leading to the inadequate perfusion of other organs. When this occurs for more than a few minutes, the myocardium is depleted of oxygen and energy substrates. Chest compressions can help in the delivery of oxygen and these substrates. When a therapeutic current is applied to the chest wall, it can effectively reset the chaotic stimuli by placing the myocytes in a refractory state. This allows the SA node to resume pacing the heart and to depolarize myocytes in an organized, consecutive pattern.

INDICATIONS

Cardioversion or defibrillation is used in both elective and emergency situations, depending on the rhythm and the hemodynamic stability of the patient. Electrical cardioversion or defibrillation in conjunction with CPR is the method of choice to help a hemodynamically unstable heart return to a normal sinus rhythm. The indications for emergency synchronized electrical cardioversion include any hemodynamically unstable patient with supraventricular tachycardia, atrial flutter, atrial fibrillation, or monomorphic ventricular tachycardia with a pulse. When the rhythm is too rapid, QRS complexes may not be detected, and a shock will not be delivered. These rhythms require

Left bundle branch block

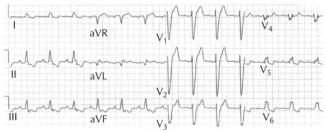

(A) Electrocardiogram showing left bundle branch block. It was recorded from a 73-year-old man. Note that the QRS complex is diffusely widened and is notched in leads V_3, V_4, V_5, and V_6. Note also that the T wave is directed opposite to the QRS complex. This is an example of a secondary T-wave change.

Ventricular preexcitation

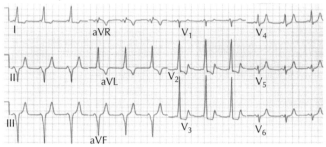

(B) ECG showing ventricular preexcitation. It is recorded from a 28-year-old woman. Note the short PR interval (0.9 seconds) and the widened QRS complex (0.134 seconds). The initial portion of the QRS complex appears slurred. This is referred to as a *delta wave*. This combination of short PR interval and widened QRS complex with a delta wave is characteristic of ventricular preexcitation. Note also that the T wave is abnormal, another example of a secondary T-wave change.

Ventricular premature beats

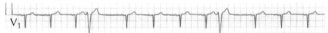

(C) Ventricular premature beats recorded from a 30-year-old man with no known heart disease.

ECG changes of left ventricular hypertrophy

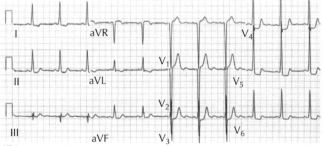

(D) Example of the ECG changes of left ventricular hypertrophy. It is recorded from an 83-year-old woman with aortic stenosis and insufficiency. Note the increase in QRS amplitude, the slight increase in QRS duration to 100 ms, and the ST-segment and T-wave changes.

FIGURE 8.1 QRS complex

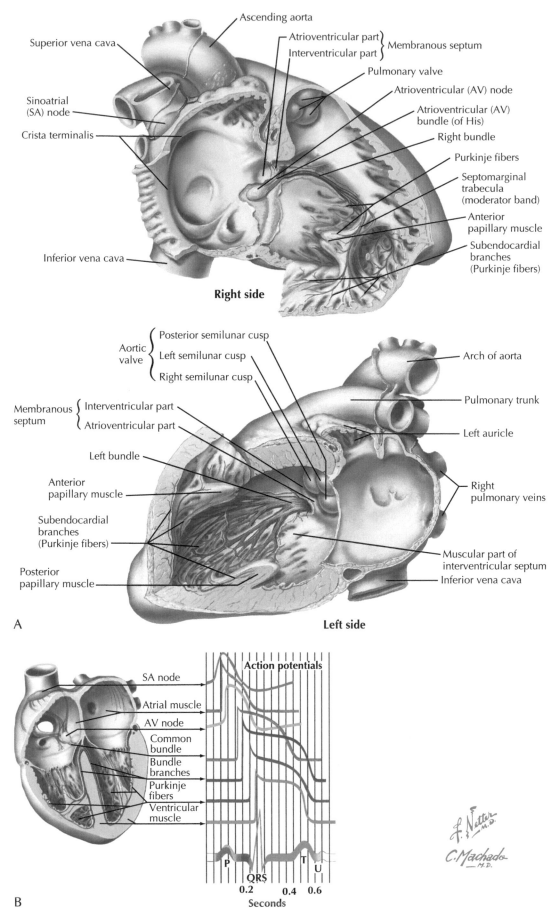

FIGURE 8.2 A, Conducting system of the heart. **B,** Action potentials recorded at each point in the conducting system.

unsynchronized high-energy shocks. The indications for emergency defibrillation include ventricular fibrillation and pulseless ventricular tachycardia.

CONTRAINDICATIONS

Cardioversion or defibrillation is contraindicated in patients with dysrhythmias that are already in a homogeneous depolarized state, such as in those caused by enhanced automaticity from digitalis toxicity, catecholamine-induced arrhythmia, and severe hypothermia. In these patients, the delivery of external energy will be ineffective and can lead to ventricular tachycardia, ventricular fibrillation, or asystole.

Ventricular tachycardia in a patient who is hemodynamically stable with a pulse is a contraindication to defibrillation. Defibrillation is also contraindicated in the presence of pulseless electrical activity and asystole because the myocardial tissues are unable to respond to the electrical impulses. A good rule of thumb is that any patient with a pulse should *not* be defibrillated. Metal objects on the patient's skin, including medication-releasing agents, are not contraindications to defibrillation, although they should be removed if possible.

METHODS

There are two methods of converting and treating arrhythmias for those who are stable (normotensive with a pulse). The first is a pharmacological approach. Many pharmacological agents work with the cells' biochemistry to convert rhythms or to control the heart rate until cardioversion can be successfully and safely completed.

Sometimes the arrhythmia is recalcitrant to medications and requires the second approach: synchronized electrical cardioversion.

Manual External Defibrillator

In 1957, Kouwenhoven was credited for developing the first closed-chest defibrillator that delivered shocks to an adult heart. Now used in conjunction with electrocardiography, a defibrillator requires the clinician to place paddles or pads on the skin of a patient to deliver an electrical current across the thorax to the heart. Three anteroposterior pads are used. This is a potentially fast and effective way to convert a hemodynamically unstable rhythm to a normal sinus rhythm. Its appropriate use depends on the health care provider being able to diagnose the correct rhythm;

therefore the manual external defibrillator is only found in ambulances, hospitals, and other health care institutions.

Manual Internal Defibrillator

The manual internal defibrillator is identical to the external version except that the charge conductors are placed in direct contact with the heart. Its use is limited to a trauma-related emergency thoracotomy or in the operating room.

Automated External Defibrillator

The AED is the most common type of defibrillator found in public locations because it is programmed to automatically identify cardiac arrhythmias. Two self-adhesive pads are applied to the victim's chest, and audio prompts tell first responders what to do and when to do it. When a shockable rhythm is detected, a button is pressed to deliver the appropriate shock to the victim. This device is favored over manual machines in the field and has been shown to have a sensitivity of greater than 90% and an overall specificity of more than 95% in accurately detected ventricular fibrillation.

Implantable Cardioverter-Defibrillator

First developed by Mirowski in the late 1960s, the implantable cardioverter-defibrillator (ICD) constantly monitors a patient's heart rhythm and delivers a shock when a life-threatening arrhythmia is sensed. These devices are placed for primary prevention in select patients with a history of sustained ventricular tachycardia or ventricular fibrillation. However, given the invasive nature of the procedure, ICDs are never placed in an emergency. Having an ICD is not a contraindication to the use of external or internal defibrillation, although it is recommended to place pads at least 8 cm away from the ICD to prevent conflict.

EQUIPMENT

Defibrillator or ECG monitor (AED, semiautomated external defibrillators, or standard defibrillator with monitors)
Paddles or adhesive pads
Conductive gel if using paddles
Standard cardiorespiratory monitors (blood pressure, pulse, and oxygen saturation)
Intravenous access for the administration of sedation or antiarrhythmic medication
Advanced cardiac life support medications

PROCEDURE

Obtain patient consent and perform a time out.

Unstable Ventricular Fibrillation or Ventricular Tachycardia Without a Pulse With a Manual Defibrillator

Monitor the patient's vital signs and ECG before, during, and after the procedure. In the first moments of cardiac arrest, three actions need to be immediately initiated: activating the emergency medical services system, providing CPR, and getting a manual defibrillator (Fig. 8.3, Video 8.1).

1. Turn on the defibrillator.
2. Expose the patient's chest wall.
3. Apply adhesive pads on the patient's chest wall to reduce transthoracic impedance. To help prevent electrical sparks, burns, or an electrical short circuit, transdermal medication patches should be removed. The skin should be dry, and excessive chest hair should be removed by rapidly ripping off the adhesive pads in contact with the chest hair or shaving the patient's chest.
   a. Place paddles or pads in one of four orientations: anterolateral, anteroposterior, anterior–left infrascapular, or anterior–right infrascapular. All four orientations are equally effective in delivering a successful shock. In the most common anterolateral position, one pad is placed on the right second intercostal space at the sternal border and the other on the left fourth or fifth intercostal space in the midaxillary line. Similarly, in the anteroposterior position, one pad is placed at the same right second intercostal space and the other between the tip of the left scapula and the spine.
4. Turn the selector switch on the defibrillator monitor to the appropriate position to acquire the ECG signal.
   a. Determine if the rhythm is shockable and proceed to select the appropriate energy level. If the type of waveform is unknown, set the default energy level to 200 joules (J) (see "Energy Selection").
   b. After determining the energy level for a shockable rhythm, the capacitor will charge. Once charged, clear the patient for defibrillation by stating "I'm clear, you're clear, everyone's clear." This is done because if anyone from the care team is touching the patient, the stretcher, or any piece of equipment attached to the patient, the shock may be transmitted to the care provider.
5. Press the button to deliver the shock. The patient's whole body will noticeably twitch.
   a. Once the shock is delivered, immediately resume CPR and continue until the return of spontaneous circulation.
   b. In case of cardiac arrest, if no pulse is present after 2 minutes of CPR, a second defibrillatory shock may be given. During this period, other tasks such as securing the airway, drawing blood, and inserting intravenous lines may be performed.

Energy Selection

Defibrillators can deliver energy in two main forms: biphasic or monophasic. First reported by Gurvich in 1939, biphasic waves, seen in most new devices, administer energy in two vectors. Biphasic waves defibrillate more effectively and at 60% of the energy of monophasic waveforms. Repeated defibrillation attempts predispose the myocardium to damage due to prolonged ischemia. The amount of energy needed depends on the type of arrhythmia. For unstable rhythms, the patient should receive unsynchronized defibrillation. The initial level should be set at 200 J, then 300 J, followed by 360 J, if defibrillation is unsuccessful. Each subsequent defibrillation remains at 360 J.

Synchronized Cardioversion

Unlike unsynchronized cardioversion, synchronized cardioversion requires conscious sedation and a time out. The procedure is the same as that for defibrillation, except that the machine must be set to deliver a synchronized shock and the appropriate energy level should be chosen based on the type of arrhythmia as described below.

Supraventricular Tachycardia and Atrial Flutter

Two types of atrial flutter exist, with type II requiring more energy for cardioversion. Type I arises from a single reentrant circuit in the right atrium, whereas type II is atypical and arises from a reentrant circuit in various locations. In general, atrial flutter requires lower energy levels than most arrhythmias and has higher successful cardioversion rates. For such narrow and regular arrhythmias, initial dose recommendations are 50 to 100 J. If the initial shock fails, stepwise increases in dosing may be attempted.

Atrial Fibrillation

Atrial fibrillation, the most frequent arrhythmia treated with cardioversion, is an irregularly irregular rhythm that can be electrically cardioverted with 120 to 200 J biphasic or 200 J monophasic energy. The anteroposterior electrode position yields higher success rates while requiring lower-energy shocks. Higher levels of energy may be needed for chronic atrial fibrillation. Electrical cardioversion has an overall success rate of 75% to 90%, depending on the chronicity of the arrhythmia and the left atrial size. Anticoagulation is required to prevent thromboembolism in the period after cardioversion, during which electromechanical asynchrony is present. Whether the atrial fibrillation is of new onset or chronic in nature determines when cardioversion can or even should be attempted.

Ventricular Tachycardia

Patients with sustained monomorphic ventricular tachycardia (defined as regular, wide, but morphologically uniform and stable QRS complexes with rates greater than 100 per minute) and hemodynamic compromise should undergo emergency synchronized cardioversion. Treatment of these arrhythmias requires 150 to 200 J biphasic or 360 J monophasic defibrillation.

Patients with polymorphic ventricular tachycardia with or without a pulse should undergo emergency defibrillation.

Three actions need to be initiated immediately

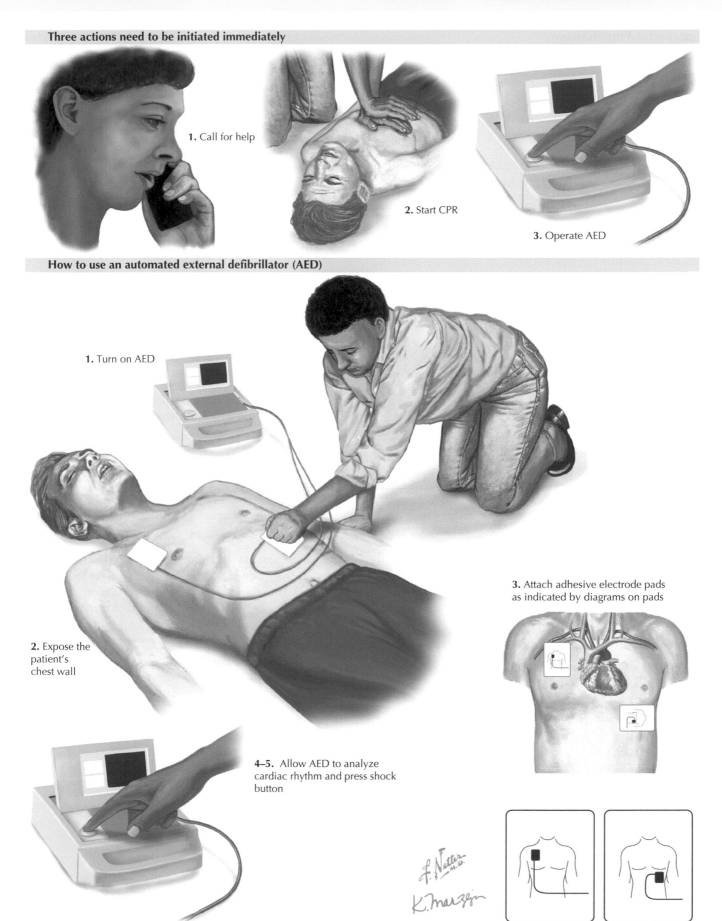

1. Call for help

2. Start CPR

3. Operate AED

How to use an automated external defibrillator (AED)

1. Turn on AED

2. Expose the patient's chest wall

3. Attach adhesive electrode pads as indicated by diagrams on pads

4–5. Allow AED to analyze cardiac rhythm and press shock button

FIGURE 8.3 Sudden cardiac arrest: steps preceding the activation of the automated external defibrillator

Ventricular Fibrillation

The recommended energy dose for a biphasic shock is an initial 120 to 200 J; for a monophasic shock it is 360 J. If unsure of the effective dose range, you may use the maximal dose. If the first shock is unsuccessful, subsequent shocks should be at least equivalent, and greater energy doses may be used.

ANATOMICAL PITFALLS

Appropriate application of cardioversion and defibrillation devices is important. Lead and paddle placement should be in the correct anatomical positions in order to avoid inappropriate stimulation.

COMPLICATIONS

The most common complications are harmless arrhythmias despite appropriately indicated cardioversion or defibrillation. The majority are atrial, ventricular, or junctional premature beats, although bradycardia, AV block, asystole, ventricular tachycardia, and ventricular fibrillation can occur.

A defibrillator delivers a fixed energy current through the chest wall, with obvious impedance by tissues. Therefore it can result in soft tissue injury, myocardial injury or necrosis, and cardiac dysrhythmias. Rarely, pulmonary edema may occur in patients with left ventricular dysfunction or transient left atrial stunning. However, with the advent of sophisticated machines and proper conductive gel or adhesive pad use, electrode placement, and technique, these complications have been drastically reduced.

CONCLUSIONS

A thorough understanding of cardioversion and defibrillation can be lifesaving. Understanding the salient anatomy and physiology and applying the best methods of treatment will maximize favorable outcomes.

Suggested Readings

2005 American Heart Association Guidelines for Cardiopulmonary Resuscitation and Emergency Cardiovascular Care. Part 7.2. Management of cardiac arrest. *Circulation.* 2005;112:IV58–IV66.

Link MS, Atkins DL, Passman RS, et al. Electrical therapies: automated external defibrillators, defibrillation, cardioversion, and pacing. Part 6. 2010 American Heart Association Guidelines for Cardiopulmonary Resuscitation and Emergency Cardiovascular Care. *Circulation.* 2010;122:S706.

Manegold JC, Israel CW, Ehrlich JR, et al. External cardioversion of atrial fibrillation in patients with implanted pacemaker or cardioverter-defibrillator systems: a randomized comparison of monophasic and biphasic shock energy application. *Eur Heart J.* 2007;28:1731–1738.

Marenco JP, Wang PJ, Link MS, et al. Improving survival from sudden cardiac arrest: the role of the automated external defibrillator. *JAMA.* 2001;285(9):1193–1200.

Neumar RW, Otto CW, Link MS, et al. Adult advanced cardiovascular life support. Part 8. *Circulation.* 2010;122(18 Suppl 3):S729–S767.

Reisinger J, Gstrein C, Winter T, et al. Optimization of initial energy for cardioversion of atrial tachyarrhythmias with biphasic shocks. *Am J Emerg Med.* 2010;28:159–165.

Sucu M, Davutoglu V, Ozer O. Electrical cardioversion. *Ann Saudi Med.* 2009;29(3):201–206.

REVIEW QUESTIONS

1. On an unmonitored unit, the nurse finds the patient unresponsive, with a rapid and weak pulse. The blood pressure is 90/50 mm Hg. A hospital-wide resuscitation response is activated. The code team arrives. A defibrillator is attached and is ready to be used. Which of the following conditions will most likely be a contraindication to cardioversion?

   A. Digitalis toxicity
   B. Hemodynamically unstable patient with supraventricular tachycardia
   C. Hemodynamically unstable patient with atrial flutter
   D. Hemodynamically unstable patient with atrial fibrillation
   E. Hemodynamically unstable patient with monomorphic ventricular tachycardia

2. In the patient described in question 1, for which of the following arrhythmias is emergency synchronized electrical cardioversion most likely indicated?

   A. Supraventricular tachycardia with a pulse and a blood pressure of 120/70 mm Hg
   B. Ventricular fibrillation
   C. Normal sinus rhythm
   D. Atrial flutter at a rate of 150 beats/min
   E. Ventricular tachycardia with no pulse
   F. Sinus arrest

3. On an unmonitored unit, the nurse finds the patient unresponsive. A hospital-wide resuscitation response is activated. The code team arrives. A defibrillator is attached and is ready to be used for synchronized cardioversion. Conscious sedation should be given for synchronized cardioversion of which of the following rhythms?

   A. Ventricular fibrillation
   B. Ventricular tachycardia with a pulse
   C. Ventricular tachycardia without a pulse
   D. Normal sinus rhythm
   E. Sinus arrest

4. In a patient with unstable atrial flutter, the initial shock to be delivered should be:

   A. Synchronized at 50 J
   B. Unsynchronized at 50 J
   C. Synchronized at 200 J
   D. Unsynchronized at 200 J
   E. First attempt should be pharmacological

Diagnostic Peritoneal Lavage

INTRODUCTION

Diagnostic peritoneal lavage (DPL) refers to the infusion of fluid into the peritoneal cavity to rapidly assess for hemoperitoneum caused by abdominal trauma. Historically, DPL was performed on an unstable patient with a high risk of intraabdominal injury. If positive, the patient would be fast tracked to the operating room for an emergency laparotomy. The use of DPL, however, has declined with the introduction of focused assessment with sonography for trauma (FAST). Although not diagnostic for blood as is DPL, FAST is highly sensitive for the presence of free fluid and is noninvasive, without the same risk of complications as DPL. Other advantages of FAST over DPL are the ability to replicate this procedure at will and the noninterference with subsequent computed tomography and magnetic resonance imaging procedures.

DPL is traditionally performed via a midline incision followed by catheter insertion in order to detect intraabdominal hemorrhage. The presence of greater than 10 mL of aspirated blood is considered positive, and emergency exploratory laparotomy is indicated to localize the injury. If there is minimal or no blood on aspiration, the next step is the introduction of lavage fluid into the peritoneal cavity, usually normal saline or lactated Ringer's solution, in order to reveal the presence of blood or enteric contents. The presence of greater than 100,000 red blood cells/mm^3 in the lavage fluid is considered positive. DPL is still used in settings without access to ultrasound, as well as for other clinical procedures (eg, cytopathology).

CLINICALLY RELEVANT ANATOMY

Incisional Anatomy

DPL is performed via a midline incision on the anterior abdominal wall (Fig. 9.1). The layers traversed are as follows.

The skin is first penetrated to enter the superficial fascia. The superficial fascia is a double layer, consisting of Camper's fascia and the inner Scarpa's fascia. The thin, membranous Scarpa's fascia extends below the inguinal ligament to fuse with the fascia lata of the thigh. Below the superficial fascia is the rectus sheath, which consists of the fused aponeuroses of the lateral abdominal muscles (Fig. 9.2). Within the rectus sheath lies the rectus abdominis muscle, which is centrally located on the anterior abdominal wall.

The rectus sheath surrounds the rectus abdominis muscle above the arcuate line but lies anterior to the muscle below the arcuate line. Above the line, the anterior layer of the sheath consists of the fused aponeuroses of the external oblique and one lamina of the internal oblique muscle; the posterior layer consists of the remaining lamina of the internal oblique aponeurosis fused with that of the tranversus abdominis muscle. Below the arcuate line, the aponeuroses of all three muscle layers are fused and lie on the anterior aspect of the rectus abdominis, with the posterior surface of the rectus abdominis lying directly on the transversalis fascia.

Deep to the rectus sheath lies the transversalis fascia, below which is a fatty layer referred to as the extraperitoneal fascia. Finally, below this fascia is the parietal peritoneum. The extraperitoneal fascia extends posteriorly around the abdominal cavity, where it may vary in thickness and enclose viscera. This fascia is surgically divided into an anterior, or preperitoneal, layer and a posterior, or retroperitoneal, layer. Viscera found in the latter portion are known as retroperitoneal organs. The extraperitoneal fascia is thicker around these organs (eg, the kidneys) for added protection.

Laparoscopically, another structure, the greater omentum, must be traversed. It is a thin, membranous, layered structure with an accumulation of fat that results in its double layer; fat accumulation can be ample in some individuals. It is a vascular structure that stretches from the greater curvature of the stomach and drapes the transverse colon while hanging without restriction in the abdominal cavity.

INDICATIONS

DPL is indicated for unstable patients who have sustained blunt abdominal trauma for examination in settings where ultrasound is not available. It is performed to diagnose the presence of blood in the intraabdominal cavity, which, if positive, will expedite transfer to the operating room for emergency exploratory laparotomy.

Currently, laparoscopic peritoneal lavage is used in other conditions to irrigate the peritoneal cavity. For example, in cases of peritonitis caused by diverticulitis or a perforated ulcer, the peritoneal cavity can be lavaged and adjunct therapy such as antibiotics can be instilled. Laparoscopy allows a visual inspection and subsequent hematological evaluation of the peritoneum, usually to determine metastatic spread of cancer into the peritoneum.

CONTRAINDICATIONS

If it appears likely that the patient will require emergency laparotomy, it is better not to delay this operation by

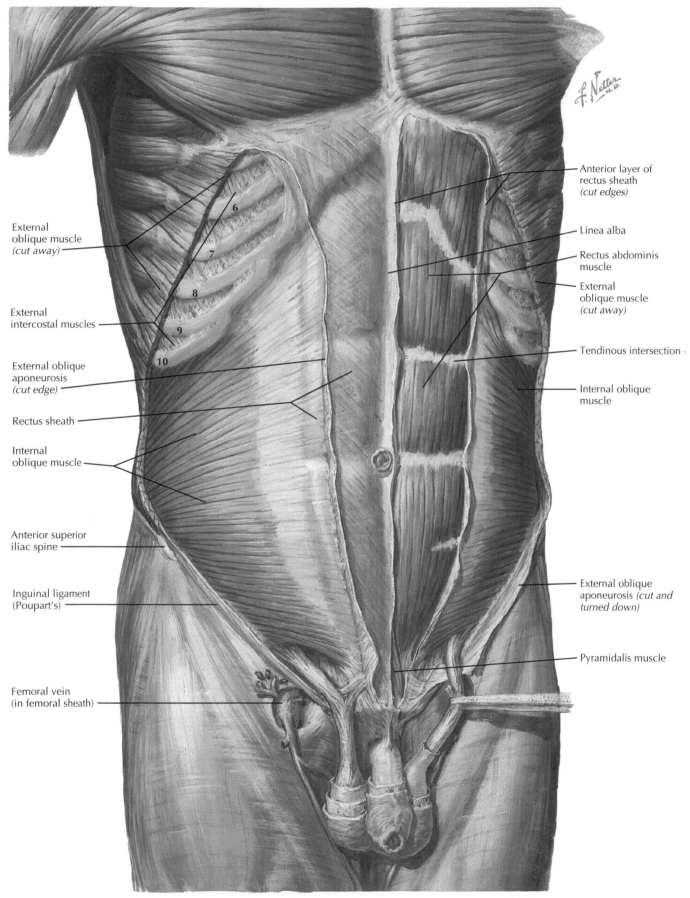

External
oblique muscle
(cut away)

External
intercostal muscles

External oblique
aponeurosis
(cut edge)

Rectus sheath

Internal
oblique muscle

Anterior superior
iliac spine

Inguinal ligament
(Poupart's)

Femoral vein
(in femoral sheath)

6

7

8

9

10

Anterior layer of
rectus sheath
(cut edges)

Linea alba

Rectus abdominis
muscle

External
oblique muscle
(cut away)

Tendinous intersection ·

Internal oblique
muscle

External oblique
aponeurosis (cut and
turned down)

Pyramidalis muscle

FIGURE 9.1 Anterior abdominal wall: intermediate dissection

Section above arcuate line

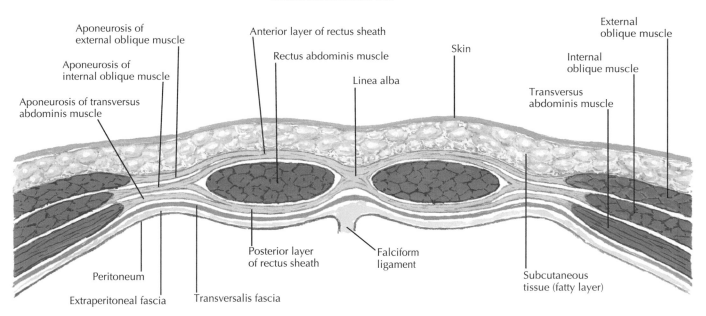

Aponeurosis of external oblique muscle

Aponeurosis of internal oblique muscle

Aponeurosis of transversus abdominis muscle

Anterior layer of rectus sheath

Rectus abdominis muscle

Linea alba

Skin

External oblique muscle

Internal oblique muscle

Transversus abdominis muscle

Posterior layer of rectus sheath

Falciform ligament

Peritoneum

Extraperitoneal fascia

Transversalis fascia

Subcutaneous tissue (fatty layer)

Aponeurosis of internal oblique muscle splits to form anterior and posterior layers of rectus sheath.
Aponeurosis of external oblique muscle joins anterior layer of sheath; aponeurosis of transversus abdominis muscle joins posterior layer. Anterior and posterior layers of rectus sheath unite medially to form linea alba.

Section below arcuate line

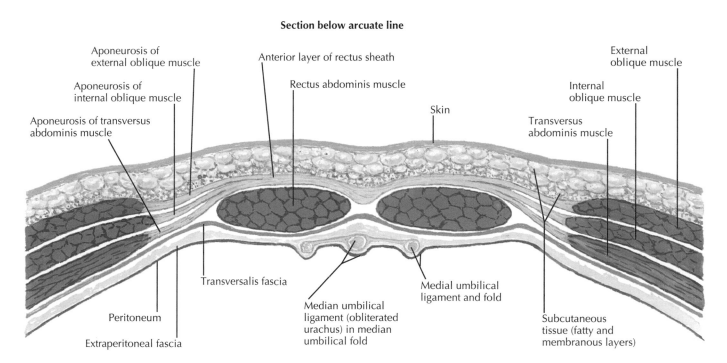

Aponeurosis of external oblique muscle

Aponeurosis of internal oblique muscle

Aponeurosis of transversus abdominis muscle

Anterior layer of rectus sheath

Rectus abdominis muscle

Skin

External oblique muscle

Internal oblique muscle

Transversus abdominis muscle

Transversalis fascia

Median umbilical ligament (obliterated urachus) in median umbilical fold

Medial umbilical ligament and fold

Peritoneum

Extraperitoneal fascia

Subcutaneous tissue (fatty and membranous layers)

Aponeurosis of internal oblique muscle does not split at this level but passes completely anterior to rectus abdominis muscle and is fused there with both aponeurosis of external oblique muscle and that of transversus abdominis muscle. Thus, posterior wall of rectus sheath is absent below arcuate line, leaving only transversalis fascia.

FIGURE 9.2 Rectus sheath: cross section

performing DPL, particularly if lavage were to be performed by an inexperienced physician. Patients with recent abdominal surgery, abdominal wall infections, morbid obesity, or coagulopathy should not undergo DPL. If ultrasound is available, it should be performed instead of DPL.

EQUIPMENT

Foley catheter
Nasogastric tube
Antiseptic preparations: chlorhexidine, iodine-based antiseptics
Drapes
Scalpel
Hemostats
Alice forceps
Toothed dissecting forceps
Retractors
Syringes
Needles (for anesthesia and J wire placement)
J wire
Intravenous (IV) lines without valves (to allow the return flow of infused solution)
Lidocaine with epinephrine
Ringer's lactate or normal saline (0.9% NaCl)
Soft-tip catheter (for entry into the peritoneal cavity)
Absorbable sutures, 4-0
Needle holder

PROCEDURE

See Fig. 9.3, Video 9.1.

Obtain patient consent and perform a time out.

1. Presurgical decompression of the bladder with a Foley catheter and of the stomach with a nasogastric tube is recommended. This is done to reduce the size of these organs and thus decrease the probability of injury (see Chapters 34 and 38).
2. Standard sterile precautions and the appropriate personal protective equipment should be used. The abdominal site should be prepared with customary skin antiseptics (chlorhexidine, iodine-based antiseptics), followed by appropriate draping.
3. Prior to incision, the skin and subcutaneous tissue through which the catheter will pass must be anesthetized with lidocaine 1% with epinephrine.
4. The Seldinger technique is used to insert the catheter into the peritoneal cavity through a midline infraumbilical incision. A small-gauge needle acts as a trocar and is inserted into the peritoneal cavity. A J wire is then introduced through the needle, pointed either left or right toward the paracolic gutters.
5. The needle is then withdrawn, leaving the J wire in place. A soft catheter is placed over the wire to be guided into the peritoneal cavity.

6. Before the catheter reaches the entry site, stab the site with a scalpel to facilitate movement through the anterior abdominal wall.
7. With gentle twisting motions of the catheter over the J wire, prod the caudally angled catheter toward either the right or left paracolic gutter. This is done to ensure entry into the peritoneal cavity.
8. Once the catheter is positioned in the peritoneal cavity, the J wire is removed. An aspirate of 10 mL of blood or enteric contents is considered positive, and emergency exploratory laparotomy is indicated.
9. If no blood is aspirated, attach valveless IV tubing to the catheter and instill 1 L of normal saline or lactated Ringer's solution. If possible, rotate the patient from side to side to ensure a thorough irrigation of the peritoneal cavity.
10. Once the fluid has been infused, lower the IV bag to below the patient's abdomen, using gravity to allow the infused fluid to return to the IV bag.
11. Once the lavage fluid has drained back into the bag (normally approximately 20% to 30% of the volume infused), send the fluid to the laboratory for analysis.

ANATOMICAL PITFALLS

DPL has a high sensitivity for intraabdominal hemorrhage, but it does not differentiate the tissue that has been damaged.

COMPLICATIONS

A false-positive tap will lead to an unnecessary exploratory laparotomy, with all the accompanying morbidity and mortality risks for that procedure. Misplacement of the catheter, usually in the preperitoneal space, can occur, or the fluid may enter the thoracic cavity in the event of a diaphragmatic rupture.

CONCLUSION

Historically, DPL was a commonly used procedure to detect intraabdominal hemorrhage or viscus rupture after blunt abdominal trauma. However, in recent years, it has been replaced by the less-invasive FAST. Consequently, the use of DPL in the emergency department has decreased dramatically.

Laparoscopic peritoneal lavage is increasingly used in the treatment of peritonitis caused by perforated peptic ulcer disease, lower grades of diverticulitis, purulent peritonitis, and in the staging of intraabdominal malignancies (colorectal, pancreatic, gastric, and ovarian tumors). DPL is not capable of diagnosing the source of hemorrhage, for example, in a solid organ or the retroperitoneum, and it may lead to an unnecessary laparotomy due to a false-positive tap.

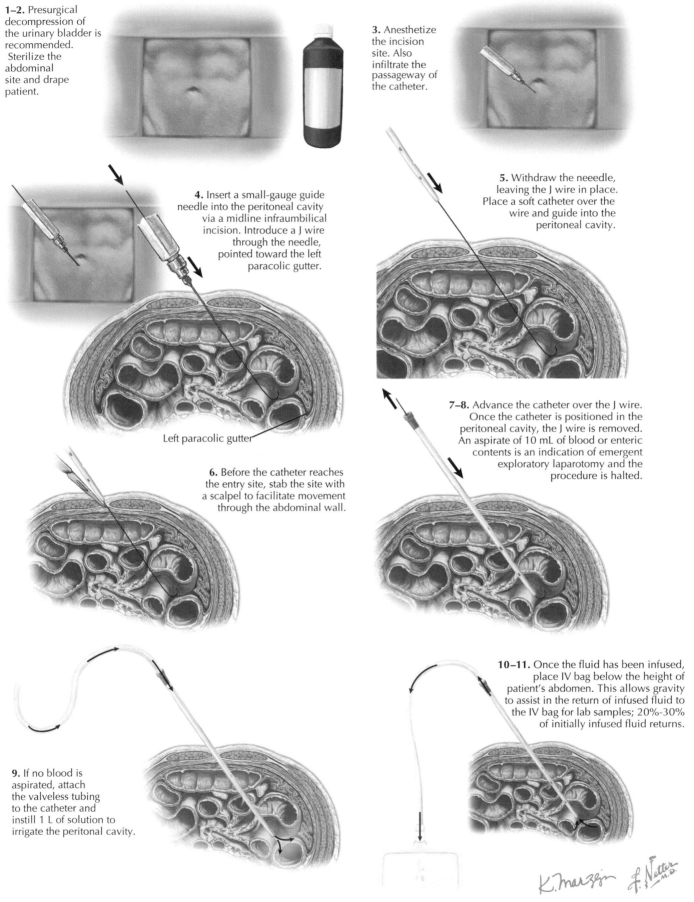

1–2. Presurgical decompression of the urinary bladder is recommended. Sterilize the abdominal site and drape patient.

3. Anesthetize the incision site. Also infiltrate the passageway of the catheter.

4. Insert a small-gauge guide needle into the peritoneal cavity via a midline infraumbilical incision. Introduce a J wire through the needle, pointed toward the left paracolic gutter.

Left paracolic gutter

5. Withdraw the neeedle, leaving the J wire in place. Place a soft catheter over the wire and guide into the peritoneal cavity.

6. Before the catheter reaches the entry site, stab the site with a scalpel to facilitate movement through the abdominal wall.

7–8. Advance the catheter over the J wire. Once the catheter is positioned in the peritoneal cavity, the J wire is removed. An aspirate of 10 mL of blood or enteric contents is an indication of emergent exploratory laparotomy and the procedure is halted.

9. If no blood is aspirated, attach the valveless tubing to the catheter and instill 1 L of solution to irrigate the peritonal cavity.

10–11. Once the fluid has been infused, place IV bag below the height of patient's abdomen. This allows gravity to assist in the return of infused fluid to the IV bag for lab samples; 20%-30% of initially infused fluid returns.

FIGURE 9.3 Diagnostic peritoneal lavage

Suggested Readings

Barnett RE, Love KM, Sepulveda EA, Cheadle WG. Small bowel trauma: current approach to diagnosis and management. *Am Surg.* 2014;80(12):1183–1191.

Sinnatamby CS. *Last's Anatomy: Regional and Applied.* St. Louis: Elsevier; 2006.

REVIEW QUESTIONS

1. The decision is made by emergency department surgeons to perform an exploratory laparotomy on a 32-year-old woman with severe abdominal pain. Where would the incision most likely be made to separate the left and right rectus sheaths?

   A. Midaxillary line
   B. Arcuate line
   C. Semilunar line
   D. Tendinous intersection
   E. Linea alba

2. A 35-year-old man is admitted to the emergency department after a severe car crash causing blunt abdominal trauma. DPL is ordered. Which of the following is the deepest layer penetrated during peritoneal lavage?

   A. Scarpa's fascia (membranous layer)
   B. Camper's fascia (fatty layer)
   C. Transversalis fascia
   D. Extraperitoneal fatty tissue
   E. External abdominal oblique fascia

3. A 35-year-old man is admitted to the emergency department after a severe car crash causing blunt abdominal trauma. The patient complains of abdominal pain. His blood pressure is 90/60 mm Hg and heart rate 101 beats/min. Which of the following is the best choice for assessment?

   A. FAST exam
   B. DPL
   C. CT with contrast
   D. CT without contrast
   E. Emergency exploratory laparotomy

4. A 35-year-old woman is admitted to the emergency department after a severe car crash causing blunt abdominal trauma. The patient complains of abdominal pain. His blood pressure is 90/60 mm Hg and heart rate 101 beats/min. In the absence of ultrasound, DPL is ordered. Which of the following conditions is a contraindication to this procedure?

   A. Pregnancy
   B. International normalized ratio of 4
   C. Hypotension
   D. Leg cellulitis
   E. History of tonsillectomy

Extended Focused Assessment With Sonography for Trauma

INTRODUCTION

Ultrasonography is an excellent noninvasive method for screening and investigating patients in a quick, cost-effective manner. This is especially true in the emergency department for patients with blunt trauma, where time is critical in attaining a good outcome. Although not as sensitive as computed tomography (CT), ultrasonography is an important initial screening tool. Acting as an extension of the trauma physical examination performed by emergency physicians and surgeons, it aids in identifying whether trauma patients can be further evaluated in the emergency department or whether they should be directly taken to the operating room for emergency exploratory laparotomy. It is not as accurate as CT, but it is faster and better than diagnostic peritoneal lavage and is superior to a physical examination alone.

An ultrasound protocol, previously known as focused abdominal sonography for trauma (FAST), was developed to evaluate patients with abdominal trauma. However, the name has since been changed to reflect the additional evaluation of extraabdominal regions such as the thoracic cavity for pneumothorax; this protocol is now called extended focused assessment with sonography for trauma (E-FAST), and it is used to assess the peritoneal, pericardial, and pleural spaces in trauma settings. The primary application of E-FAST is to identify pathological free fluid. In the setting of blunt trauma, the fluid is assumed to be blood, although it could be gastric contents, ascites, pus, bile, or urine. Unlike a CT scan, E-FAST may be easily performed multiple times at the bedside using a portable ultrasound machine, thus facilitating the prompt management of trauma patients.

CLINICALLY RELEVANT ANATOMY

The major regions examined with the original FAST protocol included the (1) hepatorenal recess and right upper quadrant, (2) perisplenic region and left upper quadrant, (3) suprapubic region, and (4) subxiphoid pericardial window (Fig. 10.1). E-FAST expands on these four views by adding bilateral thoracic views for the evaluation of pneumothorax and hemothorax. All of these views were chosen because they provide excellent windows into cavities and dependent areas where fluid may accumulate. There is minimal interference from bone or air that obscures sonographic signals. Because pericardial tamponade is the most acute, life-threatening possibility, the pericardial view is the first location to be visualized. The order of evaluation of succeeding locations is usually the hepatorenal recess (the most dependent space

for fluid accumulation in a supine patient), splenorenal recess (a location where severe hemorrhage may occur with splenic rupture), suprapubic view, and thoracic views. However, this order does not necessarily need to be followed if the mechanism of injury is known, in which case the area of suspicion can be focused on in more depth.

INDICATIONS

As noted, the primary indication for the use of E-FAST is the rapid evaluation of trauma caused by either blunt force or penetrating injury. Sonography provides a quick, noninvasive imaging modality to determine the presence of pathological intraperitoneal, intrapleural, or pericardial free fluid. In mass casualty situations, E-FAST is used to triage and prioritize patients for treatment. E-FAST can be extremely valuable in evaluating several other clinical conditions such as unexplained hypotension in either traumatic or nontraumatic settings, pregnant patients after trauma, and acute dyspnea with suspected pleural or pericardial effusion or tamponade.

CONTRAINDICATIONS

The only contraindication to the use of E-FAST is the need for immediate laparotomy. Ideally, ultrasonography should be performed before transferring the patient to the operating room to rule out pericardial tamponade, hemothorax, or pneumothorax. It is crucial for the surgeon to know which cavity should be opened first in the case of thoracoabdominal trauma, so preoperative ultrasound is highly recommended. Patients with penetrating trauma who are unstable should be taken directly to the operating theater. Unstable patients with blunt force trauma may undergo E-FAST to assess the need for surgery, but if clinical suspicion regarding the need for exploratory laparotomy is high, the patient should be taken directly to the operating room. While immediate fluid resuscitation and transfusion are not contraindications to simultaneous ultrasonography, E-FAST should not be prioritized over other resuscitation procedures.

EQUIPMENT

E-FAST includes both echocardiographic and thoracoabdominal examination, so it is ideally performed with a single transducer that can image all areas with a 3.5- to 5-MHz curvilinear or convex array probe. Occasionally, some physicians may choose to use a phased-array probe due to its better ability to capture movement.

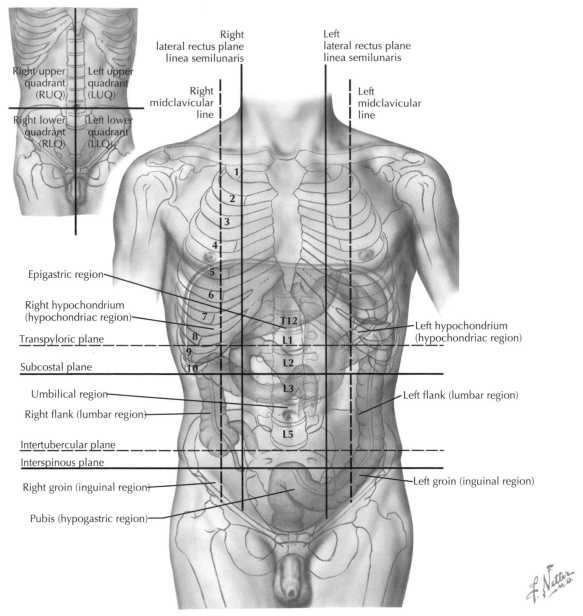

FIGURE 10.1 Regions and planes of abdomen

PROCEDURE

Perform a time out. See Videos 10-1 to 10-19.

Pericardial Examination

Examination of the pericardium and heart is performed with a subcostal or subxiphoid view (see Chapter 13, Fig. 10.2).

1. The examination is generally performed from the right side of the patient, who is placed supine.
2. Direct the transducer indicator to the patient's right.
3. Direct the transducer under the xiphoid process, angled cephalad and toward the left shoulder in a horizontal plane.
4. Apply firm pressure to the body of the transducer to have it lie flat on the patient's abdomen and allow the sound waves to pass under the xiphoid and into the pericardium.

5. Pivot, sweep, and tilt the transducer to view all four cardiac chambers and the surrounding pericardium to detect any pericardial fluid or abnormal cardiac motion.

The presence of pericardial fluid is denoted by a dark anechoic stripe separating the parietal pericardium from the visceral pericardium. The presence of pericardial fluid between the heart and pericardium is suggestive of an impending pericardial tamponade, but global wall motion abnormalities should also be evaluated so as not to confuse epicardial fat pads with effusions. Epicardial fat pads move with the heart during contraction, whereas pericardial fluid tends to remain static. Additionally, ventricular wall motion and right ventricular filling should be evaluated. Abnormalities in either of these may be interpreted as evidence of cardiac tamponade.

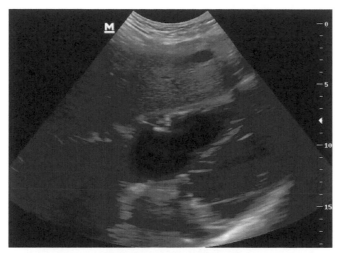

Subxiphoid view, normal

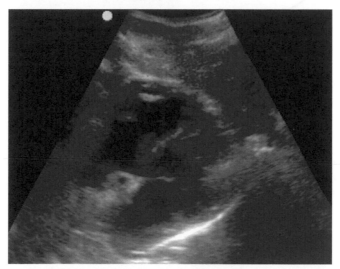

Subxiphoid view, normal

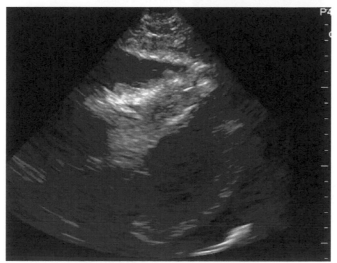

Subxiphoid view with tamponade

FIGURE 10.2 Subxiphoid cardiac view

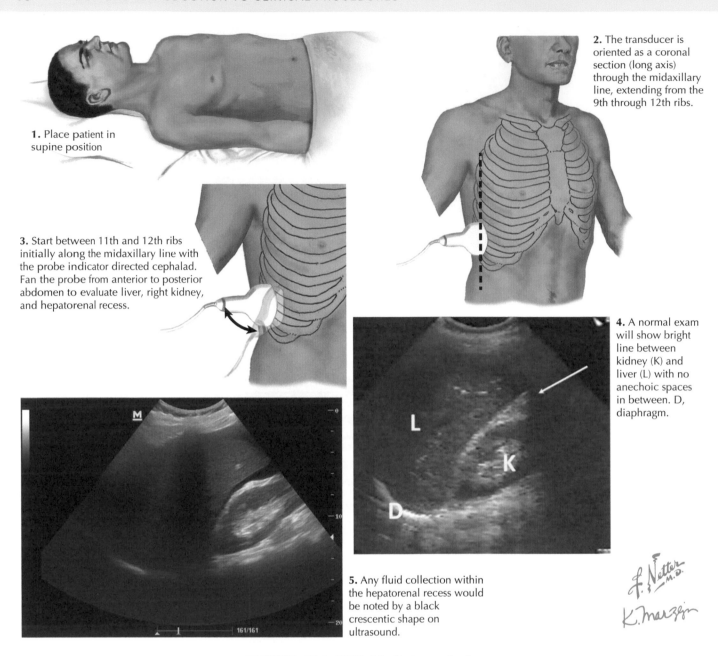

1. Place patient in supine position

2. The transducer is oriented as a coronal section (long axis) through the midaxillary line, extending from the 9th through 12th ribs.

3. Start between 11th and 12th ribs initially along the midaxillary line with the probe indicator directed cephalad. Fan the probe from anterior to posterior abdomen to evaluate liver, right kidney, and hepatorenal recess.

4. A normal exam will show bright line between kidney (K) and liver (L) with no anechoic spaces in between. D, diaphragm.

5. Any fluid collection within the hepatorenal recess would be noted by a black crescentic shape on ultrasound.

FIGURE 10.3 FAST: right flank examination

Right Flank Examination

The right upper quadrant contains the hepatorenal recess, or Morison's pouch, the most dependent space in the abdominal cavity in a supine patient (Fig. 10.3).

1. Place the patient in the supine position.
2. Orient the transducer in the coronal plane (long axis) through the midaxillary line, extending from the ninth to twelfth ribs.
3. Start between the eleventh and twelfth ribs along the midaxillary line with the probe indicator directed cephalad toward the axilla. This utilizes the liver as an acoustic window to avoid gas interference from the bowels. Addi-

tionally, cephalad angling allows evaluation of the pleural or subphrenic spaces if the patient is breathing deeply.

4. Fan the probe from the anterior to the posterior abdomen to evaluate the liver, right kidney, and hepatorenal recess.

   a. A bright line should be noted between the kidney and liver with no anechoic spaces between.

   b. Any fluid collection within the hepatorenal recess would be seen as a black crescentic shape on ultrasound. The hepatodiaphragmatic space, subdiaphragmatic recess, and liver should also be evaluated for any free fluid or hepatic injury.

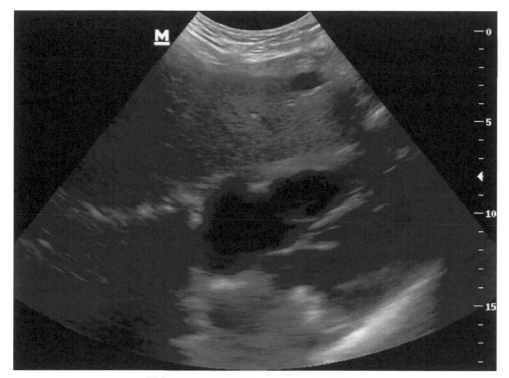

FIGURE 10.4 Left upper quadrant view

Left Flank Examination

The left flank (or splenorenal recess) examination is often the most difficult examination to perform during E-FAST because the spleen, used as the acoustic window, is much smaller and more posterosuperior compared with the liver in the right flank. As a result, bowel gas and rib shadowing interfere more in this view (Fig. 10.4). However, due to the vascular nature of the spleen, the left flank examination is crucial in E-FAST. Splenic injury may result in profuse internal hemorrhaging and be life threatening.

1. Place the patient in the supine position.
2. The transducer is directed toward the axilla and oriented in the coronal plane (long axis) through the body in the midaxillary to posterior axillary line extending from the ninth to twelfth ribs.
3. The transducer is angled cephalad in the long axis to allow anterior to posterior scanning by fanning the probe.
4. Identify the interface of the spleen and left kidney. As with the hepatorenal space, a bright line should be noted between the left kidney and spleen with no anechoic spaces in between. Any fluid collection between these two structures would be seen as a black crescentic shape on ultrasound.
5. Also evaluate the spleen for its integrity and any possible signs of damage.
6. Evaluate the left diaphragmatic and subdiaphragmatic recesses as well.

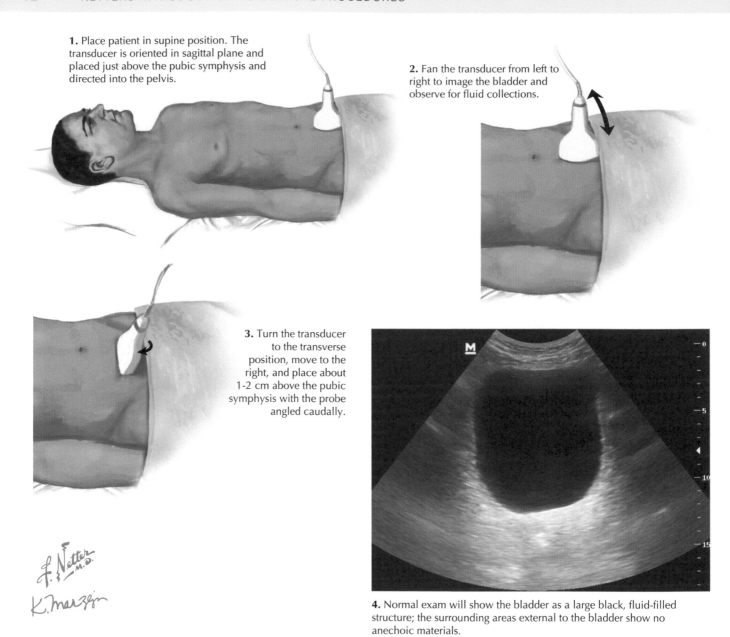

1. Place patient in supine position. The transducer is oriented in sagittal plane and placed just above the pubic symphysis and directed into the pelvis.

2. Fan the transducer from left to right to image the bladder and observe for fluid collections.

3. Turn the transducer to the transverse position, move to the right, and place about 1-2 cm above the pubic symphysis with the probe angled caudally.

4. Normal exam will show the bladder as a large black, fluid-filled structure; the surrounding areas external to the bladder show no anechoic materials.

FIGURE 10.5 E-FAST: suprapubic examination

Suprapubic Examination

The pelvic region also holds dependent areas where free fluid may accumulate. In females, the rectouterine pouch, or the pouch of Douglas, is the cul-de-sac where free fluid may accumulate in a supine patient. In males, free fluid accumulation may occur in the rectovesical pouch (Fig. 10.5).

1. When the patient is in the supine position, urine in the bladder helps create an acoustic window. Place the transducer in the sagittal plane with the indicator oriented toward the patient's head, just above the symphysis pubis and directed into the pelvis.
2. Fan the transducer to image the bladder and look for fluid collections posterior to the bladder in males and the uterus in females.
3. In the transverse plane with the indicator oriented toward the patient's right, place the transducer about 1 to 2 cm above the symphysis pubis with the probe angled caudally into the pelvis. The urinary bladder should appear as a black fluid-filled structure, while the surrounding regions should show no signs of anechoic material.
4. Fluid collections in these potential dependent spaces are anechoic and external to the bladder. Women of reproductive age may have trace amounts of physiologic free pelvic fluid, but the examiner should err on the side of caution in any case of blunt pelvic trauma.

1. Place patient in supine position.

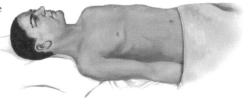

2. The field depth is set to a lower level to allow proper visualization of the pleural space between the visceral and parietal pleurae and evaluation of the pleurae sliding on one another. Absence of pleural sliding implies the presence of pneumothoraces.

Diagram of normal long-axis view

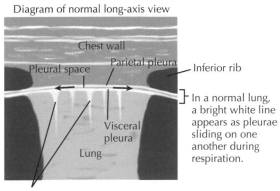

Chest wall

Pleural space   Parietal pleura   Inferior rib

In a normal lung, a bright white line appears as pleurae sliding on one another during respiration.

Visceral pleura

Lung

Comet tails also appear in normal lung function

3. Place the transducer in a longitudinal position, typically between the second through fourth intercostal spaces along the midclavicular line. Repeat on the other side to rule out pneumothoraces in either pleural space.

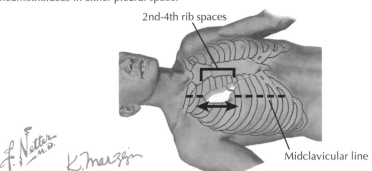

2nd-4th rib spaces

Midclavicular line

FIGURE 10.6 E-FAST: thoracic examination

Normal Lung

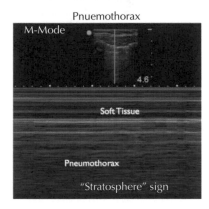

Normal Lung

M-Mode

6.5

Soft Tissue

Pleural Line

Normal Lung

"Seashore" sign

Pnuemothorax

M-Mode

4.6

Soft Tissue

Pneumothorax

"Stratosphere" sign

Thoracic Examination

E-FAST (Fig. 10.6) includes a more detailed examination of the pleurae than the original FAST. While the right and left flank examinations allow partial evaluation of the pleural spaces, examination of the thorax is done to identify pneumothorax, which may not be seen on flank examination. Hemothorax appears as anechoic free fluid between the pleurae. However, to identify pneumothorax, a higher-frequency linear probe (5 to 12 MHz) is used for the thoracic examination.

1. With the patient in the supine position, orient the transducer indicator toward the patient's head.
2. Set the field depth to a lower level to allow proper visualization of the pleural space between the visceral and parietal pleurae and evaluation of the pleurae sliding on one another. Absence of pleural sliding implies the presence of a pneumothorax.
3. Typically the probe is placed between the second and fourth intercostal spaces at the midclavicular line or in the fourth through sixth intercostal spaces at the midaxillary line. Examine bilaterally to rule out pneumothorax on either side.

ANATOMICAL PITFALLS

Sonography cannot evaluate the retroperitoneum and fails to distinguish solid organ injury. During the examination of the left and right flanks, the inferior pole of the kidney is not seen. Hence, a detailed examination of the kidneys should be performed in the case of lower abdominal injury. This is important because sometimes free fluid first accumulates close to the inferior pole of the kidneys. Patients with delayed presentation after thoracoabdominal trauma may not have the classic sonographic findings of hemorrhage because clotted blood has variable echogenicity.

COMPLICATIONS

There are no complications associated with ultrasonography for the rapid assessment of trauma patients. As discussed, limitations of E-FAST include variable operator experience and reduced sensitivity for solid organ injury and retroperitoneal hemorrhage.

CONCLUSION

E-FAST is a noninvasive investigation that can be rapidly performed at the bedside of a patient with trauma or who is hypotensive. Because it is noninvasive and does not involve ionizing radiation, E-FAST may be serially repeated as needed, aiding the clinician in management decisions. The original FAST focused on assessing the pericardium, the right and left flanks, and the pelvic region, areas most prone to either life-threatening conditions (eg, cardiac tamponade) or intraperitoneal free fluid accumulation, a sign of intraabdominal organ injury or hemorrhage. E-FAST expands on FAST by more thoroughly investigating the pleural cavities with a high-frequency linear transducer to look for pneumothorax. While not sensitive for intraperitoneal hemorrhage or solid organ injury, the effectiveness of E-FAST aids in the clinical decision-making process. The sensitivity of E-FAST may be increased with improved operator training and serial examinations to monitor the patient for changes.

Suggested Readings

American College of Emergency Physicians. Emergency ultrasound imaging criteria compendium. *Ann Emerg Med*. 2006;48:487–510.

Blaivas M, DeBehnke D, Phelan MB. Potential errors in the diagnosis of pericardial effusion on trauma ultrasound for penetrating injuries. *Acad Emerg Med*. 2000;11:1261–1266.

Branny SW, Wolfe RE, Moore EE, et al. Quantitative sensitivity of ultrasound in detecting free intraperitoneal fluid. *J Trauma*. 1995;39:375–380.

McGahan PJ, Richards JR, Bair AE, Rose JS. Ultrasound detection of blunt urological trauma: a 6-year study. *Injury*. 2005;36:762–770.

McGahan JP, Rose J, Coates TL, Wisner DH, Newberry P. Use of ultrasonography in the patient with acute abdominal trauma. *J Ultrasound Med*. 1997;16:653–662.

Natarajan B, Gupta PK, Cemaj S, Sorensen M, Hatzoudis GI, Forse RA. FAST scan: is it worth doing in hemodynamically stable blunt trauma patients. *Surgery*. 2010;148:695–700.

Ormsby EL, Geng J, McGahan JP, Richards JR. Pelvic free fluid: clinical importance for reproductive age women with blunt abdominal trauma. *Ultrasound Obstet Gynecol*. 2005;26:271–278.

Rose JS. Ultrasound in abdominal trauma. *Emerg Med Clin North Am*. 2004;22:581–599.

Scott-Conner CEH, Dawson DL. FAST examination for trauma. In: *Operative Anatomy*. 3rd ed. Philadelphia: Lippincott Williams & Wilkins; 2009:277–280.

Sirlin CB, Casola G, Brown MA, et al. US of blunt abdominal trauma: importance of free pelvic fluid in women of reproductive age. *Radiology*. 2001;219:229–235.

Stengel D, Bauwens K, Sehouli J, et al. Emergency ultrasound-based algorithms for diagnosing blunt abdominal trauma. *Cochrane Database Syst Rev*. 2008;2005(2):CD004446.

US Department of Defense. *Emergency War Surgery, Third United States Revision*. United States: Prepper Press; 2004:17.3–17.6.

REVIEW QUESTIONS

1. A 45-year-old man is admitted unconscious to the emergency department after a severe car crash. E-FAST is performed, and a dark anechoic stripe separating the parietal pericardium from the visceral pericardium is noted. In which of the following positions should the transducer be placed in order to best visualize this condition?
   - A. Under the xiphoid process, angled cephalad and toward the left shoulder in a horizontal plane
   - B. Parasternal long-axis view
   - C. Parasternal short-axis view
   - D. Suprasternal approach
   - E. Parasternal short- and long-axis views

2. A 48-year-old woman is admitted to the hospital with a distended abdomen. A CT scan shows evidence of ascites. In which of the following locations will an ultrasound most likely confirm the presence of ascitic fluid with the patient in the supine position?
   - A. Subphrenic recess
   - B. Hepatorenal recess (pouch of Morison)
   - C. Rectouterine recess (pouch of Douglas)
   - D. Vesicouterine recess
   - E. Subhepatic recess

3. A 45-year-old woman is admitted to the hospital after her automobile left the highway in a rainstorm and hit a tree. She had been wearing a seat belt. On radiographic examination, there are fractures of the ninth and tenth ribs on the left side and evidence of intraabdominal bleeding. Physical examination reveals hypovolemic shock and progressive hypotension. Which of the following organs was most likely injured to result in these clinical signs?
   - A. Liver
   - B. Pancreas
   - C. Left kidney
   - D. Spleen
   - E. Ileum

4. A 21-year-old football player is admitted to the emergency department with intense back pain. Physical examination shows that his left lower back is bruised and swollen. He complains of sharp pain during respiration. A radiograph reveals a fracture of the eleventh rib on the left side. Which of the following organs would be most likely to have sustained injury?
   - A. Spleen
   - B. Lung
   - C. Kidney
   - D. Liver
   - E. Pancreas

5. A 25-year-old man is admitted to the emergency department with a bullet wound in the neck just above the middle of the right clavicle and first rib. E-FAST reveals collapse of the right lung and a tension pneumothorax. Which of the following is the typical ultrasonographic finding for the diagnosis of pneumothorax?
   - A. Absence of pleural sliding
   - B. Presence of A lines
   - C. Presence of B lines
   - D. Presence of E lines
   - E. Presence of lung pulse

Fasciotomy

INTRODUCTION

Major muscle groups have fascial membranes that surround and encapsulate them. As a result, the muscle groups are divided into compartments. When an increase in pressure occurs within these compartments, possibly due to edema or hemorrhage, the neurovascular structures within the compartment become compressed and the viability of the tissue in the space is compromised. This is known as compartment syndrome. Fasciotomy is a surgical procedure indicated for the treatment of compartment syndrome. This limb-saving procedure, often performed in emergencies, involves cutting into the fascial compartment to relieve the increasing pressure inside.

COMPARTMENT SYNDROME

Compartment syndrome secondary to trauma, burn injuries, vascular occlusion, reperfusion injury, muscle edema, or restrictive dressings may occur inside any encapsulated fascial space. The syndrome results from a combination of increased interstitial tissue pressure along with the noncompliant nature of the fascia surrounding it. As the pressure increases within the compartment, the muscles and tissues within are subjected to decreased perfusion and consequent ischemic changes. The increasing pressure compresses venous and lymphatic outflow, which further increases compartmental pressure. This eventually blocks arterial inflow and causes nerve compression, resulting in ischemic paralysis and muscle necrosis. Muscle necrosis can be life threatening due to the systemic effects of rhabdomyolysis, including renal failure and hyperkalemia. Even if these potentially lethal conditions are managed, the necrotic muscle tends to heal with scar tissue, forming adhesions and contractures.

Early recognition, diagnosis, and treatment are paramount in the management and successful treatment of compartment syndrome. An early clinical manifestation of a tense, swollen muscle compartment is pain out of proportion to the outward appearance. Late manifestations include the loss of sensation (paresthesia), loss of pulse, pallor, and paralysis of the affected extremity.

Diagnosis may include the measurement of compartment pressures. Initially accepted as a confirmatory test for compartment syndrome, compartment pressure and perfusion pressure measurements have been scrutinized due to poor specificity and sensitivity. Mubarak and Hargens stated that an absolute tissue pressure of 30 mm Hg is the critical value at which fasciotomy should be performed because normal capillary pressure is 30 mm Hg, and a higher tissue pressure would result in tissue necrosis. Whitesides and Heckman recommended that fasciotomy be performed when the intracompartmental tissue pressure rises to within 20 mm Hg below the diastolic blood pressure. The US Department of Defense does not recommend the measurement of compartment pressures because it would be more prudent to simply perform the fasciotomy in a combat zone or emergency situation. The current consensus suggests a pressure difference of 30 mm Hg or less from the diastolic pressure as an absolute indication for surgical intervention. Studies show that peripheral nerves and muscles survive for as long as 4 hours under ischemic conditions. However, after 8 hours, the damage is irreversible.

Antibiotic prophylaxis should be given to cover skin organisms, and frequent aseptic bandage changes greatly reduce the incidence of secondary infection and further potential loss of viable tissues. If possible, the first dose of antibiotics should be given prior to the first incision.

CLINICALLY RELEVANT ANATOMY
Leg

The leg is divided into four compartments separated by fibrous fasciae: the anterior, lateral, superficial posterior, and deep posterior compartments (Figs. 11.1 and 11.2). Depending on which compartment is affected, patients present with clinical signs and symptoms specific to that area, which helps guide the treatment.

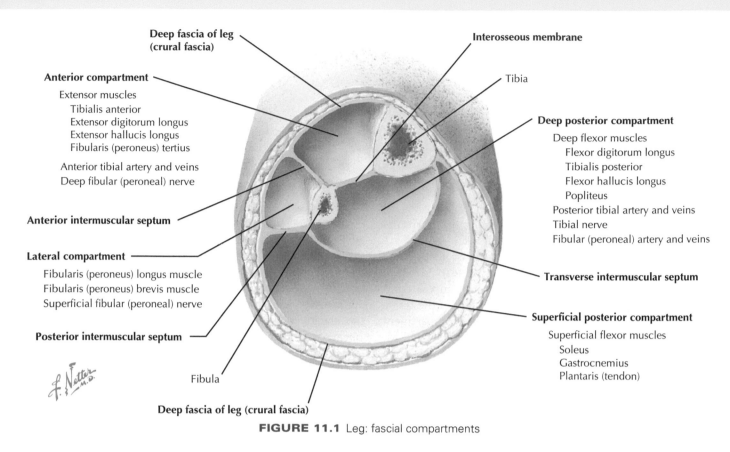

Deep fascia of leg (crural fascia)

Interosseous membrane

Tibia

Anterior compartment

Extensor muscles
Tibialis anterior
Extensor digitorum longus
Extensor hallucis longus
Fibularis (peroneus) tertius

Anterior tibial artery and veins
Deep fibular (peroneal) nerve

Anterior intermuscular septum

Lateral compartment

Fibularis (peroneus) longus muscle
Fibularis (peroneus) brevis muscle
Superficial fibular (peroneal) nerve

Posterior intermuscular septum

Fibula

Deep fascia of leg (crural fascia)

Deep posterior compartment

Deep flexor muscles
Flexor digitorum longus
Tibialis posterior
Flexor hallucis longus
Popliteus
Posterior tibial artery and veins
Tibial nerve
Fibular (peroneal) artery and veins

Transverse intermuscular septum

Superficial posterior compartment

Superficial flexor muscles
Soleus
Gastrocnemius
Plantaris (tendon)

FIGURE 11.1 Leg: fascial compartments

Anterior Compartment

The anterior compartment is bound by the tibia, fibula, interosseous membrane, anterior intermuscular septum, and deep fascia of the leg. The muscles in this compartment are responsible for dorsiflexion of the foot and include the tibialis anterior, extensor digitorum longus, peroneus tertius, and extensor hallucis longus. Innervation for the anterior compartment arises from the deep fibular (peroneal) nerve, a terminal branch of the common fibular (peroneal) nerve. The deep fibular (peroneal) nerve enters the compartment by piercing the anterior intermuscular fascial septa along with the anterior tibial vasculature, just inferior to the neck of the fibula. While providing motor innervation for the anterior compartment and dorsal foot muscles, the deep fibular (peroneal) nerve also provides sensory innervation to the first and second toes. The blood supply to the anterior compartment is primarily from the anterior tibial artery, which enters the compartment alongside the deep fibular (peroneal) nerve. It travels distally in the leg medial to the deep fibular (peroneal) nerve, becoming the dorsalis pedis artery when it crosses the ankle joint into the foot.

The anterior compartment is the most common site for acute compartment syndrome in the leg. Signs and symptoms include loss of sensation between the first two toes, loss of dorsiflexion, foot drop, claw foot, and loss of the dorsalis pedis pulse.

Lateral Compartment

The lateral compartment is bound by the fibula, anterior and posterior intermuscular septa, and deep fascia of the leg. The muscles in this compartment are responsible for foot eversion and partially for plantar flexion. The lateral compartment muscles are the peroneus longus and peroneus brevis muscles. Innervation for the lateral compartment is from the superficial fibular (peroneal) nerve, another terminal branch of the common fibular (peroneal) nerve. The superficial fibular (peroneal) nerve arises near the region where the common fibular (peroneal) nerve pierces the posterior intermuscular septum to enter the lateral compartment. As it travels down the lateral compartment, it gives off muscular branches and eventually pierces the deep fascia to supply cutaneous innervation to the lateral lower third of the leg and dorsum of the foot, with the exception of the region innervated by the deep fibular (peroneal) nerve mentioned above. The lateral compartment receives arterial supply from perforating branches of the anterior tibial artery proximally and the fibular (peroneal) artery, which runs in the deep posterior compartment.

Cross section just above middle of leg

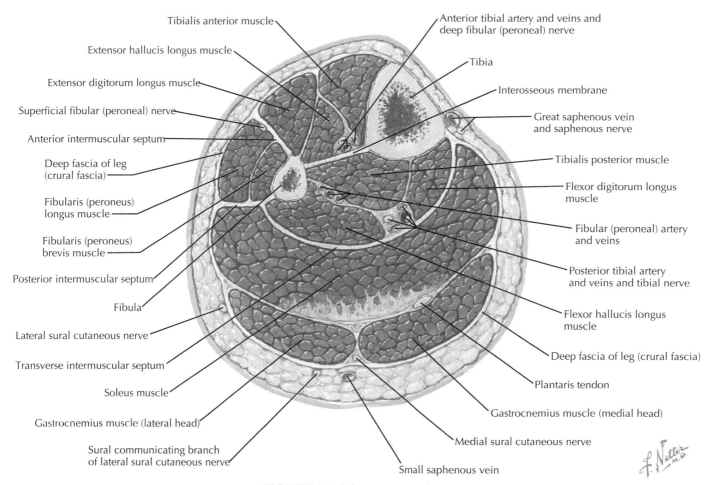

Tibialis anterior muscle

Extensor hallucis longus muscle

Extensor digitorum longus muscle

Superficial fibular (peroneal) nerve

Anterior intermuscular septum

Deep fascia of leg (crural fascia)

Fibularis (peroneus) longus muscle

Fibularis (peroneus) brevis muscle

Posterior intermuscular septum

Fibula

Lateral sural cutaneous nerve

Transverse intermuscular septum

Soleus muscle

Gastrocnemius muscle (lateral head)

Sural communicating branch of lateral sural cutaneous nerve

Anterior tibial artery and veins and deep fibular (peroneal) nerve

Tibia

Interosseous membrane

Great saphenous vein and saphenous nerve

Tibialis posterior muscle

Flexor digitorum longus muscle

Fibular (peroneal) artery and veins

Posterior tibial artery and veins and tibial nerve

Flexor hallucis longus muscle

Deep fascia of leg (crural fascia)

Plantaris tendon

Gastrocnemius muscle (medial head)

Medial sural cutaneous nerve

Small saphenous vein

FIGURE 11.2 Leg: cross section

Compartment syndrome in the anterior and deep posterior compartments may adversely affect the lateral compartment because the arteries in these two compartments also perfuse the lateral compartment. However, increased pressure within the lateral compartment specifically results in superficial fibular (peroneal) nerve deficits. Signs and symptoms of the syndrome affecting this compartment include loss of sensation over the dorsum of the foot and distal lateral leg, and weakness of eversion of the foot.

Posterior Compartment

The superficial posterior compartment contains the gastrocnemius, soleus, and plantaris muscles. Innervation for the superficial posterior compartment is provided by branches of the tibial nerve, while the arterial supply for the muscles within this compartment is branches arising from the popliteal artery proximally and the posterior tibial artery distally.

The deep posterior compartment contains the popliteus, flexor hallucis longus, flexor digitorum longus, and tibialis posterior muscles. The tibial nerve provides innervation for the posterior compartment. The major arterial supply for the posterior compartment includes the posterior tibial artery and its branches. With two major arteries and the tibial nerve traveling through the deep posterior compartment, it is imperative to diagnose and treat compartment syndrome urgently to prevent irreversible damage to the limb. Compartment syndrome in the posterior compartment results in plantar hypoesthesia, weakness in plantar flexion, and pain on dorsiflexion.

Forearm

The forearm, the most common location of compartment syndrome in the upper limb, has extensor (posterior) and flexor (anterior) compartments.

Extensor Compartment

The extensor compartment of the forearm is defined by the ulna, radius, interosseous membrane, and antebrachial fascia (Fig. 11.3). Within the compartment are the extensor muscles

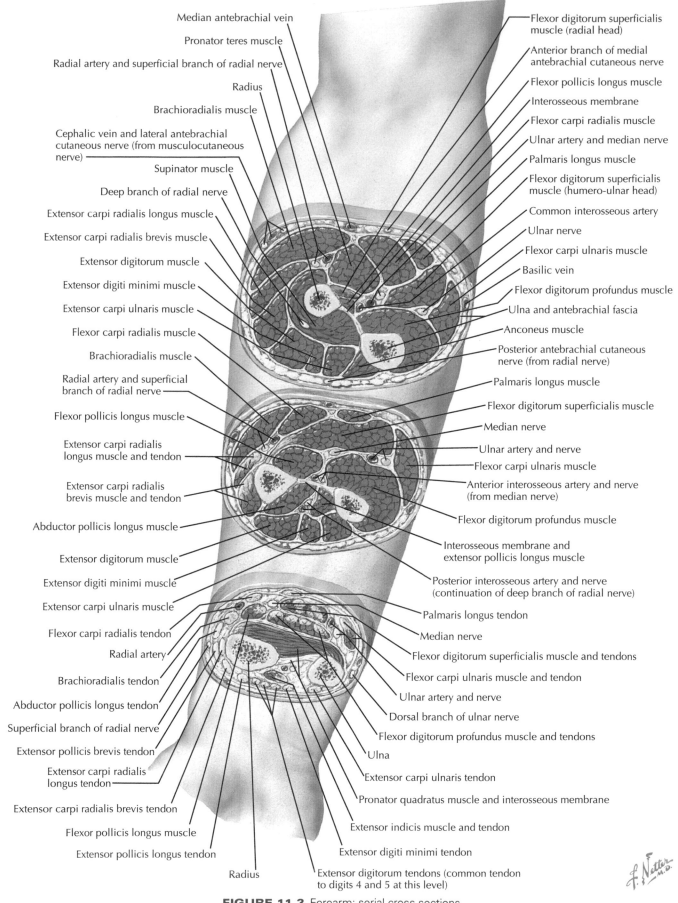

Median antebrachial vein

Pronator teres muscle

Radial artery and superficial branch of radial nerve

Radius

Brachioradialis muscle

Cephalic vein and lateral antebrachial cutaneous nerve (from musculocutaneous nerve)

Supinator muscle

Deep branch of radial nerve

Extensor carpi radialis longus muscle

Extensor carpi radialis brevis muscle

Extensor digitorum muscle

Extensor digiti minimi muscle

Extensor carpi ulnaris muscle

Flexor carpi radialis muscle

Brachioradialis muscle

Radial artery and superficial branch of radial nerve

Flexor pollicis longus muscle

Extensor carpi radialis longus muscle and tendon

Extensor carpi radialis brevis muscle and tendon

Abductor pollicis longus muscle

Extensor digitorum muscle

Extensor digiti minimi muscle

Extensor carpi ulnaris muscle

Flexor carpi radialis tendon

Radial artery

Brachioradialis tendon

Abductor pollicis longus tendon

Superficial branch of radial nerve

Extensor pollicis brevis tendon

Extensor carpi radialis longus tendon

Extensor carpi radialis brevis tendon

Flexor pollicis longus muscle

Extensor pollicis longus tendon

Radius

Flexor digitorum superficialis muscle (radial head)

Anterior branch of medial antebrachial cutaneous nerve

Flexor pollicis longus muscle

Interosseous membrane

Flexor carpi radialis muscle

Ulnar artery and median nerve

Palmaris longus muscle

Flexor digitorum superficialis muscle (humero-ulnar head)

Common interosseous artery

Ulnar nerve

Flexor carpi ulnaris muscle

Basilic vein

Flexor digitorum profundus muscle

Ulna and antebrachial fascia

Anconeus muscle

Posterior antebrachial cutaneous nerve (from radial nerve)

Palmaris longus muscle

Flexor digitorum superficialis muscle

Median nerve

Ulnar artery and nerve

Flexor carpi ulnaris muscle

Anterior interosseous artery and nerve (from median nerve)

Flexor digitorum profundus muscle

Interosseous membrane and extensor pollicis longus muscle

Posterior interosseous artery and nerve (continuation of deep branch of radial nerve)

Palmaris longus tendon

Median nerve

Flexor digitorum superficialis muscle and tendons

Flexor carpi ulnaris muscle and tendon

Ulnar artery and nerve

Dorsal branch of ulnar nerve

Flexor digitorum profundus muscle and tendons

Ulna

Extensor carpi ulnaris tendon

Pronator quadratus muscle and interosseous membrane

Extensor indicis muscle and tendon

Extensor digiti minimi tendon

Extensor digitorum tendons (common tendon to digits 4 and 5 at this level)

FIGURE 11.3 Forearm: serial cross sections

f. Netter M.D.

of the wrist and hand, such as the extensor digitorum, extensor carpi ulnaris, extensor pollicis brevis, and extensor carpi radius longus. The radial nerve and its branches innervate the muscles of these compartments, and the posterior interosseous artery provides the arterial supply. Signs and symptoms of compartment syndrome are tenderness on palpation; pain with elbow, wrist, and finger flexion; altered sensation of the dorsum of the hand; and weakened wrist extension.

Flexor Compartment

The flexor compartment is located in the anterior region of the forearm and is bound by the ulna, radius, interosseous membrane, and subcutaneous fascia. Within the compartment are the flexor and pronating muscles of the hand, such as the pronator teres, flexor carpi radialis, palmaris longus, and flexor carpi ulnaris. The ulnar and median nerves innervate the muscles of this compartment. The primary arterial supply arises from the ulnar and radial arteries.

Symptoms from compartment syndrome include paresthesias of the palm, thumb, and lateral three digits, along with pain on extension of the fingers and wrist.

INDICATIONS

The diagnosis of compartment syndrome requires a high degree of clinical suspicion. Fasciotomy is indicated when the diagnosis is suspected based on the clinical manifestations associated with compartment syndrome. These signs and symptoms are most commonly known as the "5 P's" of compartment syndrome:

- Pain
- Pallor
- Paresthesia
- Pulselessness
- Paralysis

CONTRAINDICATIONS

Fasciotomy is contraindicated when the extremity is not viable due to irreversible ischemia or traumatic injury. The duration of ischemia plays a key role in determining whether fasciotomy is contraindicated or not. If the tissue has been ischemic for more than 6 to 8 hours, reperfusion may be life threatening. Reperfusion of necrotic muscle tissue may lead to sepsis, hyperkalemia, acidosis, and acute renal failure. If the tissue has been subjected to crush injuries and profound ischemia, amputation is recommended rather than fasciotomy.

EQUIPMENT

Fasciotomy should ideally be performed in the operating room with the patient under general or regional anesthesia. However, situations will arise that will require a fasciotomy to be performed in the trauma bay of the emergency department. Severe burns to the chest can cause respiratory compromise, which will require emergent fasciotomy.

Instruments needed for fasciotomy are as follows:

Scalpel
Large, blunt dissecting scissors
Electrocautery (operating room equipment)
Sterile gown, gloves, and drapes
Wound vacuum-assisted closure (VAC) or bulky dressings

PROCEDURE

Obtain patient consent and perform a time out.

Leg Fasciotomy: Double Incision

The double-incision approach to fasciotomy is most preferred due to its ability to decompress all four compartments without the need to develop skin flaps (Fig. 11.4). The double-incision fasciotomy uses posteromedial and anterolateral longitudinal incisions. The anterolateral incision aims to release the anterior and lateral compartments, whereas the posteromedial incision is used to release the deep and superficial posterior compartments. Each incision should be at least 12 to 20 cm in length to allow full decompression and prevent the recurrence of compartment syndrome.

1. Prep the skin around the site of incision with antiseptic and drape the limb.
2. Begin with the anterolateral incision centered between the anterior tibial crest and fibula, approximately 5 cm distal to the head of the fibula and down toward the ankle. Extend the incision down into the deep fascia by dissecting subcutaneously.
3. Identify the intermuscular septum between the anterior and lateral compartments, lesser saphenous vein, and deep fibular (peroneal) nerve prior to decompressing either compartment.
4. Decompress the anterior compartment in line with the tibialis anterior muscle, from the tibial tuberosity distally to the anterior ankle, using either electrocautery or a scalpel. The incision may then be further dissected with dissecting scissors, taking care to not damage the adjacent nerve and muscular structures.
5. Release the lateral compartment with an incision from the fibular head to the lateral malleolus.
6. Make the posteromedial incision at least 2 cm posteromedial to the tibial margin, extending the incision toward the medial malleolus. The incision should not be made over or near the subcutaneous surface of the tibia, which would inadvertently expose the tibia with retraction.

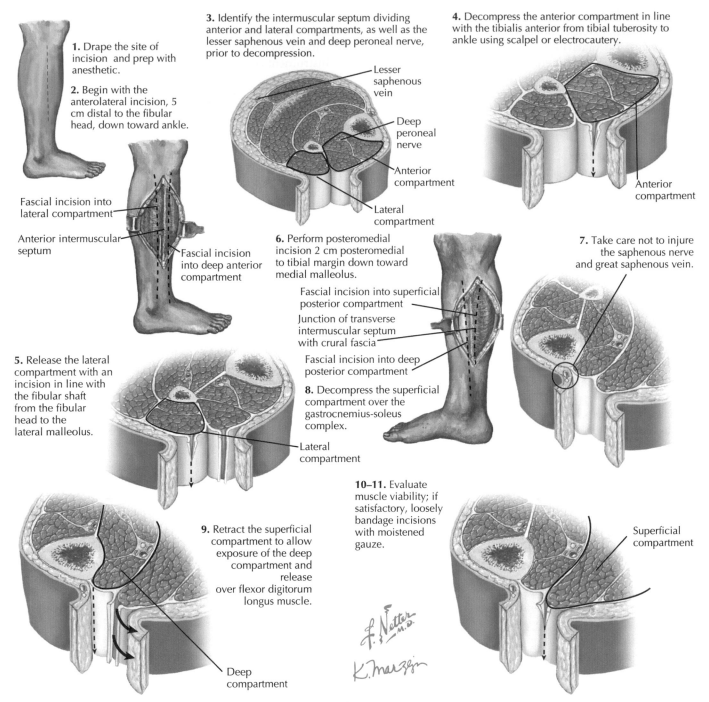

1. Drape the site of incision and prep with anesthetic.

2. Begin with the anterolateral incision, 5 cm distal to the fibular head, down toward ankle.

Fascial incision into lateral compartment

Anterior intermuscular septum

Fascial incision into deep anterior compartment

3. Identify the intermuscular septum dividing anterior and lateral compartments, as well as the lesser saphenous vein and deep peroneal nerve, prior to decompression.

Lesser saphenous vein

Deep peroneal nerve

Anterior compartment

Lateral compartment

4. Decompress the anterior compartment in line with the tibialis anterior from tibial tuberosity to ankle using scalpel or electrocautery.

Anterior compartment

5. Release the lateral compartment with an incision in line with the fibular shaft from the fibular head to the lateral malleolus.

Lateral compartment

6. Perform posteromedial incision 2 cm posteromedial to tibial margin down toward medial malleolus.

Fascial incision into superficial posterior compartment

Junction of transverse intermuscular septum with crural fascia

Fascial incision into deep posterior compartment

8. Decompress the superficial compartment over the gastrocnemius-soleus complex.

7. Take care not to injure the saphenous nerve and great saphenous vein.

9. Retract the superficial compartment to allow exposure of the deep compartment and release over flexor digitorum longus muscle.

Deep compartment

10–11. Evaluate muscle viability; if satisfactory, loosely bandage incisions with moistened gauze.

Superficial compartment

FIGURE 11.4 Leg fasciotomy: double incision

7. While making the incision and performing subcutaneous dissection, take care to not injure the saphenous nerve and vein. When identified, retract them anteriorly.

8. Release the superficial aspect of the posterior compartment over the gastrocnemius-soleus complex, using either a scalpel or cautery for incision of the fascia and dissecting scissors for further dissection.

9. Retract the superficial compartment to allow exposure of the deep compartment. Release the deep compartment over the flexor digitorum longus by dividing the attachments of the soleus muscle from the posterior tibial attachments.

10. Evaluate muscle viability after fasciotomy. If necessary, perform myomectomy to remove any ischemic or necrotic muscle tissue.

11. Dress the incisions with moistened gauze and loosely bandage in place. Interrupted sutures may be placed to approximate the edges for closure after the edema has decreased. Wound VAC systems may also be used as an adjuvant to assist in closure and prevent further edema.

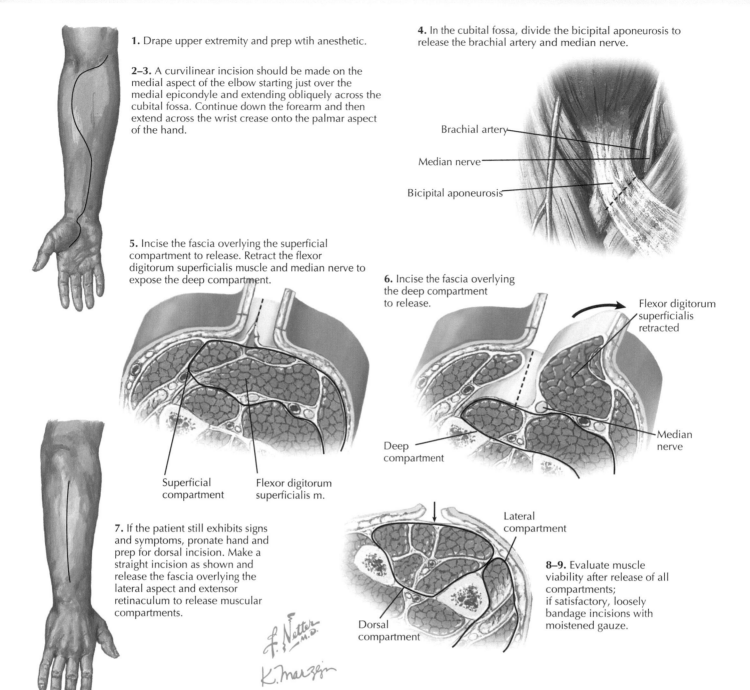

1. Drape upper extremity and prep wtih anesthetic.

2–3. A curvilinear incision should be made on the medial aspect of the elbow starting just over the medial epicondyle and extending obliquely across the cubital fossa. Continue down the forearm and then extend across the wrist crease onto the palmar aspect of the hand.

4. In the cubital fossa, divide the bicipital aponeurosis to release the brachial artery and median nerve.

Brachial artery

Median nerve

Bicipital aponeurosis

5. Incise the fascia overlying the superficial compartment to release. Retract the flexor digitorum superficialis muscle and median nerve to expose the deep compartment.

6. Incise the fascia overlying the deep compartment to release.

Flexor digitorum superficialis retracted

Superficial compartment

Flexor digitorum superficialis m.

Deep compartment

Median nerve

7. If the patient still exhibits signs and symptoms, pronate hand and prep for dorsal incision. Make a straight incision as shown and release the fascia overlying the lateral aspect and extensor retinaculum to release muscular compartments.

Lateral compartment

Dorsal compartment

8–9. Evaluate muscle viability after release of all compartments; if satisfactory, loosely bandage incisions with moistened gauze.

FIGURE 11.5 Forearm fasciotomy

Forearm Fasciotomy

Decompression of the forearm compartments involves a primary curvilinear incision to relieve pressure in the flexor compartment and a second straight dorsal incision to release the extensor compartment, if needed (Fig. 11.5).

1. Completely prepare the upper extremity from the upper arm down and drape circumferentially around the upper arm.
2. Make a curvilinear S-shaped incision on the forearm. The incision begins just over the medial epicondyle and extends obliquely across the antecubital fossa.
3. Curve the incision and continue on the ulnar aspect of the forearm, just medial to the course of the palmaris longus tendon. Extend the incision across the wrist flexion crease transversely to enter the palmar aspect of the hand between the thenar and hypothenar musculature to release the carpal tunnel as needed.
4. In the antecubital fossa, divide the bicipital aponeurosis to release the brachial artery and median nerve. This incision allows for coverage of the median nerve and prevents contractures from developing at the flexion creases.

5. Incise the fascia overlaying the flexor carpi ulnaris, flexor digitorum superficialis, and underlying neurovascular structures to release the superficial compartment. Retraction of the flexor digitorum superficialis and median nerve should expose the fascia superficial to the deep compartment.

6. Incise the flexor digitorum profundus fascia longitudinally along its full length to release the deep compartment.

7. If the dorsal and lateral compartments still exhibit manifestations of compartment syndrome after initial release, perform a second dorsal incision to decompress these compartments.

   a. Pronate the forearm and make a straight incision from the midline of the wrist proximally to the lateral epicondyle.

   b. Release the fascia overlying the lateral compartment and the extensor retinaculum to decompress both dorsal and lateral compartments.

8. Assess muscle viability after fasciotomy has released all compartments. If necessary, perform myomectomy to remove any ischemic or necrotic muscle tissue.

9. Dress the incisions with moistened gauze and loosely bandage in place. Interrupted sutures may be placed to approximate the edges for closure after the edema has decreased. Wound VAC systems may also be used as an adjuvant to assist in closure and prevent further edema.

COMPLICATIONS

The most common complication seen after fasciotomy for compartment syndrome is persistent neurologic deficits. Fasciotomy may result in iatrogenic injury (see below), but nerve damage may have been caused by the initial traumatic injury and ischemia due to increased compartmental pressures. Altered sensation at the incision site is the most common neuropathic symptom associated with fasciotomy.

Neurovascular injury is a technical complication associated with fasciotomy. Injuries to the fibular (peroneal) artery and superficial fibular (peroneal) nerve are the most common neurovascular injuries associated with emergency leg fasciotomy. Damage to the median nerve is the most common neurovascular injury seen in anterior forearm compartment fasciotomy. These injuries may be avoided by proper identification of the structures during the incision, isolating and retracting them safely, and using only blunt dissection. Incomplete fasciotomy occurs when the incision is inadequate to completely decompress the compartment(s). Other complications include reperfusion injury, tissue ischemia, wound infection, dehiscence, keloid formation, rhabdomyolysis, persistent neurological deficits, and contracture formation. All of the potential complications are associated with the risk of limb loss to amputation, sepsis, and death.

CONCLUSIONS

Acute compartment syndrome is a life-threatening condition. Failure to decompress affected compartments threatens the viability of the limb and can lead to even more severe complications. Fasciotomy is a surgical procedure used to treat acute compartment syndrome and may be limb sparing and lifesaving. It may be performed in the operating room or in an emergency setting and requires thorough knowledge of the relevant anatomy of the region to release the compartmental space and prevent neurovascular complications associated with the procedure. Clinical signs and symptoms that should raise suspicion of compartment syndrome include pain out of proportion to the external appearance, paresthesias, paralysis, pallor, and pulselessness. While compartment pressure measurements may be used to determine the need for fasciotomy, it is advised that when in doubt, the prophylactic approach should be taken, going directly to fasciotomy to prevent further complications. Antibiotic administration, regular dressing changes, and early closure aid in reducing the risks of postoperative complications.

Suggested Readings

Elliott KG, Johnstone AJ. Diagnosing acute compartment syndrome. *J Bone Joint Surg Br.* 2003;85:625–632.

Frink M, Hildebrand F, Krettek C, Brand J, Hankemeieir S. Compartment syndrome of the leg and foot. *Clin Orthop Relat Res.* 2010;468:940–950.

Kalyani BS, Fisher BE, Roberts CS, Giannoudis PV. Compartment syndrome of the forearm: a systemic review. *J Hand Surg Am.* 2011;36:535–543.

Kraugh JF, San Antonio J, Simmons JW, et al. Compartment syndrome performance improvement project is associated with increased combat casualty survival. *J Trauma Acute Care Surg.* 2013;74:259–263.

Marshall ST, Browner BD. Emergency care of musculoskeletal injuries. In: Townsend CM, Beauchamp RD, Evers BM, Mattox KL, eds. *Sabiston's Textbook of Surgery: The Biological Basis of Modern Surgical Practice.* 19th ed. Philadelphia: Elsevier; 2012:480–520.

Mubarak S, Hargens A. *Compartment Syndromes and Volkmann's Contracture.* Philadelphia: WB Saunders; 1981.

Nelson JA. Compartment pressure measurements have poor specificity for compartment syndrome in the traumatized limb. *J Emerg Med.* 2013;44:1039–1044.

Olson SA, Glasgow RR. Acute compartment syndrome in lower extremity musculoskeletal trauma. *J Am Acad Orthop Surg.* 2005;13:436–344.

Patel RV, Haddad FS. Compartment syndromes. *Br J Hosp Med (Lond).* 2005;66:583–586.

Ritenour AE, Dorlac WC, Fang R, et al. Complications after fasciotomy revision and delayed compartment release in combat patients. *J Trauma.* 2008;64:S153–S161.

Simon KB. Fasciotomy. In: Scott-Conner CEH, Dawson DL, eds. *Operative Anatomy.* 3rd ed. Philadelphia: Lippincott Williams & Wilkins; 2009:762–767.

Sise MJ, Shackford SR. Peripheral vascular injury. In: Mattox KL, Moore EE, Feliciano DV, eds. *Trauma.* 7th ed. New York: McGraw Hill; 2013:816–847.

US Department of Defense. *Emergency War Surgery, Third United States Revision.* United States: Prepper Press; 2004:22.9–22.15.

REVIEW QUESTIONS

1. Upon removal of a leg cast, a 15-year-old boy complains of numbness of the dorsum of his right foot and an inability to dorsiflex and evert his foot. Which is the most probable site of nerve compression that resulted in these symptoms?

   A. Popliteal fossa
   B. Neck of the fibula
   C. Lateral compartment of the leg
   D. Anterior compartment of the leg
   E. Medial malleolus

2. A 25-year-old woman is admitted to the emergency department after a car collision. Radiographic examination reveals a fracture at the spiral groove of the humerus. A cast is placed, and 3 days later the patient complains of severe pain over the length of her arm. On physical examination, the arm appears swollen, pale, and cool. The radial pulse is absent, and any movement of the arm causes severe pain. Which of the following conditions will most likely explain the physical findings?

A. Venous thrombosis
B. Thoracic outlet syndrome
C. Compartment syndrome
D. Raynaud's disease
E. Injury of the radial nerve

Nosebleed Management

INTRODUCTION

Even though epistaxis, or nosebleed, can occur in adulthood, it is more commonly seen in patients aged 2 to 10 years. Epistaxis is rarely a life-threatening condition because most nosebleeds are self-limited. Most episodes are isolated events, although epistaxis can occasionally become a recurrent problem.

Epistaxis most commonly occurs because of digital manipulation or a dry environment. It can be caused by trauma, foreign bodies, deviated septum, medications, chemical irritants, medical conditions, or neoplasms. A deviated septum creates turbulent airflow within the cavity, which leads to drying of the mucosa. Chemical irritants such as cocaine, inhaled corticosteroids, or oxygen delivered via a nasal cannula can irritate the nasal mucosa and result in epistaxis. Diseases that can lead to epistaxis include bleeding disorders such as von Willebrand disease and hemophilias, hypertension, alcohol abuse, thrombocytopenia, and hemorrhagic telangiectasia. Anticoagulation or antiplatelet therapy with agents such as warfarin and heparin does not directly cause epistaxis but can increase the likelihood of severe nosebleeds if they occur.

Epistaxis is categorized as either anterior or posterior based on the location of origin. Anterior bleeds make up the majority of all nosebleeds. It is estimated that 90% of anterior bleeds originate from Kiesselbach's plexus. These bleeds are usually easy to detect and control with rhinoscopy. Posterior bleeds may originate from the sphenopalatine artery, tend to be related to atherosclerosis, and are seen more often in elderly patients. Epistaxis can present as hematemesis or melena because of swallowed blood.

CLINICALLY RELEVANT ANATOMY

The nose and nasal cavity are used for the sensation of smell and as a passageway for air. To perform both of these functions, the nasal cavity has a rich blood supply (Fig. 12.1). This blood supply is derived from the branches of both the internal and external carotid arteries. The nasal septum is bilaterally symmetrical so it is supplied by the left and right branches of each artery listed below. A branch of the internal carotid artery is the ophthalmic artery, which courses along with the optic nerve and gives rise to two smaller branches, the anterior and posterior ethmoid arteries. These two branches then penetrate the roof of the nasal cavity. The anterior ethmoid artery travels through the cribriform plate as it supplies the anterior nasal septum. It continues past the nasal cavity and becomes the superior labial artery in the upper lip. The posterior ethmoid artery travels through the posterior ethmoid canal and ends in the nasal cavity. Both of these arteries bifurcate into lateral and septal branches after passing through the cribriform plate.

The external carotid artery provides blood to the nasal cavity through the maxillary and facial arteries. The maxillary artery gives rise to a terminal branch, the sphenopalatine artery, which supplies both the lateral wall of the nasal cavity and the posterior nasal septum. The facial artery gives rise to the superior labial artery, which travels up into the nasal cavity and joins the anterior ethmoid artery and a terminal branch of the sphenopalatine artery. The confluence of these three main arteries in the anterior portion of the nasal septum is known as Kiesselbach's plexus or Little's area. The maxillary artery also gives rise to the descending palatine artery, which courses through the greater palatine canal and supplies the lateral aspects of the nasal cavity. This artery continues through the incisive foramen, where it also aids in the blood supply of the anterior nasal septum.

INDICATIONS

The standard order for treatment is indicated for any episode of epistaxis seen in the emergency department. These treatments involve direct pressure, topical agents, and silver nitrate cauterization. Packing of the nasopharynx is indicated only after the standard treatments have failed to control the bleeding. Packing can be accomplished using nasal tampons, thrombogenic foams and gels, or gauze moistened with epinephrine. Electrical cauterization is indicated in more serious bleeds, which usually arise from the posterior nasopharynx.

CONTRAINDICATIONS

Every patient should first be assessed for airway, breathing, and circulation (ABC). If the patient is hemodynamically unstable because of severe epistaxis, initial management must focus on resuscitation with fluids or blood products in conjunction with the application of direct pressure to the involved nostril. Further treatment must await stabilization of the patient. Definitive treatment may also take second priority in patients requiring airway management or mechanical ventilation. Posterior packing is contraindicated in the presence of nasal bone or cribriform plate fractures.

Anterolateral view

Inferior view

Major alar cartilage

Lateral crus   Medial crus

Nasal bones

Frontal process of maxilla

Lateral process of
septal nasal cartilages

Septal cartilage

Minor alar cartilage

Accessory nasal cartilage

Major alar cartilage { Lateral crus

Medial crus

Nasal septal cartilage

Anterior nasal spine of maxilla

Alar fibrofatty tissue

Alar
fibrofatty
tissue

Nasal septal
cartilage

Anterior
nasal spine
of maxilla

Nasal septum (*turned up*)

Nasal septal branch of superior labial branch
(of facial artery)

Anastomosis between posterior septal branch
of sphenopalatine artery and greater palatine
artery in incisive canal

Schematic hinge

Septal and lateral nasal
branches of posterior ethmoidal
artery

Anterior septal branch,
Anterior lateral nasal branch,
External nasal branch
of anterior
ethmoidal
artery

Posterior septal
branch of
sphenopalatine
artery

Sphenopalatine
artery

Sphenopalatine
foramen

Alar branches of
lateral nasal
branch
(of facial artery)

Posterior lateral nasal
branches of
sphenopalatine artery

Maxillary
artery

Anastomosis between
posterior septal branch
of sphenopalatine artery
and greater palatine
artery in incisive canal

Inferior
alveolar artery

External carotid
artery

Greater palatine artery

Lateral wall of nasal cavity

Lesser palatine foramen and artery

Greater palatine foramen and artery

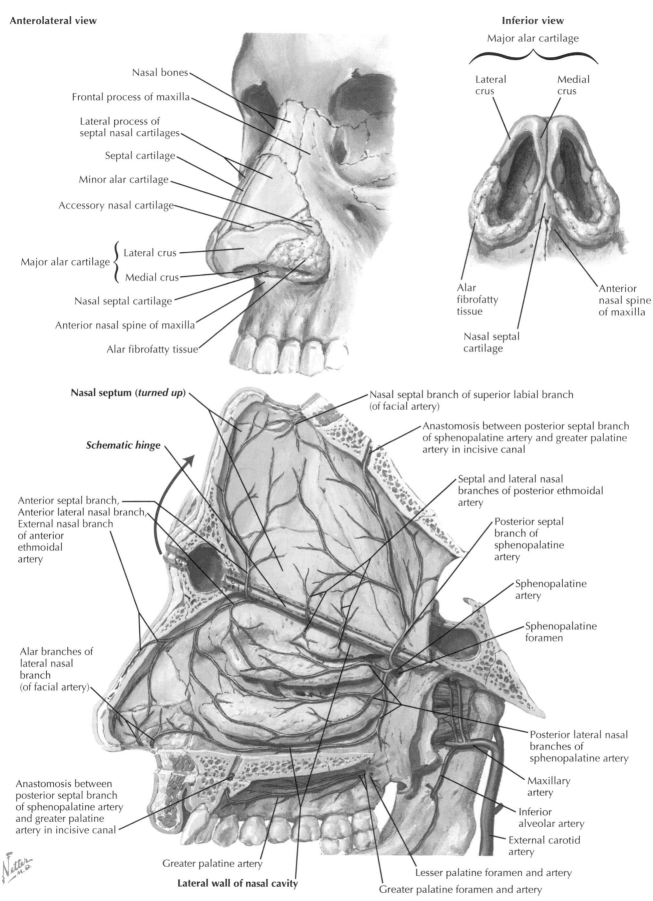

FIGURE 12.1 Anatomy of the nose

EQUIPMENT

The treatment of epistaxis typically requires minimal equipment. Local anesthetic may or may not be required, but if needed, it is advisable to use a 1:1 mixture of 0.05% oxymetazoline and 4% lidocaine. The equipment necessary for more specialized treatments typically comes in premade kits. However, for basic episodes of epistaxis, the equipment used includes the following:

Gloves
Gauze
Rhinoscope or endoscope
Cotton-tipped swabs
Anesthesia
Local vasoconstrictors
Silver nitrate

PROCEDURE

Obtain patient consent and perform a time out. See Fig. 12.2.

1. Seat the patient in an upright position with the head tilted slightly forward to reduce the venous pressure in the nasal vessels and the amount of blood that is swallowed, which can lead to nausea and hematemesis.
2. Have the patient blow his or her nose to remove any formed clots that could prevent vasoconstrictors from accessing their desired targets.
3. Once major clots have been removed, apply direct vasoconstrictors such as phenylephrine or oxymetazoline to the nasal cavity, either by a spray or with a cotton-tipped swab.
4. While the medication is acting, apply direct pressure to the origin of the bleed by squeezing the lateral walls of the nose against the septum (but avoid squeezing the nasal bones) for approximately 10 to 15 minutes. The patient should be reminded to breathe through the mouth.
5. Reassess the bleeding. If it continues, administer another application of vasoconstrictors and pressure.
6. After a round of pressure, pack the nasal cavity with gauze moistened with epinephrine (1:10,000) or phenylephrine to aid in vasoconstriction.
7. If two rounds of vasoconstrictor application and pressure with gauze packing fail to control the bleeding, the next step is chemical cauterization.
8. Locate the origin of the bleed using suction and either rhinoscopy or endoscopy. Blind cauterization can cause more damage.
9. Anesthetize the area of interest before cauterization with a 1:1 mixture of 0.05% oxymetazoline and 4% lidocaine applied with cotton-tipped swabs. Once the anesthesia has taken effect, cauterize with cotton-tipped swabs and silver nitrate.
10. If bleeding is still not controlled after cauterization, explore other treatment options, including nasal packing and balloons, arterial ligation, electrical cauterization, and embolization. Any posterior packing should always be accompanied by anterior packing.
    a. If cauterization is performed, advise the patient to use saline washes. If cauterization or packing is performed, the patient may be placed on a short course of antibiotics.
    b. If packing is placed, the patient should follow up in 2 to 3 days to have the packing removed.

ANATOMICAL PITFALLS

Cautery that does not reach the bleeding vessel or Kiesselbach's area (if involved) will not result in hemostasis. Posterior packing in the presence of a cribriform plate fracture can result in the packing being placed intracranially.

COMPLICATIONS

Complications of epistaxis include the following:
- Infection
- Septal hematoma or perforation
- Sinusitis
- Aspiration
- Toxic shock syndrome (if packing or another inserted appliance is used)
- Septal perforation associated with bilateral cautery
- Recurrent epistaxis
- Hypoxia
- Vasovagal episodes
- Hypotension
- Aspiration of balloon contents if ruptured

CONCLUSION

Epistaxis is an acute event commonly occurring from the ages of 2 to 10 years and 45 to 65 years. Most episodes are self-limited, and the prognosis is generally very good. Anatomically, the majority of cases arise from the anterior nasopharynx, where blood vessels form Kiesselbach's plexus; only a small percentage arise from the posterior blood vessels. Treatment usually only requires direct pressure, but depending upon the severity of the bleed, it may require further action such as cauterization, packing, arterial ligation, or embolization. Workup for epistaxis is usually reserved for patients with recurrent episodes or patients with a family history of blood dyscrasias such as hemophilia or coagulopathy.

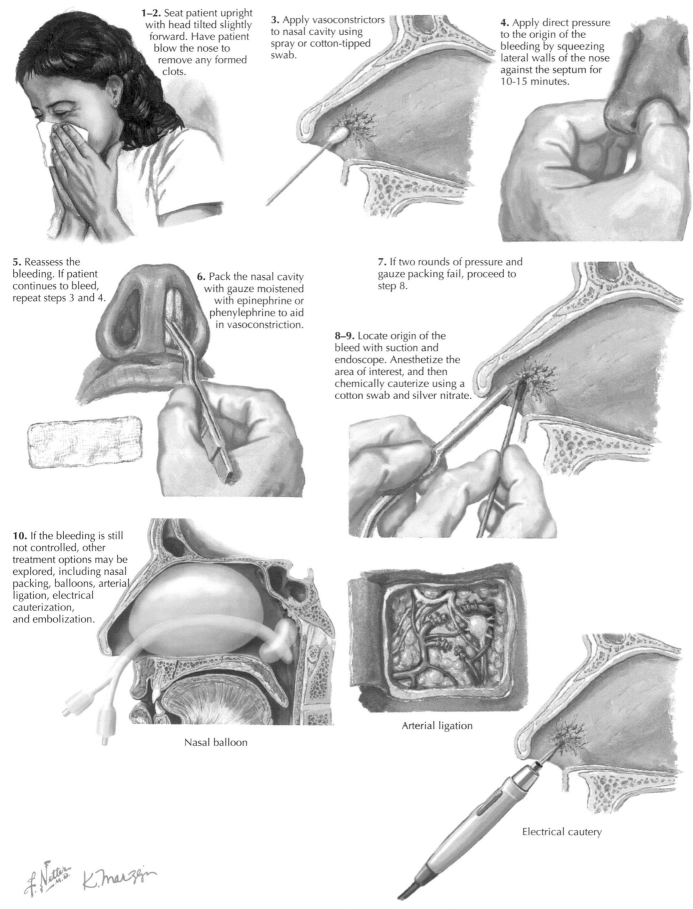

1–2. Seat patient upright with head tilted slightly forward. Have patient blow the nose to remove any formed clots.

3. Apply vasoconstrictors to nasal cavity using spray or cotton-tipped swab.

4. Apply direct pressure to the origin of the bleeding by squeezing lateral walls of the nose against the septum for 10-15 minutes.

5. Reassess the bleeding. If patient continues to bleed, repeat steps 3 and 4.

6. Pack the nasal cavity with gauze moistened with epinephrine or phenylephrine to aid in vasoconstriction.

7. If two rounds of pressure and gauze packing fail, proceed to step 8.

8–9. Locate origin of the bleed with suction and endoscope. Anesthetize the area of interest, and then chemically cauterize using a cotton swab and silver nitrate.

10. If the bleeding is still not controlled, other treatment options may be explored, including nasal packing, balloons, arterial ligation, electrical cauterization, and embolization.

Nasal balloon

Arterial ligation

Electrical cautery

FIGURE 12.2 Nosebleed management

Suggested Readings

Lustig LR, Schindler JS. Ear, nose, and throat disorders. In Papadakis M, McPhee SJ, Rabow MW, eds. *Current Diagnosis and Treatment 2015*. New York: McGraw Hill; 2014.

Summers SM, Bey T. Epistaxis, nasal fractures, and rhinosinusitis. In Tintinalli J, Stapczynski J, Ma OJ, eds. *Tintinalli's Emergency Medicine: A Comprehensive Study Guide*, 7th ed. New York: McGraw Hill; 2010.

REVIEW QUESTIONS

1. A 21-year-old man was brought to the emergency department because of severe epistaxis from the nasal septum. This area, known as Kiesselbach's (or Little's) area, involves anastomoses mostly between which of the following arteries?

   A. Ascending palatine and ascending pharyngeal
   B. Posterior superior alveolar and accessory meningeal
   C. Lateral branches of posterior ethmoidal and middle meningeal
   D. Septal branches of the sphenopalatine and superior labial
   E. Descending palatine and tonsillar branches of the pharyngeal

2. A 57-year-old man was brought to the emergency department because of severe epistaxis from the nasal septum. Which of the following is the most likely cause of epistaxis?

   A. Nose picking
   B. Hypertension
   C. Hemophilia
   D. Idiopathic thrombocytopenic purpura

Pericardiocentesis

INTRODUCTION

Cardiac tamponade is a life-threatening condition that requires immediate diagnosis and treatment. Pericardiocentesis is a procedure used to drain excess fluid that accumulates in the pericardial space (sac).

Pericardial effusions can occur as a result of trauma, malignancy, infection, or myocardial rupture. When these effusions result in cardiac tamponade, there is a significant increase in pericardial pressure that inhibits the expansion of the heart. Patients can exhibit some or all of the classic Beck's triad of signs: hypotension, distended neck veins, and distant, muffled heart sounds. Electrocardiography (ECG) often shows sinus tachycardia, low voltage, PR depression, and electrical alternans. At first, compensatory mechanisms such as increased heart rate, arterial vasoconstriction, and venoconstriction help to maintain cardiac output. When these compensatory mechanisms fail, cardiac filling and cardiac output become critically diminished, resulting in shock and cardiac arrest. Removal of even a small amount of fluid from the pericardial space can help stabilize a hemodynamically unstable patient until a definitive procedure, such as a cardiac window, can be performed.

The techniques used for pericardiocentesis have evolved extensively over the years. The introduction of ultrasound-guided pericardiocentesis has reduced the complication rate of this procedure. In many situations, however, the procedure may need to be performed with a traditional blind approach, though only if ultrasound is unavailable. It is important to have a strong clinical understanding of the relevant anatomy encountered in this procedure when using ultrasound guidance or traditional landmark techniques.

CLINICALLY RELEVANT ANATOMY

The pericardium and heart are located in the middle mediastinum (Fig. 13.1). The pericardial sac is a two-layered membrane that surrounds the heart (Fig. 13.2). The outer parietal layer of the pericardium consists of fibrous tissue made up of collagen and elastin. This outer layer adheres to the great vessels superiorly, the central tendon of the diaphragm inferiorly, and the sternum anteriorly. The inner visceral layer is the serous part of the pericardium and adheres to the epicardium. Between the visceral and parietal pericardial layers, serous fluid (15 to 50 mL) acts as a shock absorber for deceleration forces and as a lubricant for frictionless cardiac movement.

The pericardium is extensively innervated by thoracic visceral afferent fibers and, to a lesser extent, the phrenic nerve.

As a result, inflammation in this area can cause severe pain. In additions, several vital structures share a close anatomical relationship with the heart and thus must be considered when performing pericardiocentesis (see Fig. 13.2). The pleura, lungs, diaphragm, and liver are all at risk.

Electrocardiographic Changes

ECG-guided pericardiocentesis is outdated. However, constant monitoring is needed because cardiac arrhythmias can occur that may need to be treated immediately. This monitoring is carried out by attaching an alligator clip from one of the precordial EGG leads to the distal end of the needle used to perform the pericardiocentesis. If the needle comes into contact with the pericardium immediately overlying the heart, ST or PR segment elevation can be seen when no fluid is present in the pericardial sac. If the needle comes into contact with the ventricular myocardium, there is marked ST segment elevation in the presence of multiple, wide-complex ventricular ectopic beats. If this pattern is seen, the needle should be withdrawn several millimeters. ECG findings are limited in patients with previous myocardial infarction that has formed scar tissue and in those with a metastatic tumor. These problem areas are electrically silent

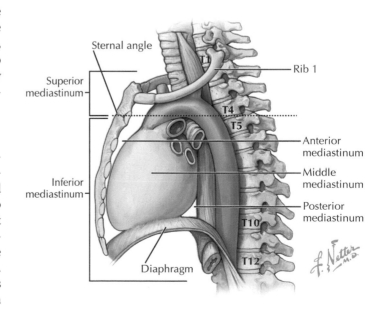

FIGURE 13.1 Pericardium and heart in middle mediastinum just posterior to the sternum. Note the relationship between the sternum, diaphragm, and heart.

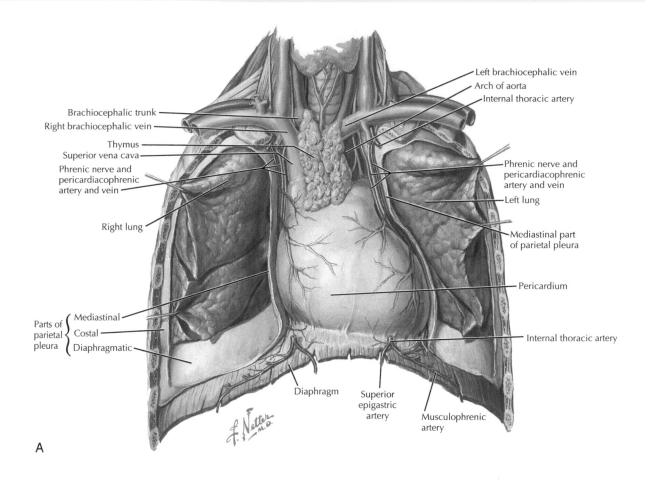

Left brachiocephalic vein
Arch of aorta
Internal thoracic artery
Brachiocephalic trunk
Right brachiocephalic vein
Thymus
Superior vena cava
Phrenic nerve and pericardiacophrenic artery and vein
Phrenic nerve and pericardiacophrenic artery and vein
Left lung
Right lung
Mediastinal part of parietal pleura
Pericardium
Parts of parietal pleura { Mediastinal Costal Diaphragmatic
Internal thoracic artery
Diaphragm
Superior epigastric artery
Musculophrenic artery

A

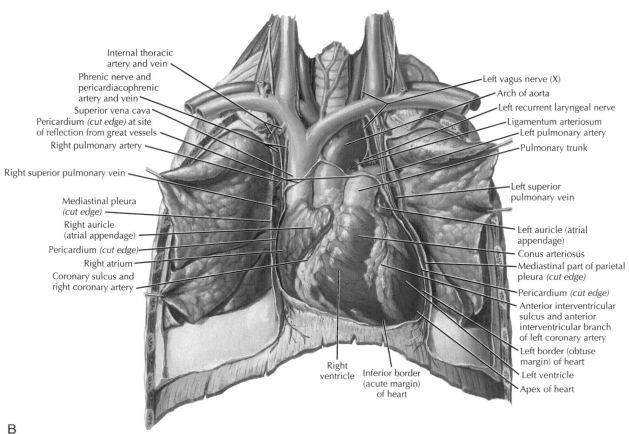

Internal thoracic artery and vein
Phrenic nerve and pericardiacophrenic artery and vein
Superior vena cava
Pericardium (cut edge) at site of reflection from great vessels
Right pulmonary artery
Right superior pulmonary vein
Mediastinal pleura (cut edge)
Right auricle (atrial appendage)
Pericardium (cut edge)
Right atrium
Coronary sulcus and right coronary artery
Left vagus nerve (X)
Arch of aorta
Left recurrent laryngeal nerve
Ligamentum arteriosum
Left pulmonary artery
Pulmonary trunk
Left superior pulmonary vein
Left auricle (atrial appendage)
Conus arteriosus
Mediastinal part of parietal pleura (cut edge)
Pericardium (cut edge)
Anterior interventricular sulcus and anterior interventricular branch of left coronary artery
Left border (obtuse margin) of heart
Left ventricle
Apex of heart
Right ventricle
Inferior border (acute margin) of heart

B

FIGURE 13.2 A, Pericardial sac surrounds the heart and is innervated by the phrenic nerve. **B,** Pericardium is removed and the anterior portion of the heart exposed.

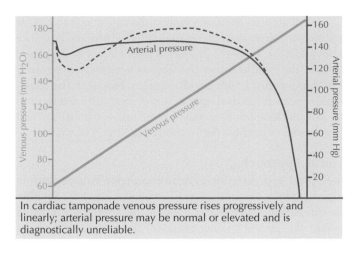

In cardiac tamponade venous pressure rises progressively and linearly; arterial pressure may be normal or elevated and is diagnostically unreliable.

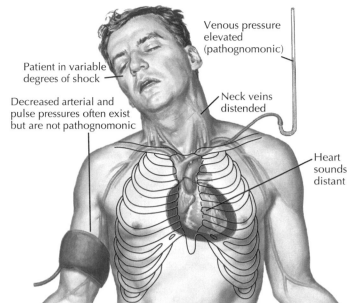

FIGURE 13.3 Parasternal pericardiocentesis technique

and may not show the current-of-injury pattern when a needle perforates the area.

INDICATIONS

Pericardiocentesis can be used for both diagnostic and therapeutic purposes.

Diagnostic Pericardiocentesis

Diagnostic pericardiocentesis is a nonemergent procedure used to aspirate fluid for analysis. Pericardial fluid aids in the diagnosis of malignancies and viral or bacterial pericarditis. The pH of the fluid can help distinguish an inflammatory from a noninflammatory process. The fluid can be cultured for bacterial infections or examined for neoplastic cells.

Therapeutic Pericardiocentesis

Therapeutic pericardiocentesis may be an emergency or a nonemergency procedure. In nonemergency situations, pericardiocentesis can be used for palliative or prophylactic measures. Tamponade in emergency situations, including cardiac arrest, pulseless electrical activity, hypotension refractory to fluid resuscitation, or traumatic hemorrhagic effusions, requires therapeutic drainage (Fig. 13.3). Although some experts recommend that patients with traumatic cardiac tamponade should be treated with emergency thoracotomy, pericardiocentesis can provide temporary relief until a more definitive procedure can be performed. Aspiration of as little as 10 to 50 mL of pericardial fluid can significantly improve cardiac output. However, the rate of reaccumulation of blood in traumatic hemorrhagic tamponade prevents pericardiocentesis from being a definitive treatment. A thoracotomy should follow immediately after pericardiocentesis for traumatic cardiac tamponade.

CONTRAINDICATIONS

There are no absolute contraindications to performing a pericardiocentesis in hemodynamically unstable patients. Thrombocytopenia and anticoagulant therapy are relative contraindications in patients who present with pericardial effusions that have not progressed to tamponade. Other relative contraindications include thoracoabdominal surgery, prosthetic heart valves, cardiac pacemakers, and poor facilities for cardiorespiratory resuscitation.

EQUIPMENT

60-mL syringe
18-gauge spinal needle
Dilator
8-Fr pigtail catheter
J-tipped guide wire
10-mL syringe, 25-gauge needle
Local anesthetic (1% to 2% lidocaine)
Antiseptic solution
Sterile drapes
Sterile gown and gloves
Ultrasound

PROCEDURE

See Video 13.1.

Obtain patient consent if possible and perform a time out. Don appropriate personal protective equipment. The procedure should be performed under sterile conditions.

Parasternal Approach

Ultrasound-guided pericardiocentesis using the parasternal method provides the most stable and controlled approach. It avoids important structures such as the diaphragm, phrenic nerve, and liver. In emergencies when ultrasound is not readily available, a traditional blind approach can still be used. The following steps describe the ultrasound-guided parasternal approach for pericardiocentesis (Fig. 13.4).

1. Monitor the patient's vital signs (blood pressure, heart rate, and respiratory rate) and electrocardiogram before, during, and after the procedure.
   a. If a central venous line is already in place (see Chapter 3), central venous pressure can also be monitored.
   b. In nonemergency situations, the size, distribution, and hemodynamic effect of the effusion should be assessed by ultrasound.
2. Use the ultrasound transducer to locate an entry site where the fluid collection is maximal and closest to the transducer. For the parasternal approach, this should be in the fifth intercostal space adjacent to the sternum. Care should be taken to avoid injury to the internal thoracic artery, which lies just lateral to the entry site.
3. Prepare the anterior chest wall and the upper part of the abdomen with chlorhexidine solution and a sterile drape.
4. Administer local anesthetic (lidocaine 1% to 2%) at the entry site.
5. Advance the needle over the superior border of the rib to avoid the neurovascular bundle that lies at its inferior border.
6. After introducing the sheathed needle at the predetermined entry site, use ultrasound to guide the needle safely through the different tissue layers toward the fluid collection. Aspirate during needle advancement to determine when the fluid has been reached.
7. Once the needle has reached the fluid, push the needle 2 mm farther and advance the sheath over the needle. The needle can then be withdrawn.
8. Injection of agitated saline can be used to confirm the proper placement of the sheath. If bubbles are seen on ultrasound within the pericardial space, the sheath is in the correct position.
9. Advance a J-tipped guide wire through the sheath and into the pericardial space. Remove the sheath, leaving the guide wire in place.
10. Advance a dilator over the guide wire, remove the dilator, then advance a smooth-walled pigtail catheter over the wire into the pericardial space.
11. Remove the guide wire and leave the drainage catheter connected to a bag to drain the pericardial fluid.

Alternative Methods
Subxiphoid Approach
A subxiphoid approach for pericardiocentesis is recommended when echocardiography cannot be readily used. The needle is inserted at a 45-degree angle between the xiphisternum and the left costal margin in the transverse plane, directed toward the left shoulder. The needle traverses the skin, superficial fascia, anterior rectus sheath, and left rectus abdominis muscle. It then passes through the posterior rectus sheath, over the diaphragm, and through the fibrous pericardium.

The subxiphoid approach is the safest approach to use for pericardiocentesis in an emergency when ultrasound guidance is not available. There is a decreased risk of injury to the pleura because the needle enters the fibrous pericardium where it is in direct contact with the diaphragm. However, the subxiphoid approach has the highest rates of morbidity and mortality. Risks include injury to the phrenic nerve, diaphragm, and liver, as well as possible perforation of the colon or stomach.

Apical Approach
The apical approach for pericardiocentesis is used only in nonemergency circumstances. The needle is inserted within the intercostal space, 1 cm outside the apex beat, directed toward the patient's right shoulder. The pericardial sac lies superficially in this area and has a relatively large transverse diameter. Important structures, including the pleura, are absent in this space.

The apical approach has various advantages over the parasternal and subxiphoid approaches, in addition to the superficial location of the pericardial sac. Unlike the right ventricle, the left ventricle is less prone to serious punctures because of its thicker walls. Overall, the apical approach provides a decreased risk of injuring the pleura, myocardium, liver, or lung.

ANATOMICAL PITFALLS
Xiphoid Process
Palpation of the xiphoid process in the subxiphoid approach can sometimes be difficult. The costal margin, which is readily detected on examination, should be used to predict the location of the xiphoid process.

Pericardium
The pericardial sac can stretch to accommodate 2 to 3 L of fluid. Chronic accumulation of fluid leads to a gradual increase in intrapericardial pressure, whereas an acute accumulation of as little as 100 mL can lead to a sudden increase in the pressure. This can result in cardiac tamponade and a sudden drop in cardiac output. The pericardial sac is also extensively innervated by the phrenic nerve. Because of this innervation, when the pericardium is touched with a needle, the patient experiences severe pain.

Liver
The left lobe of the liver shares a close anatomical relationship with the xiphisternum. When using the subxiphoid approach, it is important to enter at an angle of 45 degrees relative to the horizontal plane to avoid injury to the liver. Entering at angles less than 45 degrees can injure the liver and the stomach. When advanced at the appropriate angle, the needle will enter the diaphragmatic pericardium, avoiding the diaphragm and contents of the abdominal cavity.

Right Ventricle and Marginal Artery
The thin-walled right ventricle can be encountered during the subxiphoid and parasternal approaches. With the subxiphoid approach, the needle enters the pericardial sac at its diaphragmatic surface, which covers the acute angle of the

1. Monitor patient's vital signs.

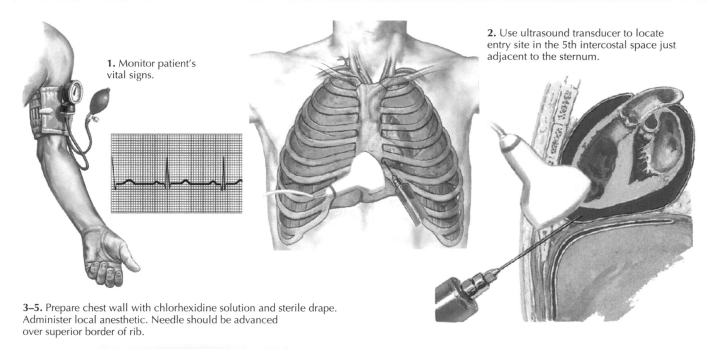

2. Use ultrasound transducer to locate entry site in the 5th intercostal space just adjacent to the sternum.

3–5. Prepare chest wall with chlorhexidine solution and sterile drape. Administer local anesthetic. Needle should be advanced over superior border of rib.

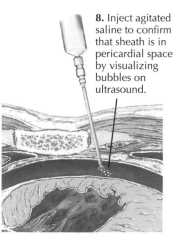

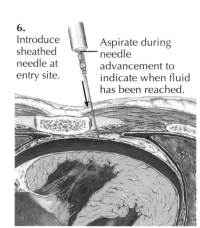

6. Introduce sheathed needle at entry site.

Aspirate during needle advancement to indicate when fluid has been reached.

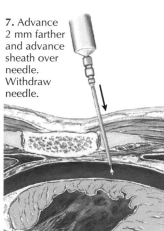

7. Advance 2 mm farther and advance sheath over needle. Withdraw needle.

8. Inject agitated saline to confirm that sheath is in pericardial space by visualizing bubbles on ultrasound.

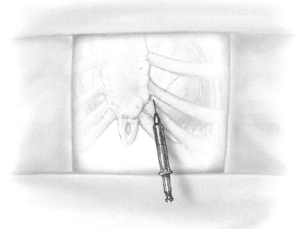

9. Advance J-tipped guide wire through sheath and into pericardial space.

Remove sheath, leaving guide wire.

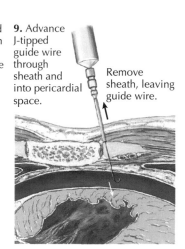

10. Advance smooth-walled pigtail catheter over guide wire.

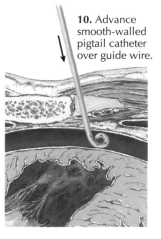

11. Remove guide wire and connect drainage catheter to an external drainage bag to drain pericardial fluid.

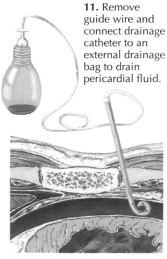

FIGURE 13.4 Pericardiocentesis

right ventricle, along which the marginal artery courses. The close relationship between the diaphragmatic pericardium, right ventricle, and marginal artery leads to an increased risk of right ventricular perforation and injury to the marginal artery.

Direction of Needle

During the subxiphoid approach, if the needle is directed toward the tip of the left scapula, the right ventricle is at a greater risk of perforation. With the apical approach, piercing the left ventricle can lead to a risk of ventricular fibrillation. The needle should always be inserted and removed in one plane. Any lateral motion can lacerate the various structures that are traversed.

COMPLICATIONS

Pericardiocentesis is often performed under stressful emergency situations, in many cases blindly, and the physician should be aware of the potential complications. Ultrasound guidance has significantly reduced the complication rate of pericardiocentesis. Current studies report complication rates as low as 4%, compared with 20% to 40% in previous studies of blind pericardiocentesis.

The most common complication of pericardiocentesis is a dry tap, which occurs when the needle is blocked by thrombus or a skin plug. During a parasternal approach, probing of the anterior costal cartilage can also block the needle. Dry taps are often resolved by repositioning or irrigating the needle. In some cases, the pericardial effusion may be located posterolaterally and would be difficult to tap through a subxiphoid or parasternal approach. An apical approach may help avoid a dry tap in that situation.

Ventricular and coronary vessel lacerations are uncommon complications of pericardiocentesis. The right ventricle is perforated more often than the left ventricle and atrium. The potential consequences of these perforations are hemopericardium and death. With the subxiphoid and parasternal approaches, the right coronary artery is at risk of injury, especially when the needle is not angled toward the tip of the left scapula in the subxiphoid approach.

Cardiac arrhythmias can be a serious complication of pericardiocentesis. Ventricular fibrillation has been known to result from puncture of the right or left ventricle. However, the incidence of serious arrhythmias is extremely low. Although premature ventricular contractions are common when the needle enters the pericardium, serious arrhythmias remain a rare complication.

Pneumothorax and pneumopericardium have been reported when using the apical and parasternal approaches. However, clinical consequences of these complications are uncommon. Other rare complications of pericardiocentesis include hemothorax, arterial bleeding, infection, and abdominal or shoulder pain.

CONCLUSION

Pericardiocentesis performed by an emergency physician can be a lifesaving procedure. By relieving the pressure within the pericardial space, patients with life-threatening cardiac tamponade can be stabilized. Needle pericardiocentesis can be used both in an emergency therapeutic setting and for diagnostic purposes. Although no procedure is without complications, a complete knowledge of the relevant anatomy and procedural techniques can help minimize morbidity.

Suggested Readings

Callahan J, Seward J, Tajik A. Cardiac tamponade: pericardiocentesis directed by two-dimensional echocardiography. *Mayo Clin Proc.* 1985;60:344–347.

Fitch MT, Nicks BA, Pariyadath M, et al. Videos in clinical medicine. Emergency pericardiocentesis. *N Engl J Med.* 2012;366:e17.

Imazio M, Adler Y. Management of pericardial effusion. *Eur Heart J.* 2013;34:1186–1197.

Krikorian JG, Hancock EW. Pericardiocentesis. *Am J Med.* 1978;65:808–814.

Lee TH, Ouellet JF, Cook M, et al. Pericardiocentesis in trauma: a systematic review. *J Trauma Acute Care Surg.* 2013;75:543–549.

Loukas M, Walters A, Boon JM, et al. Pericardiocentesis: a clinical anatomy review. *Clin Anat.* 2012;25:872–881.

Maisch B, Seferović PM, Ristić AD, et al. Guidelines on the diagnosis and management of pericardial diseases: executive summary. Task Force on the Diagnosis and Management of Pericardial Diseases of the European Society of Cardiology. *Eur Heart J.* 2004;25:587–610.

Tsang TS, Emroquez-Sarano M, Freeman WK, et al. Consecutive 1127 therapeutic echocardiographically guided pericardiocenteses: clinical profile, practice patterns, and outcomes spanning 21 years. *Mayo Clin Proc.* 2002;77:429–436.

Tsang TS, Freeman WK, Sinak LJ, Seward JB. Echocardiographically guided pericardiocentesis: evolution and state-of-the-art technique. *Mayo Clin Proc.* 1998;73:647–652.

REVIEW QUESTIONS

1. A 35-year-old man is admitted to the hospital with severe chest pain, dyspnea, tachycardia, cough, and fever. Radiographic examination reveals significant pericardial effusion. When pericardiocentesis is performed, the needle is inserted using the subxiphoid approach. The needle passes too deeply, piercing the visceral pericardium and enters the heart. Which of the following chambers would be the first to be penetrated by the needle?

   A. Right ventricle
   B. Left ventricle
   C. Right atrium
   D. Left atrium
   E. Left cardiac apex

2. A 42-year-old woman is admitted to the emergency department after a fall from the balcony of her apartment. On physical examination, there is an absence of heart sounds, reduced systolic pressure, and engorged jugular veins. Which of the following procedures can alleviate this condition?

   A. Chest tube insertion superior to the rib
   B. Central venous line
   C. Nasogastric tube
   D. Thoracocentesis
   E. Pericardiocentesis

3. A 52-year-old patient is admitted to the hospital with severe chest pain. Electrocardiographic and radiographic examinations provide evidence of a significant myocardial infarction and cardiac tamponade. An emergency pericardiocentesis is performed. At which of the following locations will the needle best be inserted to relieve the tamponade?

   A. Right seventh intercostal space in the midaxillary line
   B. Left fifth intercostal space in the midclavicular line
   C. Right third intercostal space, 1 inch lateral to the sternum
   D. Left sixth intercostal space, ½ inch lateral to the sternum
   E. Triangle of auscultation

4. For the patient in Question 3, which of the following is the most likely complication that may occur during the procedure?

   A. Dry tap
   B. Coronary vessel lacerations
   C. Ventricular tachycardia
   D. Pneumothorax
   E. Abdominal and shoulder pain

5. A 27-year-old man suffered a small-caliber bullet wound to the chest in the region of the third intercostal space, several centimeters to the left of the sternum. The patient is admitted to the emergency department, and a preliminary notation of "Beck's triad" is entered on the patient's chart. Which of the following are features of this triad?

   A. There is injury to the left pulmonary artery, left primary bronchus, and esophagus.
   B. The patient has bleeding into the pleural cavity, a collapsed lung, and mediastinal shift to the right side of the thorax.
   C. The patient has a small, quiet heart; decreased pulse pressure; and increased central venous pressure.
   D. The man is suffering from marked diastolic emptying, dyspnea, and dilation of the aortic arch.
   E. The left lung has collapsed, paradoxical respiration is present, and there is a mediastinal shift of the heart and trachea to the left.

Central Venous Catheterization

INTRODUCTION

In a patient who is hypovolemic and/or critically ill, establishing vascular access and providing resuscitation, as well as taking appropriate cervical spine precautions in trauma cases, are the foundations of management after airway and breathing are ensured. A variety of vascular access procedures may be used in the critically ill patient. Although peripheral access should be attempted first, if this is unobtainable, central venous access should be attempted. Central venous access allows fluid resuscitation and permits the measurement of hemodynamic variables and the delivery of medications and nutritional support.

Central venous access may be readily performed at reliable sites easily identified by surface anatomy—namely the jugular, subclavian, and femoral veins.

CLINICALLY RELEVANT ANATOMY

A thorough knowledge of the relevant anatomy is important in performing central venous catheterization. Understanding the venous anatomy and nearby anatomical landmarks aids in quickly locating the commonly used vessels and in avoiding possible complications involving adjacent structures.

Subclavian Vein

The subclavian vein is a direct continuation of the axillary vein (Fig. 14.1A). It extends from the outer border of the first rib to the medial border of the anterior scalene muscle, where the subclavian vein joins the internal jugular vein to become the brachiocephalic vein before draining directly into the superior vena cava. The subclavian vein lies posterior to the medial third of the clavicle and subclavius muscle, anteroinferior to the subclavian artery, anterior to the anterior scalene muscle and phrenic nerve, and superior to the first rib and pleura. The intimate relationship between the medial third of the clavicle and the subclavian vein serves as a useful landmark for the placement of central venous lines into this vein.

Internal Jugular Vein

Central venous catheterization may be performed on both the external and internal jugular veins. The internal jugular vein arises at the cranial base in the jugular foramen. It collects venous blood primarily from inside the skull and travels in the neck within the carotid sheath deep to the sternocleidomastoid muscle to unite distally with the subclavian vein posterior to the sternal edge of the clavicle. Within the carotid sheath, the internal jugular vein is anterolateral to the carotid artery and vagus nerve.

Anatomical landmarks for locating the internal jugular vein include the sternal notch, sternocleidomastoid muscle, and clavicle. The two heads of the sternocleidomastoid muscle and the clavicle form the apex of a small triangle where the internal jugular vein is located (Fig. 14.1B).

Femoral Vein

The femoral vein also serves as a site for central venous catheterization. This vein has less complex anatomy than that of the neck and shoulder seen with the internal jugular and subclavian veins, respectively, so the femoral vein may be easily cannulated in any patient who has a femoral artery pulse, with minimal risk of life-threatening complications. The femoral vein is a direct continuation of the popliteal vein and becomes the external iliac vein at the level of the inguinal ligament. Lateral to the femoral vein, the femoral artery accompanies the vein within the femoral sheath, whereas the lymphatic vessels travel medially with the vein. The femoral vein also receives venous drainage from the deep femoral and great saphenous veins before crossing the inguinal ligament to become the external iliac vein (Fig. 14.1C). Central venous catheterization of the femoral vein should be performed close to the inguinal ligament because the relationship of the artery and vein changes distally in the thigh, where the femoral artery may take an anterior position.

INDICATIONS

The most common indications for central venous catheterization include the need for central venous pressure monitoring; routine or emergency venous access; serial blood draws; the administration of medications, some of which can only be administered via a central line; and invasive venous interventions such as transvenous pacemakers and hemodialysis. The use of central venous catheters permits the careful monitoring of oxygen saturation and cardiac parameters. This often plays a primary role in the care of critically ill patients.

Poor peripheral venous access is an indication for central venous catheterization. Although large-bore peripheral intravenous (IV) access may be used for rapid volume resuscitation, the use of central venous catheters for the rapid delivery of fluids is common in patients with hypothermia and severe hemorrhagic shock when peripheral access is unobtainable. Other conditions making peripheral access difficult include a history of IV substance abuse, major burns, certain chronic medical

A. Subclavian vein anatomy

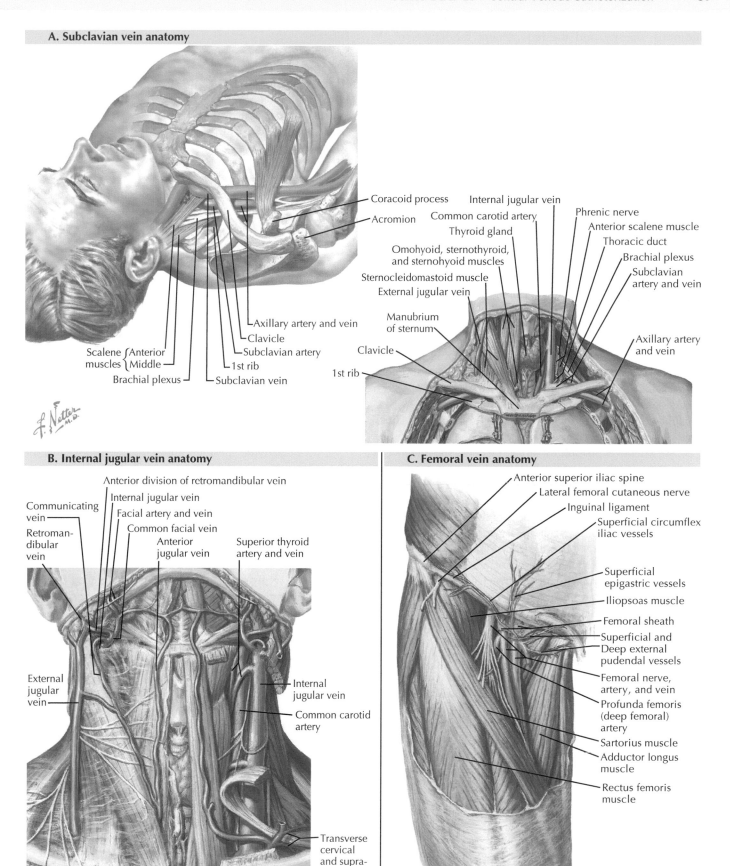

B. Internal jugular vein anatomy

C. Femoral vein anatomy

FIGURE 14.1 Subclavian vein **(A)**, internal jugular vein **(B)**, and femoral vein **(C)** anatomy

conditions, obesity, and the requirement for long-term IV therapy. The use of central venous catheterization in cardiopulmonary resuscitation remains controversial. However, the use of intraosseous devices is gaining more favor in patients in extremis who require rapid resuscitation. The purported benefits are the relative ease and speed of cannulation of the central venous vessels for the rapid administration of medications. Because of the risk of phlebitis when delivered through peripheral lines, certain noxious medications are preferentially delivered by central venous catheterization, such as vasopressors, chemotherapeutic agents, and parenteral nutrition.

CONTRAINDICATIONS

Most contraindications to central venous catheterization are relative and are based on urgency and the availability of alternatives to IV access. The major relative contraindications include coagulopathy, anatomical distortion, vasculitis, local cellulitis, prior long-term venous cannulation, prior injections of sclerosing agents, the presence of another device, vascular injury proximal to the insertion site, the need for mobility, and antibiotic hypersensitivity (if using antibiotic-impregnated catheters). Morbid obesity is also a frequent impediment to central venous catheterization because the surface landmarks may be obscured or hidden, and the excess adipose tissue may make catheterization difficult, often requiring a steeper angle of insertion. Ultrasound guidance can overcome this difficulty and should be used for access whenever possible for all central lines. The presence of panniculitis near the site of the femoral vein also poses a problem. Catheterization in patients who are uncooperative or combative poses a risk of mechanical complications. Uncooperative patients should be sedated before placing the catheter.

For central venous catheterization, coagulopathy and thrombocytopenia are the contraindications of most concern, although the relative risk of significant hemorrhaging is low. In patients with severe coagulopathy, fresh frozen plasma or platelets may be administered to correct the coagulopathy and reduce the risk of bleeding. With proper technique, however, correction of the coagulopathy is often unnecessary.

EQUIPMENT

As with any invasive procedure, central venous access should be undertaken in a sterile environment. Local anesthetics should always be used whenever possible, especially in a conscious patient.

In the hospital setting, central venous catheterization equipment comes prepackaged in kits. However, it may be necessary to gather the appropriate equipment to place the central line, including the following:

Sterile gowns and gloves
Iodine or other sterile preparatory solution
Sterile drapes
Ultrasound (with a linear high-frequency probe)
Inline disposable central line manometer (if available)
Sterile ultrasonography probe cover
Finder/introducer needles and syringes
Guide wire

Dilators
Scalpel (#10 or #11)
IV catheter and tubing
10-mL saline flushes
End caps
Suture material
Sterile gauze and dressings
10 mL lidocaine 1%

PROCEDURE

All materials, including ultrasonography equipment, should be readily available to perform central venous catheterization at the bedside. Obtain consent from the patient and perform a time out. The bed should be elevated to the level of the operator. The following techniques are based on each specific location.

Subclavian Vein

See Fig. 14.2.

1. Place the patient in a supine position. The Trendelenburg position does not significantly affect subclavian vein filling, but it may aid in preventing air embolus during the procedure.
2. Keep the ipsilateral arm in an adducted position to reduce any anatomical distortion or overlap of the clavicle on the vessel.
3. Apply an antiseptic solution such as chlorhexidine from the neck to the chest just above the internipple line; this allows the operator access to an alternative target site if the initial site cannot be cannulated.
4. Allow the skin preparation solution to dry before draping the patient with full sterile drapes. A sterile gown, gloves, hat, and masks should be worn to prevent infection.
5. Either an infraclavicular or a supraclavicular approach may be taken. With the infraclavicular approach, a small sandbag or rolled towel may be placed between the scapulae to retract the shoulder, which positions the vein closer to the clavicle.
6. Apply local anesthetic to the region before infiltration of the skin with the introducer needle.
7. Using ultrasound guidance, locate the subclavian vein and introduce the needle with the bevel pointed inferomedially or directed toward the contralateral clavicular head. A finger may be placed on the sternal notch and the thumb on the costoclavicular junction to serve as references for the direction the needle should travel.
8. If using the supraclavicular approach, rotate the patient's head and neck away from the site to allow the introducer needle to be placed along the lateral border of the clavicular head of the sternocleidomastoid muscle. The needle should be inserted superiorly and behind the clavicle, just lateral to the sternocleidomastoid's clavicular head.
9. Introduce the needle horizontally to avoid a pneumothorax.
10. Apply negative pressure with the attached syringe; dark blood will appear in the syringe when the vessel is penetrated. If using an inline manometer, check the pressure to ensure the correct vessel was cannulated.

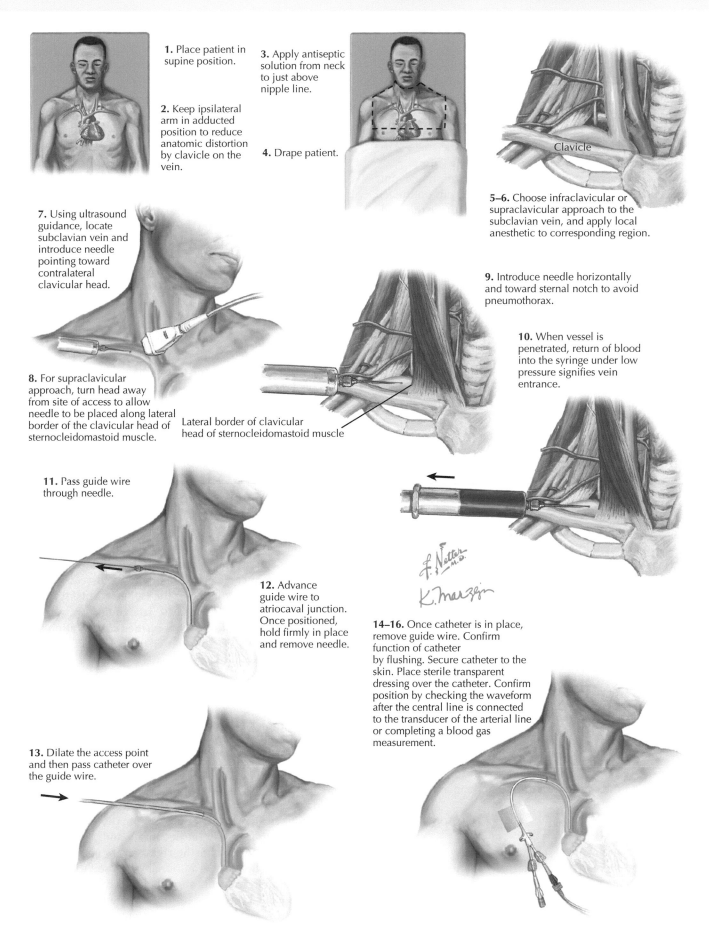

1. Place patient in supine position.

2. Keep ipsilateral arm in adducted position to reduce anatomic distortion by clavicle on the vein.

3. Apply antiseptic solution from neck to just above nipple line.

4. Drape patient.

Clavicle

5–6. Choose infraclavicular or supraclavicular approach to the subclavian vein, and apply local anesthetic to corresponding region.

7. Using ultrasound guidance, locate subclavian vein and introduce needle pointing toward contralateral clavicular head.

8. For supraclavicular approach, turn head away from site of access to allow needle to be placed along lateral border of the clavicular head of sternocleidomastoid muscle.

Lateral border of clavicular head of sternocleidomastoid muscle

9. Introduce needle horizontally and toward sternal notch to avoid pneumothorax.

10. When vessel is penetrated, return of blood into the syringe under low pressure signifies vein entrance.

11. Pass guide wire through needle.

12. Advance guide wire to atriocaval junction. Once positioned, hold firmly in place and remove needle.

14–16. Once catheter is in place, remove guide wire. Confirm function of catheter by flushing. Secure catheter to the skin. Place sterile transparent dressing over the catheter. Confirm position by checking the waveform after the central line is connected to the transducer of the arterial line or completing a blood gas measurement.

13. Dilate the access point and then pass catheter over the guide wire.

FIGURE 14.2 Subclavian vein catheterization

An inline manomenter allows the removal of the needle before the wire is inserted or the dilator is used.

11. Once venous access is obtained, stabilize the needle, remove the syringe, and advance a guide wire through the needle. The guide wire should pass smoothly and easily without resistance. If resistance is met, remove the guide wire and aspirate blood again to confirm the intraluminal needle position. Reducing the angle of the needle may facilitate passage of the guide wire.

12. With subclavian access, the guide wire should only need to travel 18 cm on the right or 21 cm on the left before reaching the atriocaval junction. Once the guide wire is positioned, hold it firmly in place and remove the needle.

13. Dilate the access point with prepackaged tapered dilators, or use the scalpel to make a small incision to allow passage of the catheter over the guide wire until the wire emerges from the distal port on the catheter. Resistance to catheter placement can be overcome by advancing the catheter and wire together, but only for a short distance to avoid subclavian vein laceration. Withdrawal of the catheter and repeat dilation of the tract may also be performed if necessary.

14. Once the catheter is placed at the appropriate length, the guide wire is carefully removed. After aspirating blood from each port of the catheter to confirm correct positioning, flush each port with saline.

15. Secure the catheter in place by suturing it or the catheter anchor to the skin.

16. Place a sterile transparent dressing over the catheter. Confirm the catheter position by checking the waveform after the central line is connected to the transducer of the arterial line or completing a blood gas measurement. A chest radiograph can be done to confirm there is no pneumothorax.

Internal Jugular Vein

See Figs. 14.3 and 14.4.

1. The patient should be positioned in a supine Trendelenburg position with the bed elevated to the level of the clinician.
2. Turn the patient's head away from the insertion site.
3. Place a towel roll under the scapula to accentuate the landmarks.
4. The internal jugular vein should be located by ultrasound when available. The procedure then follows the same steps as described for the subclavian vein.
5. Alternatively, the internal jugular vein can be found by identifying the carotid artery by palpation and cannulating lateral to it.

Femoral Vein

1. Place the patient in a supine position with the target lower limb abducted and externally rotated to open the femoral triangle.
2. The reverse Trendelenburg position may be used to increase femoral vein filling from the inferior vena cava.
3. Elevate the buttock with rolled sheets or a pillow to allow for better exposure.

4. Prepare the skin widely with antiseptic solution. The skin prep solution should be allowed to dry before draping the patient with full sterile drapes large enough to cover the entire patient.
5. The femoral vein should be located by ultrasound if available. The procedure then follows the same steps as described for the subclavian vein.
6. Alternatively, the femoral vein may be located by palpating the femoral artery pulse and introducing the needle approximately 1 cm medial to the pulse at a 45-degree angle in a cephalic direction toward the umbilicus (see Fig. 14.3). Ideally, the femoral artery pulse should be palpated 2 cm beneath the inguinal ligament. Pressure from palpation may compress the femoral vein and impede cannulation, so the pressure should be released while keeping the fingers on the skin over the artery to serve as a visual reference to the underlying anatomy.

ANATOMICAL PITFALLS

For each site, understanding the regional relationships is critical. Anatomical pitfalls associated with the internal jugular vein include cannulating the nearby medially located carotid artery and injury to the cupula of the lung, which is superior to the clavicle. Injury to the subclavian artery or lung pleura is a potential danger during subclavian vein puncture. Attempted cannulation of the femoral vein may injure the laterally located femoral artery or nerve. The importance of aiming medially to the femoral artery pulse cannot be overstated.

COMPLICATIONS

Complications with central venous catheterization are classified as immediate or delayed. Bleeding and hematoma formation are the most common immediate complications, usually a result of coagulopathy or damage to the vein wall. Vascular injury may also include arterial puncture and vessel damage by the guide wire or kinking of the catheter while it is being threaded into the vein. Immediate recognition and management of vascular injury prevents further complications. The thoracic duct may also be injured with left subclavian or internal jugular vein lines; this may be avoided by using the vessels on the right.

Other life-threatening immediate complications are arrhythmias, air emboli, and hemothorax or pneumothorax. Arrhythmias may occur if the catheter or guide wire is threaded too far into the atrium, but this may be prevented by placing the patient on an electrocardiographic monitor before the procedure and retracting the wire or catheter if a change is seen on the monitor. Placing the patient in the Trendelenburg position before the procedure may prevent air emboli. If air embolus does occur, the patient should be placed in the left lateral decubitus and Trendelenburg position to trap the air in the right ventricular apex while aspiration is performed. Additionally, resuscitation maneuvers and adrenergic agents should aid in embolus reabsorption. Pleural puncture may result in a pneumothorax or, in extreme cases, hemothorax. The patient with an iatrogenic pneumothorax should be closely monitored for tension pneumothorax.

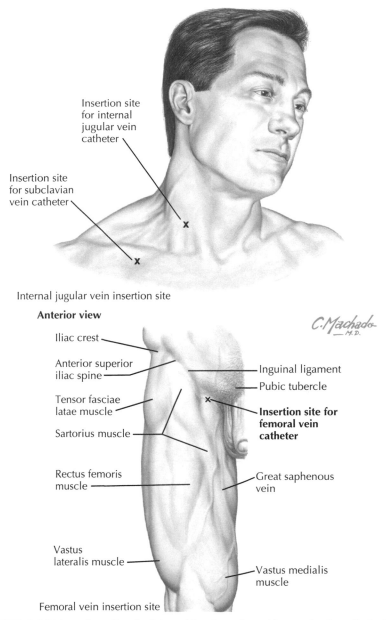

Insertion site
for internal
jugular vein
catheter

Insertion site
for subclavian
vein catheter

x

x

Internal jugular vein insertion site

Anterior view

C. Machado
— M.D.

Iliac crest

Anterior superior
iliac spine

Inguinal ligament

Pubic tubercle

×

**Insertion site for
femoral vein
catheter**

Tensor fasciae
latae muscle

Sartorius muscle

Rectus femoris
muscle

Great saphenous
vein

Vastus
lateralis muscle

Vastus medialis
muscle

Femoral vein insertion site

FIGURE 14.3 Insertion sites for internal jugular vein and femoral vein catheterization

Another complication is the unintended canalization of the associated artery. Ultrasound greatly reduces this risk but does not completely eliminate it, especially in patients with low flow states and hypotension. As noted above, in addition to performing a blood gas analysis or checking for arterial waveforms may help confirm placement.

Delayed complications include catheter-associated infections, venous thrombosis, and pulmonary emboli. Infection is the most common delayed complication and occurs more frequently with prolonged catheter placement, unsterile technique, or improper cleaning of the site. If an infection occurs, the catheter should be removed immediately and blood cultures should be taken. Empiric antibiotic therapy, including coverage for *Pseudomonas aeruginosa,* is administered until the culture and sensitivity results are available. Catheter-associated thrombosis should be treated with catheter removal and the standard venous thrombosis protocol.

Complications due to infection may be reduced with various preventive measures, including proper hand hygiene, maximal barrier precautions, early removal of unnecessary catheters, and use of antibiotic-impregnated catheters. Immediate complications may be reduced with appropriate operator training, limiting the number of attempts, confirmatory testing, and use of ultrasound guidance.

CONCLUSION

Obtaining vascular access is important for any patient who is critically ill with a need for IV access. When a peripheral line is unobtainable or inappropriate for the patient's condition, central venous or intraosseous access should be obtained. Common indications for central venous access include the administration of medications or fluid, hemodynamic monitoring, plasmapheresis, hemodialysis, poor peripheral access, and the placement of invasive venous

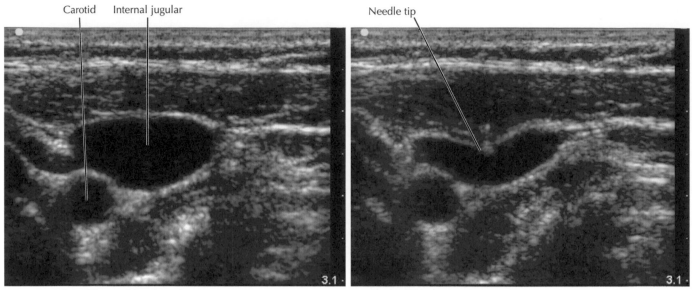

Carotid   Internal jugular

Needle tip

Transverse view of internal jugular vein

Tenting (needle compressing anterior internal jugular wall)

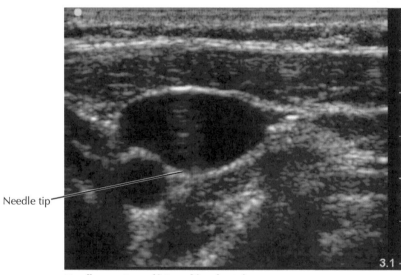

Needle tip

Needle puncture of internal jugular vein

FIGURE 14.4 Imaging of the internal jugular vein

devices. Most contraindications to central venous catheterization are relative, including coagulopathy. Central venous catheters may be placed in the subclavian, internal jugular, or femoral vein. The use of sterile technique, inline manometers, and ultrasonography, along with appropriate operator training and thorough knowledge of the anatomy and technique, will reduce complications associated with the insertion of a central venous line.

Suggested Readings

Adams BD, Lyon ML, DeFlorio PT. Central venous catheterizations and central venous pressure monitoring. In: Roberts JR, Hedges JR, eds. *Clinical procedures in emergency medicine.* 5th ed. Philadelphia: Saunders; 2010:374–410.

Doerfler ME, Kaufman B, Goldenberg AS. Central venous catheter placement in patients with disorders of hemostasis. *Chest.* 1996;110:185–188.

Ely EW, Hite RD, Baker AM, et al. Venous air embolism from central venous catheterization: a need for increased physician awareness. *Crit Care Med.* 1999;27:2113–2117.

Hilty WM, Hudson PA, Levitt MA, Hall JB. Real-time ultrasound-guided femoral vein catheterization during cardiopulmonary resuscitation. *Ann Emerg Med.* 1997;29:331–336.

McGee DC, Gould MK. Preventing complications of central venous catheterization. *N Engl J Med.* 2003;348:1123–1133.

Mumtaz H, Williams V, Hauer-Jensen M, et al. Central venous catheter placement in patients with disorders of hemostasis. *Am J Surg.* 2000;180:503–505.

Polderman KH, Girbes AJ. Central venous catheter use. Part 1. Mechanical complications. *Intensive Care Med.* 2002;28:1–17.

Rivers EP, Martin GB, Smithline H, et al. The clinical implications of continuous central venous oxygen saturation during human CPR. *Ann Emerg Med.* 1992;21:1094–1101.

Rupp SM, Apfelbaum JL, Blitt C, et al. Practice guidelines for central venous access: a report by the American Society of Anesthesiologists Task Force on Central Venous Access. *Anesthesiology.* 2012;116:539–573.

Stone MB, Price DD, Anderson BS. Ultrasonographic investigation of the effect of reverse Trendelenburg on the cross-sectional area of the femoral vein. *J Emerg Med.* 2006;30:211–213.

US Department of Defense. *Emergency war surgery, Third United States Revision.* United States: Prepper Press; 2004:8.1–8.3.

REVIEW QUESTIONS

1. A 29-year-old woman is examined in the emergency department after falling from her balcony. Radiographic examination reveals that she has a fractured clavicle, with associated internal bleeding. Which of the following vessels is most likely to be injured in clavicular fractures?

   A. Subclavian artery
   B. Cephalic vein
   C. Lateral thoracic artery
   D. Subclavian vein
   E. Internal thoracic artery

2. A 28-year-old man is admitted unconscious to the emergency department after a severe car crash. He has several deep lacerations and is bleeding profusely. A central venous line is placed in his right subclavian vein using a supraclavicular approach. Which of the following is the best landmark at which the needle should be inserted to access the subclavian vein during this procedure?

   A. Superiorly and behind the clavicle, just lateral to the clavicular head of the sternocleidomastoid muscle
   B. Superiorly and behind the clavicle, just medial to the clavicular head of the sternocleidomastoid muscle
   C. Inferiorly and behind the clavicle, just lateral to the clavicular head of the sternocleidomastoid muscle
   D. Inferiorly and behind the clavicle, just medial to the sternal head of the sternocleidomastoid muscle
   E. Superiorly and behind the clavicle, just lateral to the sternal head of the sternocleidomastoid muscle

3. A 28-year-old man is admitted unconscious to the emergency department after a severe car crash. He has several deep lacerations and is bleeding profusely. A central venous line is placed in his right femoral vein. With palpation of the femoral artery pulse, which of the following is the best approach for introducing the needle to access the femoral vein during this procedure?

   A. 1 cm medial to the femoral artery pulse, at a 45-degree angle in a cephalic direction toward the umbilicus
   B. 1 cm lateral to the femoral artery pulse, at a 45-degree angle in a cephalic direction toward the umbilicus
   C. 3 cm lateral to the femoral artery pulse, at a 45-degree angle in a caudal direction toward the knee
   D. 1 cm medial to the femoral artery pulse, at a 45-degree angle in a caudal direction toward the anterior superior iliac spine
   E. 1 cm lateral to the femoral artery pulse, at a 45-degree angle in a cephalic direction toward the anterior superior iliac spine

Peripheral Arterial Line Placement

INTRODUCTION

The proper placement of a peripheral arterial line (PAL) is essential to the competent care of patients in the emergency department and intensive care unit. The procedure, clinically known as a "PAL" or an "art line," allows the health care provider to access arterial blood for diagnostic purposes. The PAL also offers several advantages over the traditional noninvasive techniques of blood pressure monitoring. Intraarterial blood pressure measurement is more accurate than indirect blood pressure monitoring. In addition, when an indwelling arterial cannula is placed, the continuous monitoring of mean arterial pressure in real time becomes possible. For patients being treated with continuous intravenous infusion of vasoactive drugs, the PAL allows the effective monitoring of rapid fluctuations in blood pressure.

CLINICALLY RELEVANT ANATOMY

The PAL may be placed in the radial, ulnar, brachial, axillary, femoral, posterior tibial, or dorsalis pedis arteries. However, the most common sites in adults are the radial and femoral arteries, with the former preferred due to its consistent anatomy, ease of access, and low rate of complications (Figs. 15.1 and 15.2). The measurement of mean arterial pressure is consistently accurate with both radial and femoral arterial cannulation. In neonates, the PAL is most often placed in either the radial or posterior tibial artery. In older infants, the radial, posterior tibial, or femoral artery may be used.

The radial artery usually originates near the cubital fossa as a branch of the brachial artery (Fig. 15.3). After leaving the cubital fossa, the vessel runs distally along the lateral aspect of the forearm. During its course in the distal forearm, the radial artery is located lateral to the tendon of the flexor carpi radialis. The artery then enters the "anatomical snuffbox" at the wrist before continuing its course through the heads of the first dorsal interosseous muscle (see Fig. 15.2). It passes anteriorly between the heads of the adductor pollicis muscle, at which point it becomes the deep palmar arch (see Fig. 15.2).

INDICATIONS

The placement of a PAL is essential for continuous blood pressure monitoring if there is failure of indirect monitoring by noninvasive methods. It is also performed if frequent sampling of arterial blood is necessary for analysis. A PAL may also be placed for exchange transfusion in infants and neonates if catheterization of the umbilical artery is not possible for clinical or technical reasons.

CONTRAINDICATIONS

The placement of a PAL is not indicated when the pulse is absent at the site of insertion. In cases of Buerger disease (thromboangiitis obliterans), full-thickness burns, inadequate circulation to the extremity, Raynaud phenomenon, limb malformation, uncorrected coagulopathy, or local skin infection, an unaffected site should be sought.

EQUIPMENT

Radial artery catheterization kit, including an introducer needle, catheter, feeding tube assembly, and guide wire with an actuating lever
1% lidocaine without epinephrine
Sterile towels
Tape
Pressure transducer

PROCEDURE
Ultrasound

Several organizations now recommend using ultrasound for the insertion of PALs, and it should be used whenever available. It allows imaging of the artery to be cannulated in real time. Once the artery has been identified, catheterization is attempted as either a one-person or two-person procedure. The latter has the advantage that the practitioner inserting the line is able to use both hands.

Allen Test

Before insertion of a PAL in the radial artery, it is necessary to ensure adequate collateral circulation. Traditionally, this has been done by performing the Allen test, a simple noninvasive bedside procedure. The provider places his or her thumbs on the medial and lateral sides of the anterior aspect of the patient's wrist, temporarily occluding both radial and ulnar arteries. The patient is asked to clench the fist for 30 seconds. After the patient opens the hand and the palm is seen to be pale, the provider releases the ulnar side of the wrist. If color returns to the entire palm within 5 seconds or less, there is a sufficient collateral circulation.

However, the validity of the Allen test is controversial. Several authors report ischemic injury to the hand after radial artery cannulation despite a normal Allen test. Other studies have demonstrated poor correlation of actual distal blood flow with Allen test results. Many experts therefore suggest that Doppler evaluation of collateral flow should be conducted in patients determined to have a high risk of complications resulting from PAL insertion in the radial artery.

Palmar view

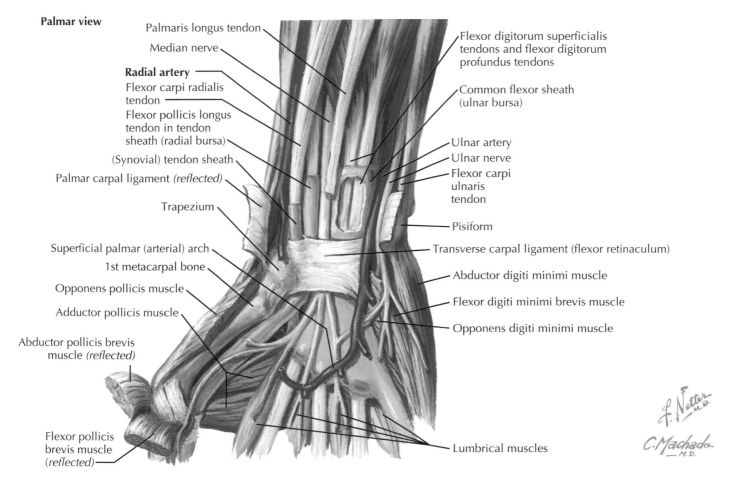

Palmaris longus tendon

Median nerve

Radial artery

Flexor carpi radialis tendon

Flexor pollicis longus tendon in tendon sheath (radial bursa)

(Synovial) tendon sheath

Palmar carpal ligament *(reflected)*

Trapezium

Superficial palmar (arterial) arch

1st metacarpal bone

Opponens pollicis muscle

Adductor pollicis muscle

Abductor pollicis brevis muscle *(reflected)*

Flexor pollicis brevis muscle *(reflected)*

Flexor digitorum superficialis tendons and flexor digitorum profundus tendons

Common flexor sheath (ulnar bursa)

Ulnar artery

Ulnar nerve

Flexor carpi ulnaris tendon

Pisiform

Transverse carpal ligament (flexor retinaculum)

Abductor digiti minimi muscle

Flexor digiti minimi brevis muscle

Opponens digiti minimi muscle

Lumbrical muscles

FIGURE 15.1 Arrangement of tendons, vessels, and nerves at the wrist

Lateral (radial) view

*Snuffbox contents (superficial to deep)

Radial nerve (dorsal digital branch)
Cephalic vein branches *(cut away)*
Radial artery and branches
Scaphoid bone

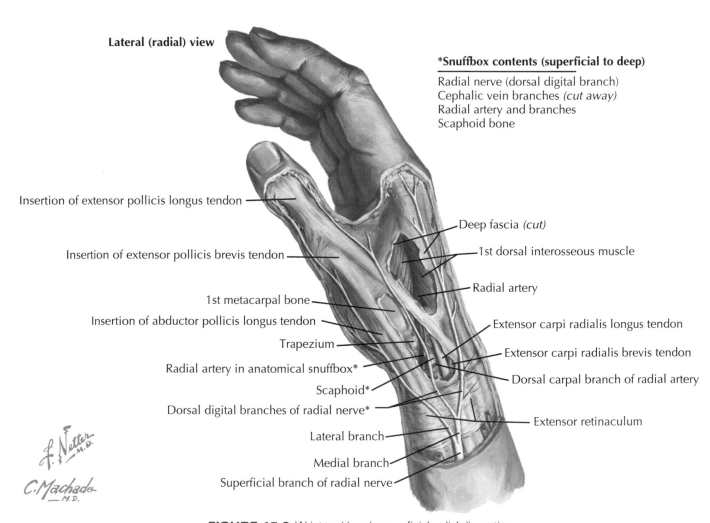

Insertion of extensor pollicis longus tendon

Insertion of extensor pollicis brevis tendon

1st metacarpal bone

Insertion of abductor pollicis longus tendon

Trapezium

Radial artery in anatomical snuffbox*

Scaphoid*

Dorsal digital branches of radial nerve*

Lateral branch

Medial branch

Superficial branch of radial nerve

Deep fascia *(cut)*

1st dorsal interosseous muscle

Radial artery

Extensor carpi radialis longus tendon

Extensor carpi radialis brevis tendon

Dorsal carpal branch of radial artery

Extensor retinaculum

FIGURE 15.2 Wrist and hand: superficial radial dissection

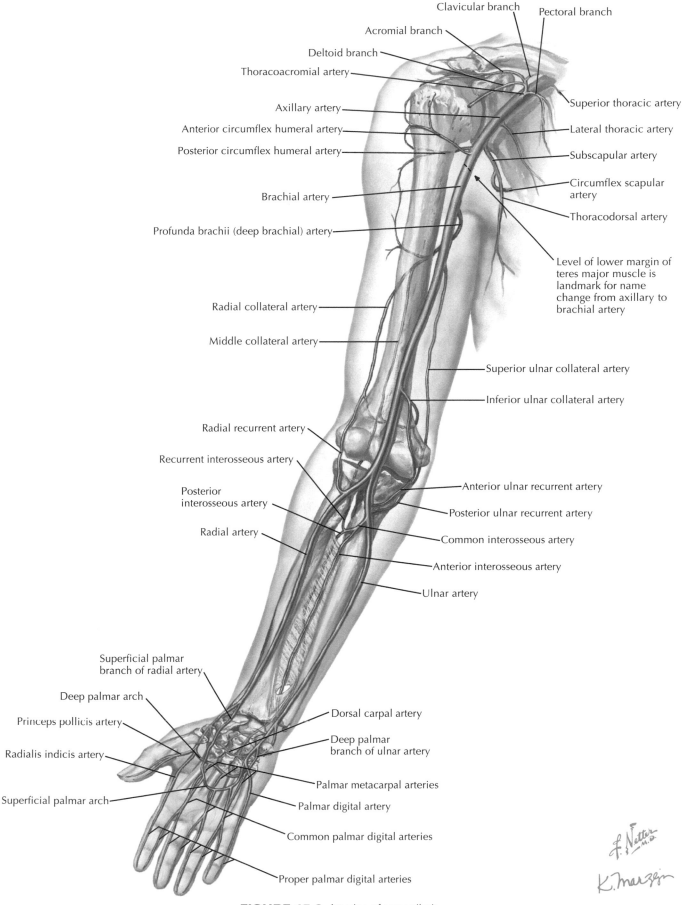

Clavicular branch
Pectoral branch
Acromial branch
Deltoid branch
Thoracoacromial artery
Axillary artery
Superior thoracic artery
Anterior circumflex humeral artery
Lateral thoracic artery
Posterior circumflex humeral artery
Subscapular artery
Circumflex scapular artery
Brachial artery
Thoracodorsal artery
Profunda brachii (deep brachial) artery
Level of lower margin of teres major muscle is landmark for name change from axillary to brachial artery
Radial collateral artery
Middle collateral artery
Superior ulnar collateral artery
Inferior ulnar collateral artery
Radial recurrent artery
Recurrent interosseous artery
Anterior ulnar recurrent artery
Posterior interosseous artery
Posterior ulnar recurrent artery
Radial artery
Common interosseous artery
Anterior interosseous artery
Ulnar artery
Superficial palmar branch of radial artery
Deep palmar arch
Dorsal carpal artery
Princeps pollicis artery
Deep palmar branch of ulnar artery
Radialis indicis artery
Palmar metacarpal arteries
Superficial palmar arch
Palmar digital artery
Common palmar digital arteries
Proper palmar digital arteries

FIGURE 15.3 Arteries of upper limb

Insertion of the Peripheral Arterial Line in the Radial Artery

In adults and children, the insertion of a PAL in the radial artery is performed percutaneously following a modified Seldinger technique. This technique is colloquially known as the over-the-wire procedure (Fig. 15.4, Video 15.1).

Obtain informed consent and perform a time out.

1. Gather a radial artery catheterization kit or the components listed above.
2. After washing the hands and performing either the Allen test or a Doppler study of blood flow, the provider should slightly extend the patient's wrist in order to better identify the intended arterial site by palpation. The wrist may be secured to an arm board with tape, if necessary.
3. Thoroughly cleanse the skin with antiseptic solution at the site of intended insertion. As the procedure may be painful in the conscious patient, lidocaine (1%, without epinephrine) may be injected around the site. In addition to relieving pain, this step may also help reduce vascular spasm.
4. Insert the needle at an angle of approximately 30 to 45 degrees and puncture the artery in a slight lateral to medial direction so that the artery can be stabilized against the tendon of the flexor carpi radialis.
5. At this point, carefully stabilize the introducer needle and advance the guide wire using the actuating lever. The guide wire should be advanced into the lumen of the radial artery.
6. Once the guide wire has been inserted as far as possible, push the needle and catheter assembly an additional 1 to 2 mm.
7. While holding the wire in place, remove the needle and advance the catheter over the needle into the lumen of the artery.
8. Remove the guide wire while holding the catheter firmly in place. Once this step has been completed, monitor the hub of the assembly for free-flowing blood.
9. Finally, attach a pressure transducer to the catheter's T-connecter. Observe the monitor for a good arterial waveform, remembering that transient arterial spasm may cause initial dampening of the waveform.

ANATOMICAL PITFALLS

The radial artery is medial to the tendon of the brachioradialis muscle and lateral to the flexor carpi radialis muscle. The median nerve is usually located between the tendons of the palmaris longus and flexor carpi radialis muscles. During the placement of a PAL, great caution is necessary to avoid piercing these nearby structures.

COMPLICATIONS

When properly performed, this procedure is exceedingly safe, resulting in major complications in less than 1% of cases. Although rare, several of these complications may be serious. They include infection, sepsis, ischemia, nerve damage, compartment syndrome, thrombosis, pseudoaneurysm, arteriovenous fistula, and air embolism. More common complications are less severe and include temporary occlusion due to arterial spasm, hematoma, and bleeding. Careful technique may reduce some or all of these complications.

The best treatment for infection is prevention. Be sure to liberally apply antiseptic to the intended site of cannulation. Special caution should be taken to avoid allowing air into the catheter, as this may cause air embolism. Hematomas may be treated with the rest, ice, compression, and elevation method. In the event of bleeding, pressure should be applied until it stops.

CONCLUSIONS

The PAL is widely accepted as the gold standard for the measurement of mean arterial pressure in both critically and chronically ill patients. It permits repeated access for arterial blood gas analysis. This relatively simple technique holds great utility due to its low risk of complications and significant clinical contributions. While many arteries can be used for the placement of a PAL, the radial artery is by far the most common choice. The practitioner must be prepared to be flexible and creative in site selection in order to tailor this intervention to the individual needs and complexities of each patient.

1–2. Obtain an appropriate radial artery catheterization kit. Position the patient by extending the wrist slightly to better identify the intended arterial site. Secure arm to an arm board if necessary.

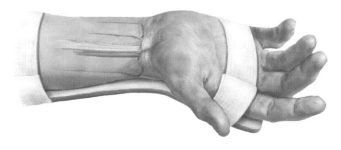

3. Cleanse the skin with antiseptic solution at the intended site of insertion. Puncture the artery in a slight lateral to medial direction. This allows the artery to be stabilized against the flexor carpi radialis tendon. Insert the cannula at a 30- to 45-degree angle.

Radial artery   Flexor carpi radialis tendon

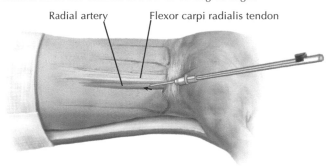

4. Carefully stabilize the introducer needle and advance the guide wire into the lumen of the radial artery using the actuating lever.

Actuating lever moves guide wire forward

Introducer needle within catheter

Guide wire

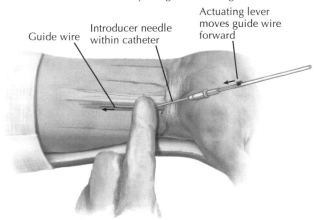

5. Once the guide wire has been inserted as far as possible, push the needle and catheter assembly an additional 1-2 cm.

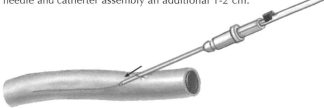

6. While holding the introducer needle in place, advance the catheter into the lumen of the artery.

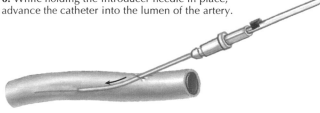

7. While holding the catheter firmly in place, remove the needle, guide wire, and feeding assembly. Monitor the hub for free-flowing blood.

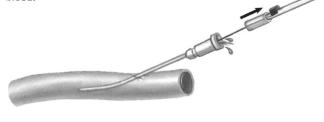

8. Attach the pressure transducer to the T-connector and observe the monitor for a good pulse wave.

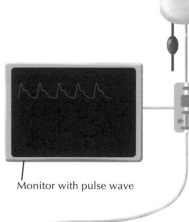

Pressure bag

Transducer

Monitor with pulse wave

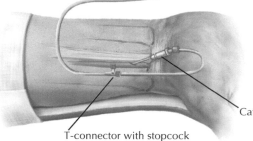

Catheter hub

T-connector with stopcock

FIGURE 15.4 Peripheral arterial line placement

Suggested Readings

American Institute of Ultrasound in Medicine. *Use of Ultrasound to Guide Vascular Access Procedures*. Guidel: AIUM Pract; 2012.

Babu SC, Laskowski IA, Morasch MD, Maun D. Arteriovenous fistulas. Available at http://emedicine.medscape.com/article/459842-treatment; 2013.

Canning PD, Linscott MS. Femoral artery cannulation. Available at http://e medicine.medscape.com/article/80412-overview; 2012.

Jaffe R, Samuels S, Schmiesing C, Golianu B. *Anesthesiologist's Manual of Surgical Procedures*. 4th ed. Philadelphia: Lippincott Williams & Wilkins; 2009.

Milzman D, Janchar T. Arterial puncture and cannulation. In: Roberts J, Hedges J, eds. *Clinical Procedures in Emergency Medicine*. 5th ed. Philadelphia: Elsevier; 2010:349–363.

Scheer B, Perel A, Pfeiffer UJ. Clinical review: complications and risk factors of peripheral arterial catheters used for haemodynamic monitoring in anaesthesia and intensive care medicine. *Crit Care*. 2002;6:199–204.

The Royal Children's Hospital Melbourne. Clinical guidelines: peripheral arterial access of the neonate in neonatal intensive care. Available at http://www.rch.org.au/uploadedFiles/Main/Content/neonatal_rch/clinical_ practice_guidelines/NICU Peripheral Arterial Line Final.pdf; 2013.

Thompson S, Hirschberg A. Allen's test re-examined. *Crit Care Med*. 1988;16:915.

Wilkins R. Radial artery cannulation and ischaemic damage: a review. *Anesthesia*. 1985;40:896–899.

REVIEW QUESTIONS

1. While working out with weights, a 28-year-old woman experiences severe pain in her chest. The pain is referred to the anterior chest wall and radiates to the mandible and her left arm. She feels dizzy, and after 10 minutes collapses and loses consciousness. A physician happens to be near her and immediately tries to palpate her radial pulse. The radial artery lies between two tendons near the wrist, which are useful landmarks. Which of the following is the correct pair of tendons?

   A. Flexor carpi radialis and palmaris longus
   B. Flexor carpi radialis and brachioradialis
   C. Brachioradialis and flexor pollicis longus
   D. Flexor pollicis longus and flexor digitorum superficialis
   E. Flexor pollicis longus and flexor digitorum profundus

2. A 59-year-old woman is admitted to the hospital in shock. On physical examination, several lacerations are noted in her forearm, and her radial pulse is absent. Where is the best place to identify the radial artery immediately after it crosses the wrist?

   A. Between the two heads of the first dorsal interosseous muscle
   B. In the anatomical snuffbox
   C. Below the tendon of the flexor pollicis longus
   D. Between the first and second dorsal interosseous muscles
   E. Between the first dorsal interosseous muscle and the adductor pollicis longus

3. A 22-year-old unconscious woman is admitted to the emergency department. The nurse checks the radial pulse to determine the patient's heart rate. This pulse is felt lateral to which tendon?

   A. Palmaris longus
   B. Flexor pollicis longus
   C. Flexor digitorum profundus
   D. Flexor carpi radialis
   E. Flexor digitorum superficialis

Peripheral Intravenous Cannulation

INTRODUCTION

Cannulation of the peripheral veins involves the guidance of a removable needle and a thin, sterile cannula into the superficial vessels. It is the most frequently used method for vascular access in medicine. Preferable sites for peripheral intravenous (IV) cannulation are the superficial veins of the forearm and dorsum of the hand. IV cannulation of the peripheral veins is a common requirement in emergency departments as well as in the surgical setting. Hydration, nutritional supplementation, infusion of drugs, and administration of blood transfusions all require access to the venous vasculature. Ultrasound can be used to locate veins that are not obvious to visualization or palpation alone.

CLINICALLY RELEVANT ANATOMY
Veins in the Dorsal Hand and Forearm

The dorsum of the hand and forearm offers multiple points for venous cannulation, most often at the dorsal metacarpal veins and the distal cephalic vein (Figs. 16.1 and 16.2). Blood returns from the digits via the dorsal digital veins and then via the intercapitular veins. It flows into the dorsal metacarpal veins, which are often large enough for cannulation. Venous return continues into the dorsal venous network, which interconnects the dorsal metacarpal veins. Both the cephalic and basilic veins arise from this dorsal venous arch. The cephalic vein generally arises from the radial aspect of the dorsal venous arch and continues along the lateral forearm. The basilic vein arises from the medial edge of the dorsal venous network and proceeds along the ulnar side of the wrist and medial forearm.

The cephalic vein, with its large diameter and straight path, is an ideal site for IV cannulation and is frequently used in clinical practice. Cephalic vein cannulation on the dorsal hand may be performed along the medial border of the area known as the "anatomical snuffbox." The snuffbox is bordered by the extensor pollicis brevis and abductor pollicis longus tendons on the lateral edge and the extensor pollicis longus on the medial side. The radial artery crosses deep to the cephalic vein within the anatomical snuffbox.

Veins in the Ventral Forearm

Within the forearm, large superficial veins are used for venous cannulation. From the wrist, the basilic vein travels toward the elbow medially, whereas the cephalic vein travels toward the elbow laterally. The basilic vein in children generally travels a straight route into the axillary vein, making it a common site for cannulation. The cephalic vein has many collateral branches within the arms of children, making it difficult to use in clinical practice. The median antebrachial vein runs superficially along the ventral forearm and then splits into the median basilic vein and median cephalic vein before entering the cubital fossa. Approximately 70% of individuals have anatomical variations of the median cubital vein. Common variations include "H" and "M" patterns, with cephalic and basilic veins forming the sides and the median cubital vein in the middle. The median cubital vein is the most superficial structure within the cubital fossa and is separated from the brachial artery and median nerve by the bicipital aponeurosis.

INDICATIONS

Peripheral IV cannulation has many indications, including intermittent or continuous drug administration, fluid administration, parenteral nutrition, and blood sampling. Peripheral access should be implemented when central venous access is not necessary, because it is a simpler, safer alternative to central venous cannulation. The decision to use a given cannulation site is based on several factors, including patient position and comfort, urgency of the need for cannulation, duration of IV treatment, gauge of the needle, and ease of venous access.

Cannulation at the dorsum of the hand should be attempted before using more proximal sites in the cubital fossa. This allows for increased patient comfort and increased mobility of the arm. Furthermore, veins on the dorsum of the hand are usually easily palpated and readily visible. When managing trauma, however, the median cubital vein is preferred when large-bore needles are required to administer large amounts of IV fluids. It is also larger in diameter and easily palpated, facilitating rapid cannulation.

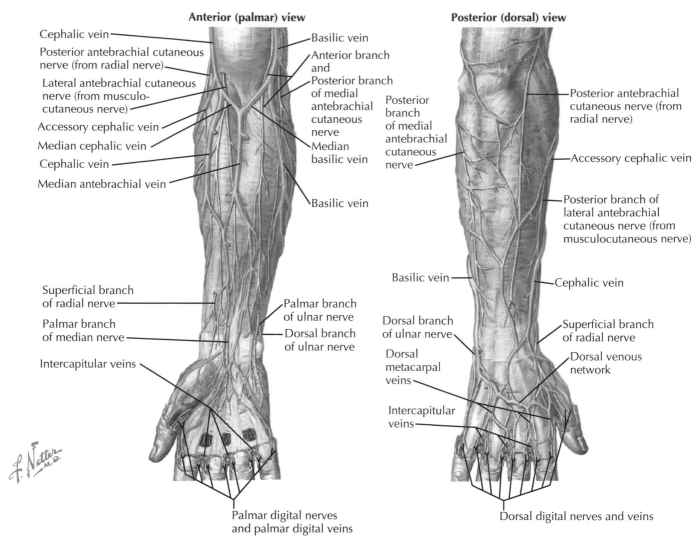

Anterior (palmar) view

Cephalic vein

Posterior antebrachial cutaneous nerve (from radial nerve)

Lateral antebrachial cutaneous nerve (from musculo-cutaneous nerve)

Accessory cephalic vein

Median cephalic vein

Cephalic vein

Median antebrachial vein

Basilic vein

Anterior branch and

Posterior branch of medial antebrachial cutaneous nerve

Median basilic vein

Basilic vein

Superficial branch of radial nerve

Palmar branch of median nerve

Intercapitular veins

Palmar branch of ulnar nerve

Dorsal branch of ulnar nerve

Palmar digital nerves and palmar digital veins

Posterior (dorsal) view

Posterior branch of medial antebrachial cutaneous nerve

Posterior antebrachial cutaneous nerve (from radial nerve)

Accessory cephalic vein

Posterior branch of lateral antebrachial cutaneous nerve (from musculocutaneous nerve)

Basilic vein

Cephalic vein

Dorsal branch of ulnar nerve

Dorsal metacarpal veins

Intercapitular veins

Superficial branch of radial nerve

Dorsal venous network

Dorsal digital nerves and veins

FIGURE 16.1 Veins of the hand and forearm. The median cubital vein is not seen in the figure and can often be a normal anatomic variant.

CONTRAINDICATIONS

Contraindications to the use of peripheral IV cannulation include skin infections or significant edema at the cannulation site. Areas over joints should be avoided to prevent patient discomfort and the risk of catheter kinking. In patients who have undergone axillary lymph node removal or mastectomy, the ipsilateral arm should be avoided to prevent the further impairment of lymphatic drainage. The same is true for an arm containing an arteriovenous fistula for renal dialysis. Cannulation can cause damage to the fistula. Palpation of the veins can help avoid the attempted cannulation of sclerotic veins, which feel firmer than normal. To prevent the risk of IV catheter-associated infections, the catheter should be replaced every 72 hours.

Posterior (dorsal) view

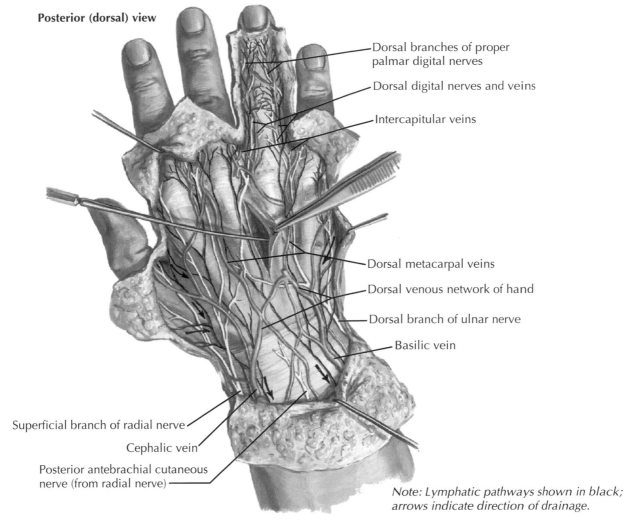

Dorsal branches of proper palmar digital nerves

Dorsal digital nerves and veins

Intercapitular veins

Dorsal metacarpal veins

Dorsal venous network of hand

Dorsal branch of ulnar nerve

Basilic vein

Superficial branch of radial nerve

Cephalic vein

Posterior antebrachial cutaneous nerve (from radial nerve)

Note: Lymphatic pathways shown in black; arrows indicate direction of drainage.

FIGURE 16.2 Veins of the hand

EQUIPMENT

Gloves
Dressing, gauze
Tourniquet
Appropriate topical anesthetic
Chlorhexidine topical preparation
Isotonic saline
Syringe of appropriate size
Luer-Lok adapter
24- to 14-gauge over-the-needle IV catheter
Saline or heparin flush
Appropriate-gauge tubing
Catheter tubing cap
Ultrasound
High-frequency linear probe
Transducing gel

PROCEDURE

Obtain patient consent and perform a time out.

Preparation

Preparation of the patient should include attempts to minimize anxiety as the associated sympathetic stimulation can lead to vasoconstriction and difficulty in accessing the superficial veins. Providers should wash their hands before and after contacting the patient and wear gloves along with appropriate personal protective equipment.

Landmark Approach

See Fig. 16.3.

1. Apply a tourniquet to the arm to inhibit venous return.
2. Ask the patient to open and close the fist to increase venous blood flow against the tourniquet and promote venous dilation.
   a. Keeping the patient's hand below the level of the heart allows gravity to assist in venous dilation.
   b. A warm compress applied to the area to be cannulated may facilitate further venous dilation, if necessary.
3. Clean the site of cannulation with topical chlorhexidine, and do not touch the site once sterile.
4. If appropriate, apply 1% to 2% lidocaine to the site or a topical local anesthetic cream.
5. Remove the cap of the needle carefully.
6. With the nondominant hand, hold the patient's hand or forearm distal to the site of cannulation and pull the skin taut with the thumb, applying tension in the direction of the vessel. This will help secure the vessel during the procedure.
7. Angle the needle to the surface of the skin at approximately 30 degrees, with the bevel facing upward.
8. Advance the needle through the skin and vessel wall.
   a. Monitor for a flashback of blood into the chamber proximal to the needle, indicating penetration into the vessel.
9. After confirming the flashback of blood, stop advancing and lower the angle of the needle parallel to the skin.
10. Stabilize the needle and advance the surrounding catheter with the index finger.
11. Remove the needle from the catheter slowly, watching for the flow of blood out of the cannula.
12. Apply pressure to the vein proximally to prevent blood from leaking out of the open end of the catheter.
13. The needle should never be readvanced once withdrawal is started because it may shear off the catheter and cause emboli.
14. Remove the tourniquet.
15. Flush the cannula with IV saline to confirm patency and an adequate flow rate for the administration of therapy.
16. Attach appropriate tubing for IV fluid infusion or drug administration.
17. If not administering IV therapy immediately, cap the end of the cannula and administer a saline or heparin flush to help keep the vessel patent.
18. Protect the cannula site with sterile, clear polyurethane dressing and secure an extra few inches of the tubing with adhesive dressing in the event that tugging on the IV line occurs.

Ultrasound-Guided Placement

See Fig. 16.4.

1. Choose a high-frequency linear probe (5 to 13 MHz) appropriate for the area of imaging and attach the probe to the device.
2. Cover the probe with a sterile covering and apply sterile transducer gel to the head of the probe.
3. Turn on the ultrasound machine and select the appropriate study.
   a. Manual adjustments of the gain setting may be made to ensure that the center of the vessel appears black with a white border.
4. Align the probe marker to the patient's right side, correlating with the left side of the ultrasound screen.
5. Begin scanning in the transverse plane to localize the appropriate vein.
6. After localizing the vein, some operators may want to rotate the transducer to run longitudinally with the vessel before inserting the needle.
7. Follow the procedure as described above for landmark cannulation.
8. When observing the needle in the transverse plane, it is important to recognize that the needle is perpendicular to the plane of imaging and will appear as a single bright dot. Beneath the needle is an anechoic shadow, which should not be confused with the needle itself.
9. Follow the tip of the needle through the vessel wall by fanning the probe in the direction of the needle.
10. In the longitudinal plane, the entire length of the needle and catheter can be viewed as they travel parallel to the plane of imaging into the vessel.
11. Stabilizing the transducer over the vessel is critical to maintaining a view of both the vein and needle during puncture.
12. Confirm entrance of the needle into the vessel by noting blood in the flashback chamber.
13. Follow the procedure outlined above for advancing and securing the catheter.

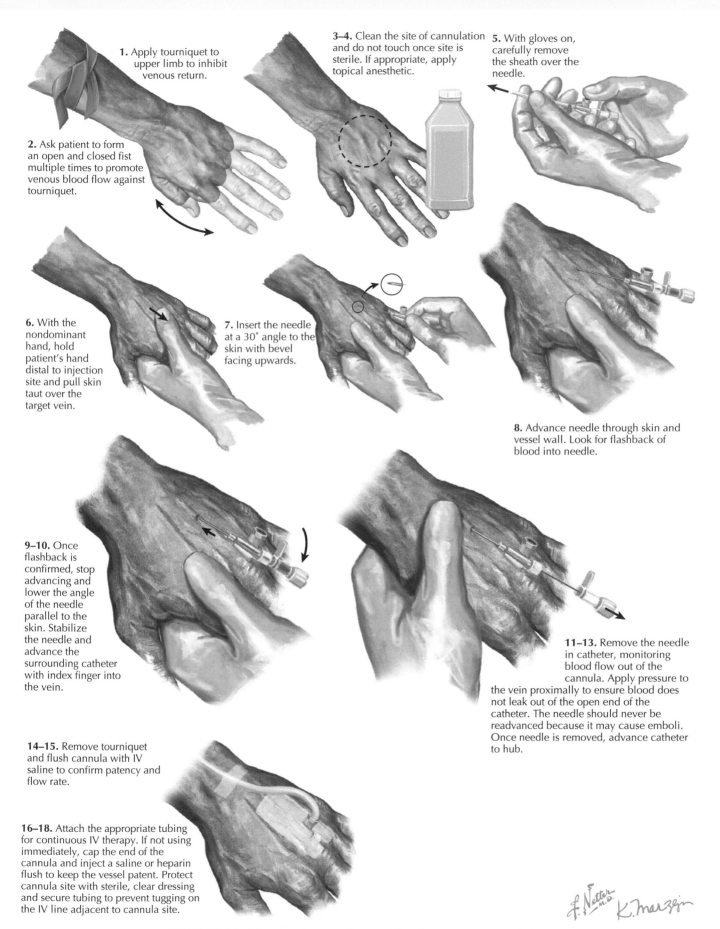

1. Apply tourniquet to upper limb to inhibit venous return.

2. Ask patient to form an open and closed fist multiple times to promote venous blood flow against tourniquet.

3–4. Clean the site of cannulation and do not touch once site is sterile. If appropriate, apply topical anesthetic.

5. With gloves on, carefully remove the sheath over the needle.

6. With the nondominant hand, hold patient's hand distal to injection site and pull skin taut over the target vein.

7. Insert the needle at a 30° angle to the skin with bevel facing upwards.

8. Advance needle through skin and vessel wall. Look for flashback of blood into needle.

9–10. Once flashback is confirmed, stop advancing and lower the angle of the needle parallel to the skin. Stabilize the needle and advance the surrounding catheter with index finger into the vein.

11–13. Remove the needle in catheter, monitoring blood flow out of the cannula. Apply pressure to the vein proximally to ensure blood does not leak out of the open end of the catheter. The needle should never be readvanced because it may cause emboli. Once needle is removed, advance catheter to hub.

14–15. Remove tourniquet and flush cannula with IV saline to confirm patency and flow rate.

16–18. Attach the appropriate tubing for continuous IV therapy. If not using immediately, cap the end of the cannula and inject a saline or heparin flush to keep the vessel patent. Protect cannula site with sterile, clear dressing and secure tubing to prevent tugging on the IV line adjacent to cannula site.

FIGURE 16.3 Landmark approach to peripheral intravenous cannulation

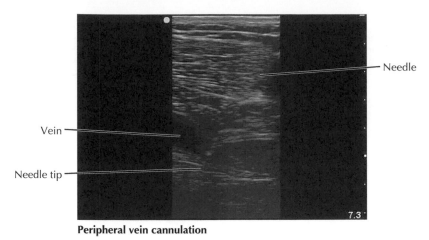

Peripheral vein cannulation

FIGURE 16.4 Ultrasound view of venous cannulation

ANATOMICAL PITFALLS

When selecting a site for cannulation, consideration should be given to relevant structures underlying the superficial veins. Needle injury to any nearby structures represents a major concern. Anatomical variations increase this risk and must be considered before beginning the procedure. If veins of the upper extremity are not accessible, the greater and lesser saphenous veins and the dorsal veins of the foot can be used for cannulation in adults and children. However, cannulation of the lower limbs increases the risk of complications such as venous thrombosis in adults.

Dorsal Hand

The radial artery and terminal portion of the superficial radial nerve run near the area of the anatomical snuffbox. The radial artery most often crosses deep to the cephalic vein within the snuffbox at a point 8 mm distal to the styloid process. An aberrant radial artery is seen in 0.8% to 1% of cases. Of particular concern is an aberrant radial artery traveling superficial to the tendons that form the anatomical snuffbox, leading to misidentification of the artery as a superficial vein. Accidental cannulation of the radial artery at this site occurs at a rate of 0.5%. Accidental arterial cannulation is indicated by bright-red blood with a greater degree of backflow after puncture. If in doubt (especially in patients with hypotension or hypothermia, and in low-flow states), remove the catheter and apply pressure. An ultrasound transducer measurement showing pulsatile backflow in the cannula with an arterial pressure wave, along with measurement of blood gas content, may confirm the incorrect location of the catheter. The damage from accidental arterial cannulation is largely a result of the therapy being infused. Symptoms include pain, thrombosis, vascular insufficiency leading to ischemic cell death, and gangrene.

Injury to the terminal branches of the superficial radial nerve is also possible within the anatomical snuffbox. The superficial radial nerve provides sensation to the first digit and web space, the second digit, and the lateral side of the third digit. Injury to these terminal branches during cannulation may present as acute pain radiating along the proximal and posterior arm, with loss of sensation in any of the innervated areas. If symptoms persist, the patient should be referred to a hand surgeon.

Ventral Forearm

Arterial vessels within the ventral forearm, which lie deep to the venous system, are common areas of accidental cannulation because of their subcutaneous location. The brachial artery branches into the radial artery and ulnar artery at the neck of the radius. The radial artery travels on the lateral aspect of the forearm and branches distally on the lateral aspect of the wrist. The ulnar artery travels on the medial aspect of the forearm alongside the ulnar nerve. Within the ventral forearm, the median antebrachial vein is a common site for cannulation, where the risk of injuring the radial artery is minimal.

Patients with a superficially located radial artery are at greater risk for accidental puncture, which can cause partial occlusion, pseudoaneurysm, or hematoma, when cannulating the median antebrachial vein. Most patients have a few millimeters of distance between the median antebrachial vein and the radial artery, although a few have a variant superficial radial artery, as previously mentioned. This superficial radial artery crosses 1 mm deep to the cephalic vein, approximately 20 to 28 cm proximal to the styloid process of the radius.

COMPLICATIONS

Peripheral venous cannulation has a very low rate of complication; most complications are attributed to improper technique. The most common complications are thrombophlebitis, extravasation of fluid, and hematoma.

Thrombophlebitis, caused by irritation due to the catheter, is inflammation of the vein and formation of a blood clot. Attention to minimizing catheter movement and a smaller size significantly reduces the risk of thrombophlebitis. Cannulation of the lower extremity is correlated with a higher incidence of thrombophlebitis and is therefore avoided when possible. Cardinal signs of inflammation, including localized redness and pain of the skin overlying the vein, can signify thrombophlebitis. Treatment of phlebitis can be managed with nonsteroidal antiinflammatory drugs, warm soaks, and antibiotics as needed.

Extravasation occurs when administered fluid accumulates outside the vasculature. Depending on the therapy being administered, tissue effects may be severe. Chemotherapy agents are at particular risk of causing extravasation injury, given the toxic nature of the drugs used. When providing these drugs via peripheral IV cannulation, the hands and wrists are avoided because of the exposure to many nerves and tendons. Central lines are used in prolonged therapy to avoid continued cannulation of peripheral veins.

CONCLUSION

Peripheral IV cannulation is a simple procedure with a variety of indications and benefits. Complications are rare when performed by an experienced health care provider. Care should be taken to select the appropriate site for cannulation, most often the dorsal metacarpal veins, cephalic vein at the lateral wrist or forearm, and median cubital vein in the cubital fossa. The landmark method for cannulation is the most commonly used approach for the placement of a peripheral IV line. However, the increased availability of ultrasound allows for improved safety and visualization of the vasculature when necessary.

Suggested Readings

Beale EW, Behnam A. Injection injury of an aberrant superficial radial artery requiring surgical intervention. *J Hand Microsurg.* 2011;4(1):39–42.

Drake RL, Vogl W. Upper limb. In: *Gray's anatomy for students.* 3rd ed. Philadelphia: Churchill Livingstone; 2014:768–783.

Dychter SS, et al. Intravenous therapy: a review of complications and economic considerations of peripheral access. *J Infusion Nurs.* 2012;35(2):84–91.

Egan G, et al. Ultrasound guidance for difficult peripheral venous access: systematic review and meta-analysis. *Emerg Med J.* 2013;30(7):521–526.

Iserson KV. Is informed consent required for the administration of intravenous contrast and similar clinical procedures? *Ann Emerg Med.* 2007;49(2):231–233.

Lake C, Beecroft CL. Extravasation injuries and accidental intra-arterial injection. *Contin Educ Anaesth Crit Care Pain.* 2010;10(4):109–113.

Lirk P, et al. Unintentional arterial puncture during cephalic vein cannulation: case report and anatomical study. *Br J Anaesth.* 2004;92(5):740–742.

Naeem R, Soueid A, Lahiri A. The dangers of intravenous cannulation within the anatomical snuffbox. *J Hand Surg (Eur Vol).* 2012;37(4):362–363.

Netter FH. Upper limb. In: *Atlas of human anatomy.* 6th ed. Philadelphia: Elsevier; 2014:402.

Ortega R, et al. Peripheral intravenous cannulation. *N Engl J Med.* 2008;359:e26.

Pikwer A, Åkeson J, Lindgren S. Complications associated with peripheral or central routes for central venous cannulation. *Anaesthesia.* 2012;67(1):65–71.

Satish N, et al. Accidental cannulation of aberrant radial artery. *Ann Card Anaesth.* 2014;17(1):76.

Scales K. Vascular access: a guide to peripheral venous cannulation. *Nurs Standard.* 2005;19(49):48–52.

Shivappagoudar VM, George B. Unintentional arterial cannulation during cephalic vein cannulation. *Indian J Anaesth.* 2013;57(3):320.

Soifer NE, et al. Prevention of peripheral venous catheter complications with an intravenous therapy team: a randomized controlled trial. *Arch Intern Med.* 1998;158:473–477.

Stone MB, et al. Needle tip visualization during ultrasound-guided vascular access: short-axis vs. long-axis approach. *Am J Emerg Med.* 2010;28(3):343–347.

Westergaard B, Classen V, Walther-Larsen S. Peripherally inserted central catheters in infants and children: indications, techniques, complications and clinical recommendations. *Acta Anaesthesiol Scand.* 2013;57(3):278–287.

REVIEW QUESTIONS

1. Laboratory studies in the outpatient clinic on a 24-year-old woman include the assessment of blood chemistry. Which of the following arteries is most likely at risk during venipuncture at the cubital fossa?

   A. Brachial
   B. Common interosseous
   C. Ulnar
   D. Anterior interosseous
   E. Radial

2. IV access is required in a 34-year-old obese female with dehydration who has "difficult" veins. Her vital signs are blood pressure, 90/60 mm Hg; pulse, 120 beats/min; respirations, 18 breaths/min; and oxygen saturation, 99%. What would be the most appropriate modality to rehydrate the patient?

   A. Oral hydration
   B. Peripheral IV
   C. Intraosseous catheter
   D. Venous cutdown
   E. Determining the cause of the dehydration

3. A 25-year-old man was an IV drug abuser, injecting himself with heroin for 5 years, with residual scar tissue over the usual points of venous access. The patient is admitted to the emergency department for a detoxification program requiring an IV infusion. The femoral vein in his groin is the only accessible, patent vein for IV use. Which of the following landmarks is the most reliable to identify the femoral vein?

   A. The femoral vein lies medial to the femoral artery
   B. The femoral vein lies within the femoral canal
   C. The femoral vein lies lateral to the femoral artery
   D. The femoral vein lies directly medial to the femoral nerve
   E. The femoral vein lies lateral to the femoral nerve

Venous Cutdown

INTRODUCTION

Establishment of vascular access and resuscitation are crucial in the management of patients who have sustained trauma or who are hypotensive. Various vascular access procedures are available. In the past, venous cutdown was commonly used as a simple surgical technique allowing excellent venous access in children and markedly hypovolemic patients. It has fallen out of favor in recent years due to its relative morbidity, along with the increased use of the Seldinger technique and the ultrasound-guided placement of central venous and intraosseous catheters. However, venous cutdown remains an alternative technique if peripheral, central venous, or intraosseous cannulation cannot be performed in critically ill patients, in emergencies, or if equipment is not available.

CLINICALLY RELEVANT ANATOMY

A thorough knowledge of the relevant anatomy is important in accomplishing a successful venous cutdown. Understanding the venous anatomy and possible variations (Fig. 17.1) aids in the timely performance of the procedure while avoiding injury to adjacent structures.

Great Saphenous Vein

The great saphenous vein is the most commonly used vessel for a cutdown. It arises from the dorsal venous arch of the foot, ascends 2 cm anterior to the medial malleolus, and runs along the medial aspect of the leg. It crosses posterior to the medial femoral epicondyle and continues its ascent on the anteromedial surface of the thigh before entering the fascia lata through the saphenous opening to join the femoral vein in the femoral triangle, approximately 4 cm below the inguinal ligament (Fig. 17.2).

Cutdown of the great saphenous vein may be performed at two locations. The preferred site is in the groin, where the vein has a large diameter and dissection is easy. The other most commonly used site is near the ankle, a few centimeters proximal to the medial malleolus. This site is excellent for cutdowns in pediatric patients because only minimal blunt dissection is needed to isolate the vein. In addition, the area is sufficiently removed from where other resuscitative measures are performed; hence, dislodgment of the venous line is unlikely. However, caution should be exercised so as not to transect the saphenous nerve, which runs in close proximity to the distal great saphenous vein. Venous cutdown may also be performed 1 to 4 cm distal to the medial malleolus, but this location is rarely used as it has many disadvantages such as kinking of the line with ankle flexion.

Basilic Vein

In cases where the great saphenous vein may not be amenable to cutdown due to lower extremity trauma or amputation, an alternate site in the upper extremity may be used. The basilic vein is preferred. Veins from the dorsal venous network of the hand unite to form both the cephalic and basilic veins. The cephalic vein runs on the lateral (radial) aspect and the basilic vein along the medial (ulnar) aspect of the forearm (see Fig. 17.3). As the basilic vein travels proximally along the forearm, it moves anterolaterally at the mid-forearm, lateral to the medial epicondyle of the humerus. In the antecubital fossa, the median cubital vein connects the cephalic and basilic veins before they continue their separate paths, although anatomical variations exist. The basilic vein may perforate the brachial fascia at a level just above the medial epicondyle or as high as the mid–upper arm as it ascends along the medial aspect of the biceps muscle. Just distal to the axillary region, circumflex humeral veins feed into the basilic vein prior to its joining the brachial vein.

A cutdown of the basilic vein may be performed at the antecubital fossa 2 cm proximal and 2 to 3 cm lateral to the medial epicondyle. The vein there is very superficial, so after incision only minimal blunt dissection is needed to expose the vessel. Further dissection may damage the brachial artery, median nerve, and muscle bellies of the biceps brachii. A more proximal location may be used, but this is rarely done because the medial cutaneous nerve of the arm runs parallel with the basilic vein in the upper arm.

Cephalic and Brachial Veins

The cephalic and brachial veins are rarely used for venous cutdown. The cephalic vein arises from the dorsal venous network on the hand and travels along the radial aspect of the forearm in close proximity to the lateral cutaneous nerve. It ascends anteromedially across the antecubital fossa, may communicate with the basilic vein via the median cubital vein, and continues proximally on the lateral aspect of the biceps brachii muscle. Near the level of the shoulder, the cephalic vein passes superficially between the deltoid and pectoralis major muscles through the deltopectoral groove before draining into the axillary vein.

Given the cephalic vein's large diameter and superficial position, it would seem to be an excellent alternative for cutdown. However, because the lateral cutaneous nerve runs in such close proximity to the vein, blunt dissection must be performed with great care to avoid nerve damage. A cutdown

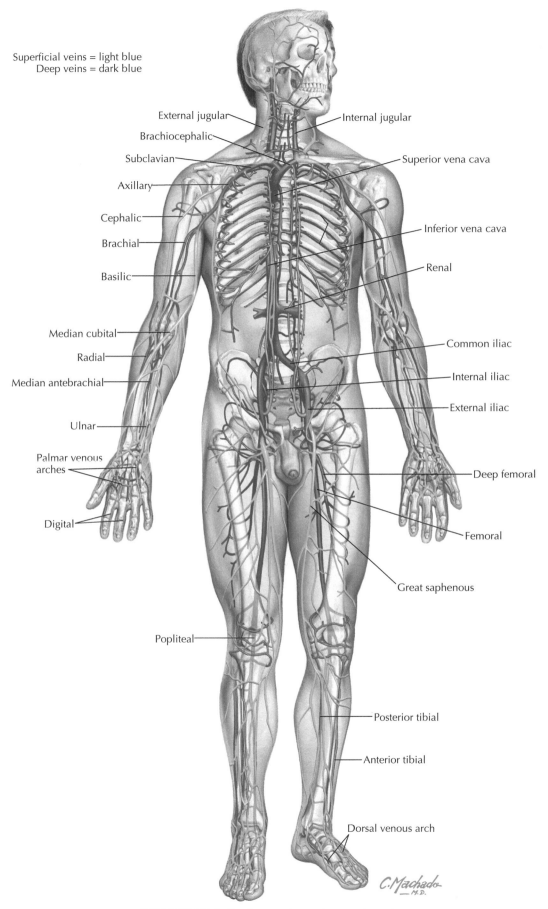

Superficial veins = light blue
Deep veins = dark blue

External jugular
Brachiocephalic
Subclavian
Axillary
Cephalic
Brachial
Basilic
Median cubital
Radial
Median antebrachial
Ulnar
Palmar venous arches
Digital

Internal jugular
Superior vena cava
Inferior vena cava
Renal
Common iliac
Internal iliac
External iliac
Deep femoral
Femoral
Great saphenous
Popliteal
Posterior tibial
Anterior tibial
Dorsal venous arch

C. Machado
M.D.

FIGURE 17.1 Cardiovascular system: major veins

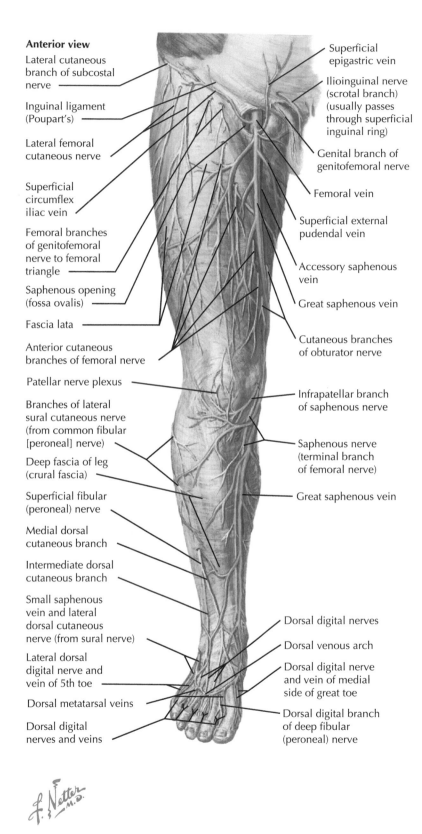

Anterior view

Lateral cutaneous branch of subcostal nerve

Inguinal ligament (Poupart's)

Lateral femoral cutaneous nerve

Superficial circumflex iliac vein

Femoral branches of genitofemoral nerve to femoral triangle

Saphenous opening (fossa ovalis)

Fascia lata

Anterior cutaneous branches of femoral nerve

Patellar nerve plexus

Branches of lateral sural cutaneous nerve (from common fibular [peroneal] nerve)

Deep fascia of leg (crural fascia)

Superficial fibular (peroneal) nerve

Medial dorsal cutaneous branch

Intermediate dorsal cutaneous branch

Small saphenous vein and lateral dorsal cutaneous nerve (from sural nerve)

Lateral dorsal digital nerve and vein of 5th toe

Dorsal metatarsal veins

Dorsal digital nerves and veins

Superficial epigastric vein

Ilioinguinal nerve (scrotal branch) (usually passes through superficial inguinal ring)

Genital branch of genitofemoral nerve

Femoral vein

Superficial external pudendal vein

Accessory saphenous vein

Great saphenous vein

Cutaneous branches of obturator nerve

Infrapatellar branch of saphenous nerve

Saphenous nerve (terminal branch of femoral nerve)

Great saphenous vein

Dorsal digital nerves

Dorsal venous arch

Dorsal digital nerve and vein of medial side of great toe

Dorsal digital branch of deep fibular (peroneal) nerve

FIGURE 17.2 Cutaneous nerves and superficial veins of the leg

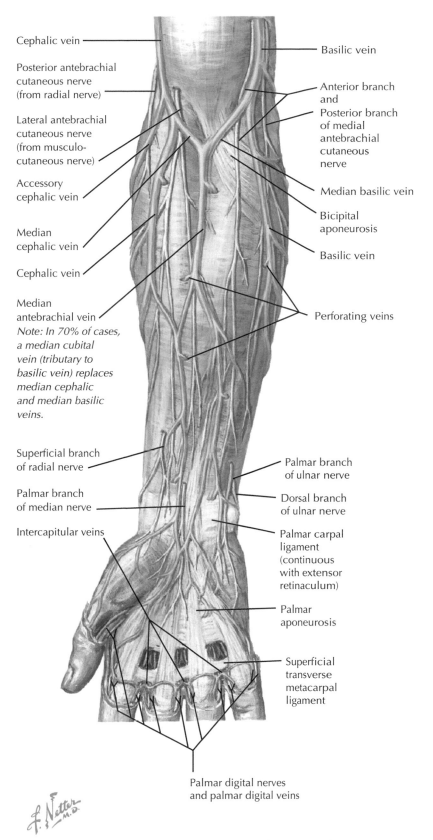

Cephalic vein

Posterior antebrachial
cutaneous nerve
(from radial nerve)

Lateral antebrachial
cutaneous nerve
(from musculo-
cutaneous nerve)

Accessory
cephalic vein

Median
cephalic vein

Cephalic vein

Median
antebrachial vein
*Note: In 70% of cases,
a median cubital
vein (tributary to
basilic vein) replaces
median cephalic
and median basilic
veins.*

Superficial branch
of radial nerve

Palmar branch
of median nerve

Intercapitular veins

Basilic vein

Anterior branch
and

Posterior branch
of medial
antebrachial
cutaneous
nerve

Median basilic vein

Bicipital
aponeurosis

Basilic vein

Perforating veins

Palmar branch
of ulnar nerve

Dorsal branch
of ulnar nerve

Palmar carpal
ligament
(continuous
with extensor
retinaculum)

Palmar
aponeurosis

Superficial
transverse
metacarpal
ligament

Palmar digital nerves
and palmar digital veins

FIGURE 17.3 Cutaneous nerves and superficial veins of the forearm

of the cephalic vein may be performed at the wrist, at the antecubital fossa near the distal flexor crease, or near the deltopectoral groove. The brachial veins are small vessels located in close proximity to the brachial artery. Unlike the cephalic and basilic veins, they are considerably deeper and require more extensive blunt dissection to cannulate. These vessels are rarely used unless other sites are unavailable and time and vessel size are not critical factors.

INDICATIONS

A venous cutdown is indicated as an alternative to peripheral and central venous access in critically ill patients where time is a factor or less invasive options are not available (eg, percutaneous venous catheterization utilizing the Seldinger technique or an interosseous procedure). It is most commonly used in small children in cases of shock or profound hypovolemia and in patients with sclerosed veins. Extensive injuries, burns, or scar tissue may make less invasive venous access procedures difficult.

CONTRAINDICATIONS

Venous cutdowns are contraindicated when a less-invasive technique for gaining venous access is available or if the procedure would delay treatment of the patient. While a cutdown may be performed within a minute by experienced clinicians, inexperienced personnel are likely to take longer. Other contraindications to venous cutdown include coagulopathy and overlying cellulitis. Coagulopathy can lead to hemorrhaging at the site of the cutdown. Overlying infection and cellulitis may pose a risk of further complications such as sepsis. Venous thrombosis is a contraindication to venous cutdowns. Finally, major blunt or penetrating trauma to the extremity at or proximal to the cutdown site is an absolute contraindication because the underlying vessels may be damaged.

EQUIPMENT

Sterile gowns, gloves, and mask
Iodine or other sterile cleansing solution
Sterile drapes
Scalpel, #10 or #11
Curved hemostat
Scissors, Metzenbaum
Self-retaining retractors
Intravenous catheter (larger than 14 gauge)
Intravenous tubing
Suture material (nylon, 4-0)
Silk tie material (2-0 or 3-0)
Sterile gauze and dressings

PROCEDURE

Obtain consent and perform a time out.

As with any surgical procedure, venous cutdown should be performed in as sterile an environment as possible, even in an emergency. Local anesthetic may or may not be required, but it is advisable in conscious patients to use 1% lidocaine as well as conscious sedation if possible. The following description is of the venous cutdown technique without guide wire assistance.

Distal Great Saphenous Vein

See Fig. 17.4.

1. Position the patient supine with the foot externally rotated, exposing the ankle. A tourniquet may be applied proximal to the ankle but is not required.
2. Prepare the skin with antiseptic solution and drape the area.
3. Locate the great saphenous vein 1 cm anterior and 1 cm superior to the medial malleolus and make a superficial transverse 2.5- to 3-cm incision through the skin to expose the vein.
4. Using the curved hemostat, bluntly dissect the subcutaneous tissue to isolate the vein from the nerve and underlying bone. Self-retaining retractors may be used to allow better visualization of the vein. Free a 2-cm section of the vein to allow silk ties to be passed underneath the exposed vein proximally and distally.
5. Ligate the vein with the distal suture, leaving the proximal ligature untied.
6. Using a hemostat, elevate the vein and place gradual traction to flatten the vessel.
7. Use a scalpel to make a 1- to 2-cm venotomy on the anterior surface of the vein and place an appropriately sized intravenous catheter into the vein. The cannula bevel should be either tapered or shortened to avoid accidental piercing of the posterior wall of the vein. Dilators may be used if the venotomy is small.
8. After cannulation, secure the catheter to the vein with the proximal tie. Attach intravenous tubing to the catheter and secure with the suture. Alternatively, the intravenous tubing may be introduced directly into the venotomy to yield higher flow rates.
9. Close the incision site with simple interrupted sutures.
10. Apply a clean sterile dressing to protect the site and tubing.

Proximal Great Saphenous Vein

The procedure for the venous cutdown near the groin is very similar to that used at the ankle.
1. The patient should be positioned supine with the foot externally rotated.
2. Prepare the skin and drape the region. Local anesthetic may be injected.
3. At a point 3 to 4 cm below the inguinal ligament, make a superficial transverse 5- to 6-cm incision medial to the midline of the thigh.
4. A self-retaining retractor may be placed while dissecting the subcutaneous tissues with hemostats. Manual dissection may also be done to expedite the procedure. If thigh muscles or deep fascia are encountered, the dissection may have gone too deep.
5. Elevate the vessel as described above, make a 1- to 2-cm venotomy on the anterior surface of the vein with the scalpel, and place the intravenous catheter into the vein. Dilators and introducers may be used if necessary.
6. Secure the catheter, close the incision, and dress the site as described above.

1–3. Position patient supine with foot externally rotated and prepare the ankle with antiseptic solution. Locate the great saphenous vein 1 cm anterior and 1 cm superior from the medial malleolus and make a transverse incision to expose the vein.

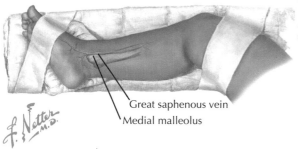

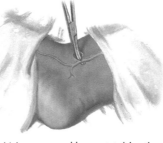

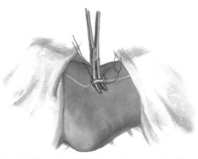

Great saphenous vein

Medial malleolus

4. Using a curved hemostat, bluntly dissect the subcutaneous tissue to isolate the vein, freeing a 2-cm section so that silk ties may be passed underneath proximally and distally.

5–6. The vein should be ligated with the distal ligature tied and the "proximal ligatue untied. Elevate with a hemostat to flatten the vessel.

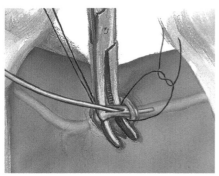

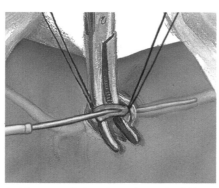

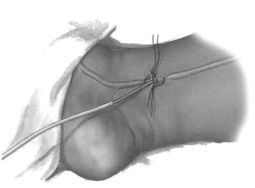

7–8. Perform a 1- to 2-cm venotomy with a scalpel, and place appropriately sized intravenous catheter in vein.

9. After cannulation, the catheter should be secured with the proximal tie. Intravenous tubing is attached to the catheter and secured with a suture.

10–11. The incision site is closed with simple interrupted sutures, and sterile dressing is applied to protect the site and tubing.

FIGURE 17.4 Venous cutdown: distal great saphenous vein

Forearm Veins

See Fig. 17.5.

1. The patient's arm should be abducted 90 degrees, flexed 90 degrees, and externally rotated to allow exposure of both cephalic and basilic veins.
2. For basilic vein cutdown, make a 3-cm superficial incision on the medial portion of the arm 2 cm proximal and 2 to 3 cm lateral to the medical epicondyle. For a cephalic vein cutdown, make a 5-cm superficial incision along the deltopectoral groove.
3. Self-retaining retractors may be placed, and blunt dissection should be carefully done to expose the vein in the subcutaneous tissues.
4. Isolate the vein from the underlying muscle or bone and elevate it to allow ligation and venotomy as described.
5. Venotomy should be no more than 50% of the vein thickness.
6. Cannulate the vein, secure the catheter, and close and dress the wound as described above.

ANATOMICAL PITFALLS

Nearby nerves and arteries are at risk in a venous cutdown. For example, a cutdown of the great saphenous vein just anterior to the medial malleolus risks injuring the saphenous nerve. Therefore, with any cutdown procedure, the regional neurovascular relationships must be keep in mind.

COMPLICATIONS

Hemorrhage

While complications with venous cutdown are rare, they still do occur. Hematoma and hemorrhage at the cutdown site are among the more common complications. If the patient has an undiagnosed coagulopathy or the venotomy was not properly closed, hemorrhage may occur.

Infection

Infection is another common complication of venous cutdown. Prior skin infection and inadequate skin preparation may lead to a severe wound infection. Additionally, phlebitis may occur as a result of the procedure. This is especially true if the catheter is left in place for a long time. Thus one management goal of a venous cutdown is early removal of the catheter as soon as alternative vascular access is available. Topical antibiotics and one dose of a prophylactic antibiotic may also be given at the time of the procedure to decrease the wound infection rate.

Neurovascular Injury

Injury to surrounding structures is the most common complication seen in venous cutdown. Nerve injury is especially common because all potential cutdown sites have peripheral nerves in close proximity to the veins. Ulnar nerve injury is a

1. The arm should be abducted, flexed, and externally rotated for maximum exposure of cephalic and basilic veins.

2. Make a 3-cm superficial incision on the medial portion of the arm, 2 cm proximal and 2-3 cm lateral to the medial epicondyle.

3. Perform blunt dissection to expose vein in subcutaneous tissue.

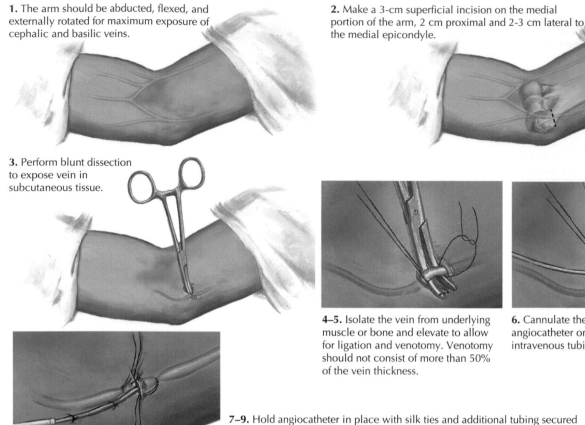

4–5. Isolate the vein from underlying muscle or bone and elevate to allow for ligation and venotomy. Venotomy should not consist of more than 50% of the vein thickness.

6. Cannulate the vein with angiocatheter or directly with intravenous tubing.

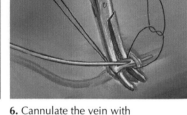

7–9. Hold angiocatheter in place with silk ties and additional tubing secured with a suture to the skin. The incision site is closed with interrupted sutures, and sterile dressing is applied to protect the site and tubing.

FIGURE 17.5 Venous cutdown: forearm veins

major complication of venous cutdown in the arm. Injuries to adjacent arteries may also occur and possibly be life threatening (eg, if the femoral artery is damaged in a proximal saphenous vein cutdown). The catheter may pierce the posterior wall of the vein. More rare complications include thrombosis and air embolus.

CONCLUSION

Obtaining vascular access is vitally important in any trauma or in a severely hypovolemic patient. While less-invasive peripheral and central venous access placement techniques are preferred, on occasion venous cutdown may be required when all else fails or other treatment modalities are not available. A cutdown may be done to gain access to several different veins, but the most common are the great saphenous and basilic veins. Clinicians working in an emergency setting should be familiar with these techniques. A thorough knowledge of the anatomy and technique will aid in reducing iatrogenic complications.

Suggested Readings

American College of Surgeons Committee on Trauma. *ATLS: Advanced Trauma Life Support for Doctors: Student Course Manual.* 8th ed. Chicago: American College of Surgeons; 2008.

Chappell S, Vilke GM, Chan TC, Harrigan RA, Ufberg JW. Peripheral venous cutdown. *J Emerg Med.* 2006;31:411–416.

Klofas E. A quicker saphenous vein cutdown and a better way to teach it. *Trauma.* 1997;43:985–987.

Krishnamurthy G, Keller MS. Vascular access in children. *Cardiovasc Intervent Radiol.* 2011;34:14–24.

Lanter PL, Williams J. Venous cutdown. In: Roberts JR, Hedges JR, eds. *Clinical Procedures in Emergency Medicine.* 5th ed. Philadelphia: Elsevier; 2010:411–417.

Taghizadeh R, Gilbert PM. Long saphenous venous cutdown revisited. *Burns.* 2006;32:267–268.

US Department of Defense. *Emergency War Surgery, Third United States Revision.* Prepper Press; 2004:8.3–8.4.

REVIEW QUESTIONS

1. A 49-year-old man underwent a venous cutdown procedure using the great saphenous vein. Postoperatively, the patient complains of pain and a lack of normal sensation on the medial surface of the leg and foot on the side where the cutdown was performed. Which nerve was most likely injured during the procedure?

   A. Common fibular (peroneal)
   B. Superficial fibular (peroneal)
   C. Lateral sural
   D. Saphenous
   E. Tibial

2. A 32-year-old woman with kidney failure required dialysis. However, a search for a suitable vein in her upper limb was unexpectedly difficult. The major vein on the lateral side of the arm was too small, and others were too delicate. Finally, a vein was found on the medial side of the arm that passed through the superficial and deep fascia to join veins running along the brachial artery. Which of the following veins was this?

   A. Basilic
   B. Lateral cubital

   C. Cephalic
   D. Medial cubital
   E. Medial antebrachial

3. A 24-year-old nurse is performing phlebotomy at the median cubital vein. She places the needle into the median cubital vein but is unable to withdraw blood. She quickly realizes that she passed the needle completely through the vein. Which of the following structures located deep to the median cubital vein has acted as a barrier and prevented her from puncturing an artery?

   A. Flexor retinaculum
   B. Pronator teres muscle
   C. Bicipital aponeurosis
   D. Brachioradialis muscle
   E. Biceps brachii tendon

Dislocated Hip Reduction

INTRODUCTION

Hip dislocation refers to a displacement of the femoral head from contact with the acetabulum, either anteriorly or posteriorly. This classification is based on where the femoral head lies in relation to the acetabulum in the coronal plane. Anterior dislocations are further classified into superior and inferior. Other classification systems are sometimes used, such as a central dislocation involving an acetabular fracture. Posterior hip dislocations are more common (85% of all dislocations) and tend to most often result from automobile accidents (high-speed trauma). Hip dislocations are also commonly seen in those with prosthetic hips and developmental dysplasias of the hip. Hip dislocations are orthopedic emergencies requiring early recognition and immediate reduction. Prompt reduction with the patient under anesthesia or sedation is necessary to prevent osteonecrosis of the femoral head.

CLINICALLY RELEVANT ANATOMY

The hip joint is a synovial ball-and-socket joint (Fig. 18.1) formed by articulation of the femoral head with the hemispherical acetabulum. Except for the rough pit in the femoral head where the ligament of the head of the femur attaches, the acetabulum and femoral head are covered with articular cartilage, which extends onto the proximal femoral neck. The cartilage is thickest anterosuperiorly on the acetabulum and anterolaterally on the femoral head, two areas that are the principal weight-bearing areas in the joint. The acetabulum is deepened by a fibrocartilaginous rim known as the labrum. This rim limits the diameter of the acetabulum and encapsulates the femoral head, thus maintaining the stability of the joint. The joint is surrounded by a fibrous capsule reinforced by the iliofemoral (the strongest), pubofemoral, ischiofemoral, and transverse acetabular ligaments. These ligaments are the main source of joint stability. The capsule is surrounded by muscles. Anteriorly, it is covered by the pectineus. Laterally, the psoas major tendon and the iliacus descend across it. More laterally, the straight head of the rectus femoris crosses the joint. Superiorly, it is covered by the rectus femoris medially and the gluteus minimus laterally. Inferiorly, the pectineus and the obturator externus spiral obliquely to protect its posterior aspect. Given the architecture of the hip and the resultant stability, tremendous force is required to dislocate the joint as well as reduce such an injury.

INDICATIONS

Patients requiring hip reduction often present at the emergency department following a motor vehicle collision (Fig. 18.2). The high-energy nature of the event causing hip dislocation often results in multiple injuries. Life-threatening injuries must first be ruled out or managed. Hip dislocation, and thus the need for emergent hip reduction, should be suspected in patients who present with the lower limb held in adduction and either internally (posterior dislocation) or externally (anterior dislocation) rotated. This suspicion is confirmed by an anteroposterior pelvis radiograph. The indications for reduction include the following:
- A dislocation with or without neurological deficit when there is no associated fracture
- A dislocation with an associated fracture if no neurological deficits are present

CONTRAINDICATIONS

Closed reduction is absolutely contraindicated in patients with femoral neck fractures and open traumatic hip dislocations. In these cases, traction would result in displacement of the femoral neck fracture, further increasing the risk of osteonecrosis. Open traumatic hip dislocations are taken directly to surgery. Other contraindications include multiple failed closed reduction attempts (two to three times), irreducible hip dislocation, fragment incarcerated in the joint, increasing neurological deficit, and associated vascular injury.

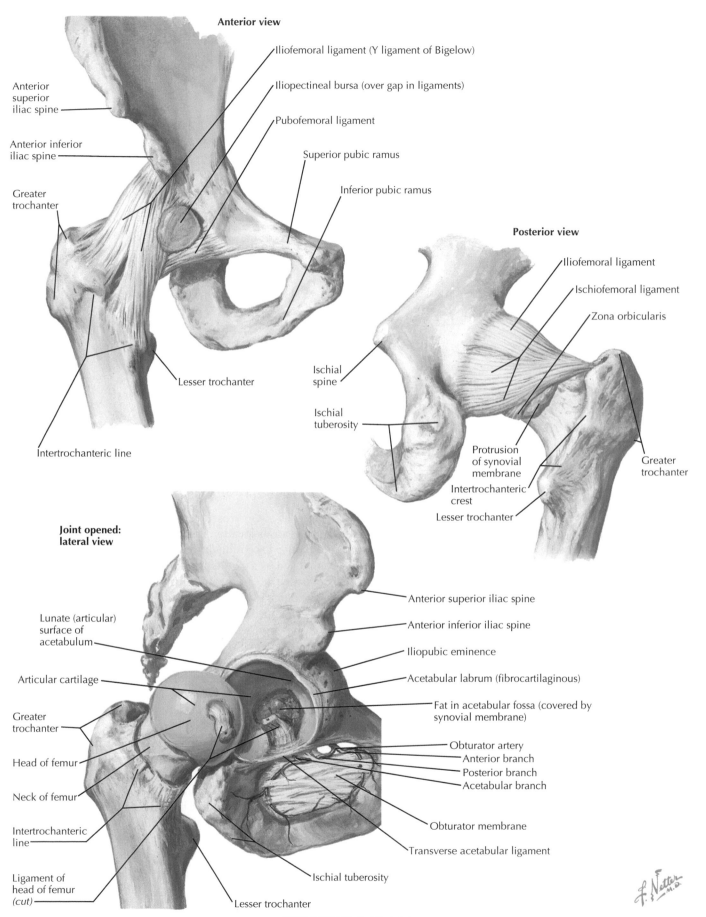

Anterior view

Anterior superior iliac spine

Anterior inferior iliac spine

Greater trochanter

Intertrochanteric line

Lesser trochanter

Iliofemoral ligament (Y ligament of Bigelow)

Iliopectineal bursa (over gap in ligaments)

Pubofemoral ligament

Superior pubic ramus

Inferior pubic ramus

Posterior view

Iliofemoral ligament

Ischiofemoral ligament

Zona orbicularis

Ischial spine

Ischial tuberosity

Protrusion of synovial membrane

Intertrochanteric crest

Lesser trochanter

Greater trochanter

Joint opened: lateral view

Lunate (articular) surface of acetabulum

Articular cartilage

Greater trochanter

Head of femur

Neck of femur

Intertrochanteric line

Ligament of head of femur (cut)

Lesser trochanter

Ischial tuberosity

Transverse acetabular ligament

Obturator membrane

Anterior superior iliac spine

Anterior inferior iliac spine

Iliopubic eminence

Acetabular labrum (fibrocartilaginous)

Fat in acetabular fossa (covered by synovial membrane)

Obturator artery

Anterior branch

Posterior branch

Acetabular branch

FIGURE 18.1 Hip joint

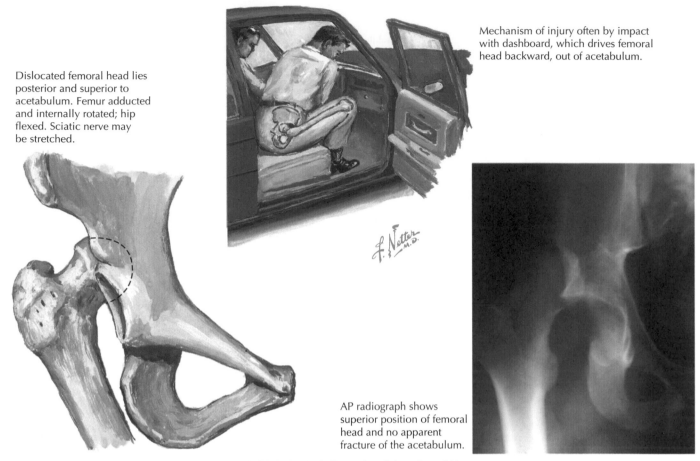

Dislocated femoral head lies posterior and superior to acetabulum. Femur adducted and internally rotated; hip flexed. Sciatic nerve may be stretched.

Mechanism of injury often by impact with dashboard, which drives femoral head backward, out of acetabulum.

AP radiograph shows superior position of femoral head and no apparent fracture of the acetabulum.

FIGURE 18.2 Posterior dislocation of hip

EQUIPMENT

Minimal equipment is needed for the emergency reduction of a dislocated joint. However, it is imperative that the surgeon understand that the mechanism by which a hip is dislocated requires a large force. Thus, to reduce the injury, an equally large force is needed to overcome the opposing forces of muscles and ligaments without causing further damage. It is therefore recommended that slow, steady, longitudinal traction be used because it tires the muscles in spasm and results in a smoother reduction.

One or two assistants, depending on the technique used
Stretcher
Oxygen supply
Bag-valve-mask device
Oxygen saturation monitor
Wall suction, suction tubing, and Yankauer suction catheter
Intravenous catheter (at least 20 gauge)
Medication as needed for sedation
Normal saline (0.9% NaCl) flushes

PROCEDURES

Obtain patient consent and perform a time out.

The best initial treatment for both anterior and posterior dislocations is reduction under sedation or general anesthesia. The reduction involves traction in line with the deformity.

An anterior dislocation can be converted into a posterior one and reduced accordingly. Posterior hip dislocations can often be reduced by a closed procedure. However, 2% to 4% may be irreducible due to the interposition of certain muscle groups. Such dislocations are corrected by open reduction through a posterior approach. If the hip is found to be clinically unstable after reduction, a femoral pin is used to hold it in longitudinal skeletal traction.

Three closed reduction techniques are used to reduce a posterior hip dislocation. The procedure selected depends on the setting and resources available at the time, as well as associated injuries. For instance, techniques that place patients in the prone position, such as the Stimson maneuver, should not be used in cases of visceral or head trauma. Similarly, lateral positioning techniques, such as the Dahners and Hundley modification of Skoff's technique, should be avoided in patients with cervical spine trauma. Techniques like the Lefkowitz maneuver that require sedation should be avoided in patients with definite or impending airway compromise. Techniques that utilize the prone position can also cause problems with airway management. Most techniques rely on an intact knee joint. However, because most dislocations are caused by trauma, the knee joint is also often affected. Thus thorough examination of the ipsilateral knee and the remainder of the pelvis and lower extremity and spine is necessary before a closed reduction is attempted.

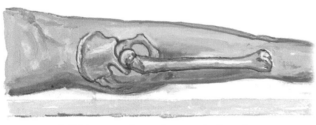

1. With appropriate pain control, place the patient in the supine position.

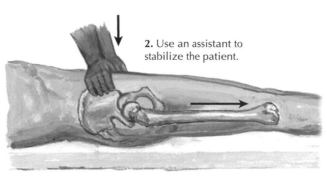

2. Use an assistant to stabilize the patient.

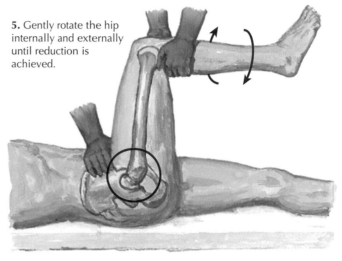

3. Apply traction to the leg in direct line with the deformity.

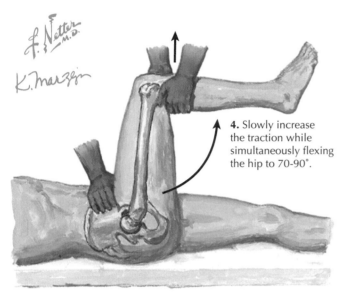

4. Slowly increase the traction while simultaneously flexing the hip to 70-90°.

5. Gently rotate the hip internally and externally until reduction is achieved.

FIGURE 18.3 Dislocated hip reduction: Allis maneuver

Allis Maneuver

See Fig. 18.3.
1. Place the patient in the supine position.
2. Have an assistant stabilize the pelvis.
3. With the patient's knee flexed, apply traction to the leg in a direct line with the deformity.
4. Slowly increase the traction force while simultaneously flexing the hip to approximately 70 to 90 degrees.
5. Gently rotate the hip internally and externally until reduction is achieved.

Bigelow and Reverse Bigelow Maneuvers

These maneuvers are associated with iatrogenic femoral neck fracture and are therefore infrequently used.
1. Place the patient in the supine position.
2. Have an assistant apply counter-traction with downward pressure on the anterior superior iliac spine.
3. Apply traction to the affected leg in the direction of the deformity.
4. Flex the hip to a minimum of 90 degrees.
5. Abduct, externally rotate, and extend the leg. In the reverse Bigelow maneuver, the leg is instead adducted, sharply internally rotated, and extended.

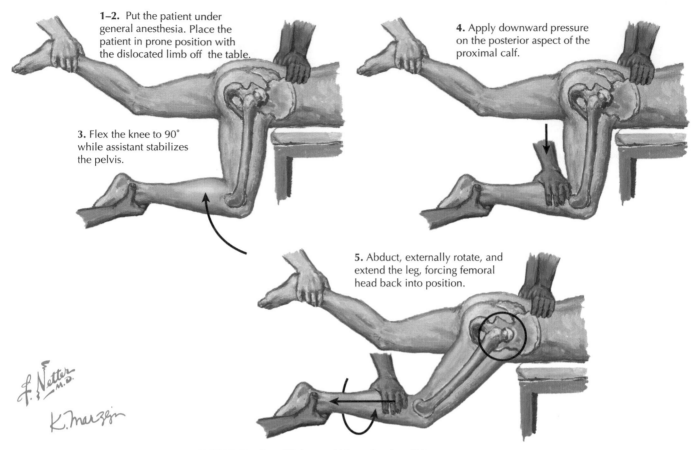

1–2. Put the patient under general anesthesia. Place the patient in prone position with the dislocated limb off the table.

3. Flex the knee to 90° while assistant stabilizes the pelvis.

4. Apply downward pressure on the posterior aspect of the proximal calf.

5. Abduct, externally rotate, and extend the leg, forcing femoral head back into position.

FIGURE 18.4 Dislocated hip reduction: Stimson maneuver

Stimson Maneuver

See Fig. 18.4.

1. Put the patient under general anesthesia.
2. Place the patient in the prone position with the dislocated limb off the side of the stretcher. In this position, the hip is flexed to 90 degrees.
3. Flex the knee to 90 degrees while an assistant stabilizes the pelvis.
4. Apply downward pressure on the posterior aspect of the proximal calf.
5. Abduct, externally rotate, and extend the leg. This will force the femoral head back into the acetabulum.

Alternate Methods

In addition to these three classical reduction techniques, other closed reduction techniques have been described.

Dahners and Hundley Modification of Skoff's Technique

1. Place the patient in the lateral position.
2. Place hospital sheets around the proximal thigh and knee of the dislocated leg.
3. Apply traction to the maximally flexed leg.

Modification of the Stimson Maneuver

This modification is not suitable for patients with multiple injuries or potential airway compromise.

1. Place the patient in the supine position.
2. Administer an intravenous muscle relaxant.
3. Place the patient into the prone position with the hip off the end of the table.
4. Flex the patient's hip to 90 degrees.
5. Place your knee on the patient's calf and apply a downward force.

Lefkowitz Maneuver

This method is used for traumatic and prosthetic dislocations.

1. Sedate the patient and place in the supine position.
2. Plant the patient's ipsilateral foot firmly on the bed.
3. Place your flexed knee under the patient's flexed knee and hip, with your other foot on a stool beside the bed.
4. Apply gentle, steady downward pressure to the ankle to reduce the hip.

East Baltimore Lift

This is a modification of the 90-90 supine position.

1. This technique requires three people.

2. Place the patient in the supine position, and have one assistant stabilize the pelvis.
3. Stand on the side of the affected hip while the other assistant stands on the opposite side, both with the knees flexed.
4. Place your arm under the patient's calf and rest it on the shoulder of the assistant.
5. The assistant should do the same with the opposite arm.
6. Control the rotation of the affected hip by holding the patient's ankle.
7. Along with the assistant, stand up straight to apply traction on the hip.

Modification of Allis Maneuver for Reduction of an Anterior-Inferior Hip Dislocation

1. Place the patient supine.
2. Apply inline femoral traction with the hip mildly flexed.
3. Gently internally rotate and adduct the hip as a lateral force is applied to the inner thigh with the use of a sheet.

Reduction of an Anterior-Superior Hip Dislocation

1. Place the patient supine.
2. Apply inline traction until the femoral head is at the level of the acetabulum.
3. Gently internally rotate the hip.

Assessment After Hip Reduction

1. Assess that the reduction has been successful by ordering a radiograph.
2. Assess hip stability by gently moving the hip through a range of motion.
3. If a posterior wall fracture is also present, assess the stability of the hip by placing it in 90 degrees flexion, 20 degrees adduction, and slight internal rotation while applying a posteriorly directed force.
4. If there is no radiographic or clinical evidence of instability, order computed tomography to confirm or rule out the presence of fragments or other injury.
5. If there is evidence of incongruity, open reduction is indicated.
6. If there is no evidence of further injury, a knee immobilizer can be placed in an effort to maintain the reduction.

ANATOMICAL PITFALLS

Anterior dislocations have the best prognosis and central dislocations the worst. The delay between dislocation and reduction directly relates to the risk of infarction of the femoral head. A delay exceeding 6 hours potentially compromises blood flow to the hip joint and therefore increases the incidence of aseptic necrosis of the femoral head from 5% to 50%.

COMPLICATIONS

The most common complications are late degenerative osteoarthritis in 75% of cases and osteonecrosis in 15%. The latter, also known as avascular necrosis of the femoral head, is the most feared complication of hip dislocation and is directly related to the time from injury to reduction. Displacement of the femoral head results in a taut force on the blood vessels, which leads to disruption of the blood supply, causing the femoral head to degenerate. Eventually the joint becomes severely arthritic. This condition is not reversible. Avascular necrosis can also occur as a complication of the hip reduction itself, the risk factor for which is forced abduction. Other complications of closed reduction include femur fracture, sciatic nerve neuropraxia, persistent subluxation, and failed closed reduction.

CONCLUSIONS

Hip dislocation is a true orthopedic emergency requiring hip reduction, provided there are no contraindications, within 6 hours of injury to avoid osteonecrosis. Because hip dislocation tends to occur in a setting of high-energy trauma such as a car collision, life-threatening conditions need to be attended to first. Once the patient is stabilized and the diagnosis of hip dislocation is confirmed, the physician should select the most appropriate reduction technique based on the type of dislocation, coexisting conditions, expertise, and available resources. Owing to the amount of force required, the closed reduction technique has associated complications such as sciatic nerve injury, femur fracture, and avascular necrosis.

Suggested Readings

Goddard NJ. Classification of traumatic hip dislocation. *Clin Orthop Relat Res.* 2000;377:11–14.

Gray H. The pelvis. In: Stranding S, ed. *Gray's Anatomy: The Anatomical Basis of Clinical Practice.* London: Elsevier; 2008.

Newton KR, Thomas du Plessis M. An unusual presentation of a traumatic posterior hip dislocation. *BMJ Case Rep.* Jun 6;2014.

Phillips AM, Konchwalla A. The pathologic features and mechanism of traumatic dislocation of the hip. *Clin Orthop Relat Res.* 2000;377: 7–10.

Rezaee A, Knipe H. Hip dislocation. Available at http://radiopaedia.org/articles/hip-dislocation.

Tile M, Helfet DL, Kellam JF. *Fractures of the Pelvis and Acetabulum*, 3rd ed. Lippincott Williams & Wilkins; 2003:534.

Yang EC, Cornwall R. Initial treatment of traumatic hip dislocations in the adult. *Clin Orthop Relat Res.* 2000;377:24–31.

Yates C, Bandy WB, Blasier RD. Traumatic dislocation of the hip in a high school football player. *J Am Phys Ther Assoc.* 2008;88(6): 780–788.

REVIEW QUESTIONS

1. A 72-year-old woman dislocated her hip when she fell down the steps to her garage. Which of the following structures is most significant in resisting hyperextension of the hip joint?
   A. Pubofemoral ligament
   B. Ischiofemoral ligament
   C. Iliofemoral ligament
   D. Negative pressure in the acetabular fossa
   E. Gluteus maximus muscle

2. A 75-year-old man is transported to the emergency department with severe pain in his right hip and thigh. A radiographic examination reveals avascular necrosis of the femoral head. Which of the following conditions most likely occurred to produce avascular necrosis in this patient?

   A. Dislocation of the hip with tearing of the ligament of the femoral head
   B. Intertrochanteric fracture of the femur
   C. Intracapsular femoral neck fracture
   D. Thrombosis of the obturator artery
   E. Comminuted fracture of the extracapsular femoral neck

3. A 42-year-old mother of three children visits the outpatient clinic complaining that her youngest son cannot walk yet. Radiographic and physical examinations reveal an unstable hip joint. Which of the following ligaments is responsible for stabilization of the hip joint in childhood?

   A. Iliofemoral
   B. Pubofemoral
   C. Ischiofemoral
   D. Ligament of the head of the femur
   E. Transverse acetabular ligament

4. A 69-year-old man was involved in a motor vehicle crash. Upon arrival at the emergency department, it is determined that he has an anterior hip dislocation with a fracture of the femoral neck. The leg is mottled and cooler than the other extremity. Which of the following will be the most likely action?

   A. Allis maneuver
   B. Have an orthopedic surgeon immediately do an open reduction with internal fixation
   C. Stimson maneuver
   D. Amputate the leg prior to gangrene setting in

Dislocated Finger Reduction

INTRODUCTION

Finger dislocation is a common medical emergency that occurs when one or more of the bones of the fingers are moved from their correct anatomical positions. The injury is typically caused by high-speed impact against the hand or hyperextension of the affected digit. Clinically, the dislocated finger presents with pain, loss of function, and occasionally tingling or numbness of the digit.

Ideally, a dislocated finger should be treated by a doctor as a medical emergency to prevent permanent disability. However, since such injuries often occur in a sports-related setting, reduction is regularly done by coaches where the injury occurred. In such cases, postreduction assessment by an emergency physician is of utmost importance. In the emergency department, digit dislocation is managed by radiographic analysis to exclude bone fracture, joint reduction after the application of appropriate anesthesia, and splinting or buddy taping of the digit.

CLINICALLY RELEVANT ANATOMY

The interphalangeal joints are hinge joints supported by a soft tissue envelope consisting of several ligaments. Each distal interphalangeal (DIP), proximal interphalangeal (PIP), and metacarpophalangeal (MCP) joint is supported by a pair of collateral and accessory collateral ligaments that attach to a palmar ligament (volar plate) (Fig. 19.1). The ulnar collateral and accessory collateral ligaments support the joint medially, whereas lateral support is provided by the radial aspects of the ligaments. The palmar ligament is a thick fibrous band of connective tissue that tapers toward its proximal attachment, thereby allowing folding of the ligament during flexion. During extension, the ligament is tense, preventing hyperextension of the digits. Dorsal to the MP and PIP joints is the central slip of the extensor tendon, which inserts into the base of the middle phalanx. A medial or lateral dislocation of the digit implies a failure of the collateral ligaments with partial disruption of the palmar ligament, whereas a dorsal dislocation results from failure of the palmar ligament proper. Volar dislocations occur where there is injury to the overlying central slip.

INDICATIONS

Radiographic evaluation of the hand is important and should include anteroposterior, lateral, and oblique views. A true lateral view is useful in excluding joint fractures that may be less visible on an anteroposterior view, particularly fractures associated with a torn palmar plate. After any additional injury to the hand is excluded, anesthesia is often necessary to facilitate adequate examination and reduction of the dislocation. This is typically achieved through a finger or wrist block or with intravenous regional anesthesia (Bier block) at the discretion of the clinician.

CONTRAINDICATIONS

Contraindications to dislocated finger reduction that require the consultation of a specialist include the following:
- Digital nerve or vessel compromise
- Associated fracture
- Open joint dislocation
- Ligamentous or volar plate rupture
- Joint instability
- Inability to reduce the dislocation

Proximal Interphalangeal Joint
Dorsal PIP Dislocations

Dislocations of the PIP joints of the second to fifth digits are the most common dislocations of the hand (Fig. 19.2). They often arise from sporting injuries involving high-speed impact against the distal phalanges, resulting in dorsal or lateral displacement of one or more bones of the joint. In the more frequently seen dorsal dislocation of the PIP joint, the palmar ligament is usually impaired, and the middle phalanx is shifted over the dorsal aspect of the proximal phalanx. Once a dislocation is diagnosed, further examination of the affected joint should be performed only after successful reduction. Examination of the joint then includes hyperextension to assess the palmar ligament and application of stress to the ulnar and radial collateral ligaments to test their integrity. Injuries to the PIP joints are generally more likely to heal poorly and result in disability. It is therefore advisable to refer such cases for orthopedic follow-up and hand therapy after emergency care is complete.

Palmar and Lateral PIP Dislocations

A palmar or volar dislocation of any joint in the hand is uncommon and often difficult to reduce. Such a dislocation is typically associated with disruption of the central slip of the extensor tendons and generally carries a poor prognosis. Even when managed carefully, a volar dislocation may heal with reduced joint mobility. When reduction has been

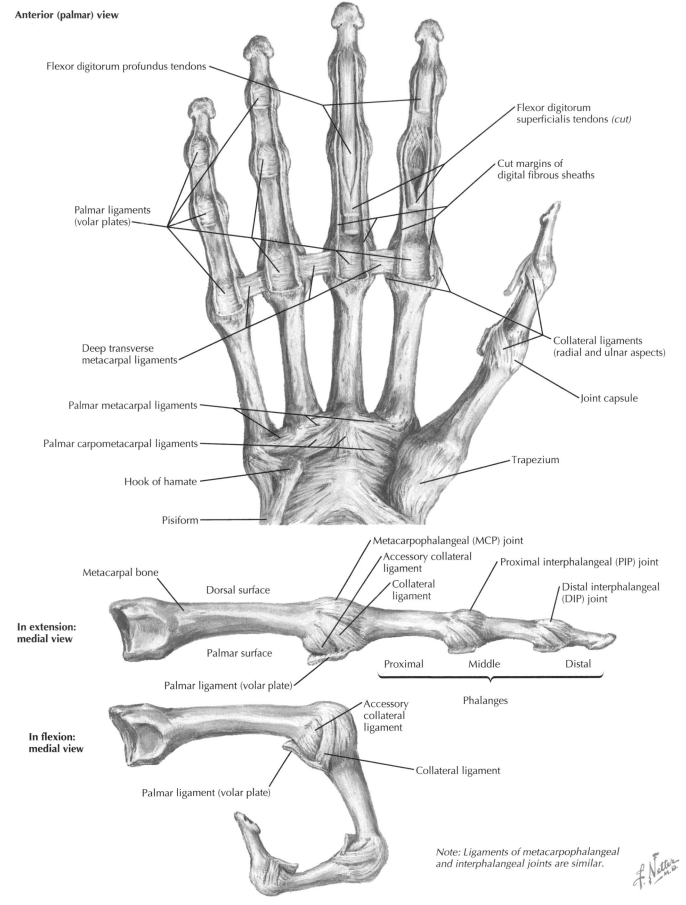

Anterior (palmar) view

Flexor digitorum profundus tendons

Flexor digitorum superficialis tendons (cut)

Cut margins of digital fibrous sheaths

Palmar ligaments (volar plates)

Collateral ligaments (radial and ulnar aspects)

Deep transverse metacarpal ligaments

Joint capsule

Palmar metacarpal ligaments

Palmar carpometacarpal ligaments

Trapezium

Hook of hamate

Pisiform

Metacarpophalangeal (MCP) joint

Accessory collateral ligament

Proximal interphalangeal (PIP) joint

Metacarpal bone

Dorsal surface

Collateral ligament

Distal interphalangeal (DIP) joint

In extension: medial view

Palmar surface

Proximal   Middle   Distal

Palmar ligament (volar plate)

Phalanges

In flexion: medial view

Accessory collateral ligament

Collateral ligament

Palmar ligament (volar plate)

Note: Ligaments of metacarpophalangeal and interphalangeal joints are similar.

FIGURE 19.1 Metacarpophalangeal and interphalangeal ligaments

Proximal Interphalangeal Joint Dislocations

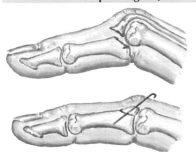

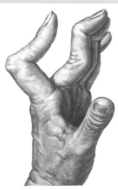

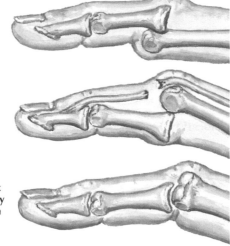

Dorsal dislocation
(most common)

Palmar dislocation
(uncommon) causes
**boutonnière
deformity.** Central
slip of extensor
tendon often torn,
requiring open
fixation, followed
by dorsal splinting.

**Rotational
dislocation** (rare)

Volar dislocation of middle phalanx with
avulsion of central slip of extensor tendon,
with or without bone fragment. Failure to
recognize and properly treat this condition
results in boutonnière deformity and
severely restricted function.

Boutonnière deformity of index
finger with **swan-neck deformity**
of other fingers in a patient with
rheumatoid arthritis

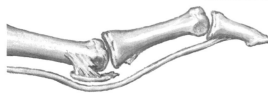

Dorsal dislocation of proximal interphalangeal joint
with disruption of volar plate and collateral ligament
may result in **swan-neck deformity** and compensatory flexion deformity of distal interphalangeal joint.

Defect	Comment
Coach's finger	Dorsal dislocation of the joint
Boutonnière deformity	Dislocation or avulsion fracture of middle phalanx; failure to treat may cause deformity and chronic pain
Rotational	Rare dislocation
Swan-neck deformity	Dorsal dislocation with disruption of palmar (volar) and collateral ligaments

Carpometacarpal and Metacarpophalangeal Injuries Other Than Fracture: Thumb Ligament Injury and Dislocation

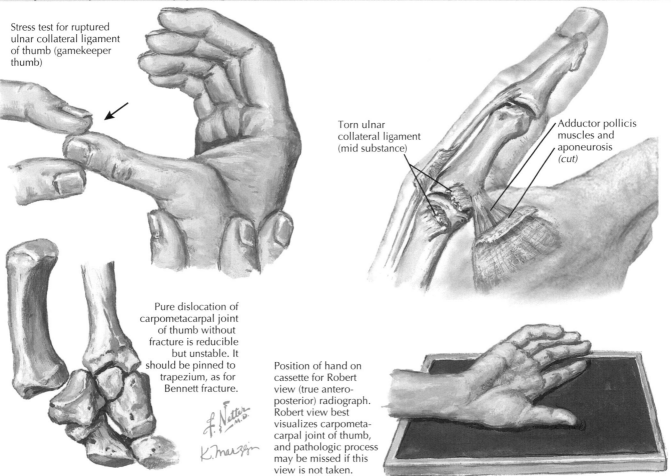

Stress test for ruptured
ulnar collateral ligament
of thumb (gamekeeper
thumb)

Torn ulnar
collateral ligament
(mid substance)

Adductor pollicis
muscles and
aponeurosis
(cut)

Pure dislocation of
carpometacarpal joint
of thumb without
fracture is reducible
but unstable. It
should be pinned to
trapezium, as for
Bennett fracture.

Position of hand on
cassette for Robert
view (true antero-
posterior) radiograph.
Robert view best
visualizes carpometa-
carpal joint of thumb,
and pathologic process
may be missed if this
view is not taken.

FIGURE 19.2 Finger injury

performed prior to arrival at the emergency department, particular attention to the postreduction digit is essential in determining the type of dislocation that occurred. If a volar dislocation is misdiagnosed and splinted in a manner suitable for a dorsal PIP dislocation, inadequate healing and eventual deformation of the digit may occur.

Lateral dislocations of the PIP joint can be diagnosed with a postreduction stress test of the ulnar and radial collateral ligaments. The injury is reduced in a manner similar to that for a dorsal or volar dislocation.

EQUIPMENT

Tape
Splint

PROCEDURE

Obtain patient consent and perform a time out.

Reduction of an Interphalangeal Dislocation

See Fig. 19.3.

1. With appropriate pain control, exaggerate the existing injury by hyperextending the joint while applying slight longitudinal traction until there is distraction of the middle phalanx.
2. Apply pressure to the base of the middle phalanx while flexing the digit.
3. Splint.

Note that although simply applying longitudinal traction is often done by coaches at the site of injury, it is not a generally recommended means of effecting reduction. It may cause tightening of the surrounding soft tissues and actually prevent appropriate reduction of the joint. Closed dislocations are usually easily reduced. However, clinical indications for surgical reduction include the following:

- Irreducible dislocations (usually a volar dislocation with a fracture)
- Entrapment of the palmar plate
- Unstable condylar fractures (usually more than 30% to 40% of articular surface affected)

Metacarpophalangeal and Carpometacarpal Dislocations

Dislocations of the MCP joints are classified as either simple or complex. In a simple dislocation, there is no entrapment of soft tissue or bone. In a complex dislocation, the metacarpal head becomes ensnared by the lumbricals and flexor tendons as the palmar plate is entrapped dorsal to the metacarpal head. Clinically, a complex dislocation can be characterized by the parallel arrangement of the phalanx and metacarpal; the angle between the two bones is less acute than that seen in a simple dislocation. These must be reduced operatively. Though a simple dislocation of the MCP joint can be managed by closed

reduction, a complex MCP injury is sometimes created in the attempt.

It is important to note that using simple traction to reduce any type of MCP dislocation is unadvisable. This would likely cause a simple dislocation to develop into an irreducible one or further complicate an already irreducible injury.

Reduction of an MCP dislocation

See Fig. 19.4.

1. With appropriate pain control, place the wrist in a flexed position to allow relaxation of the flexor tendons.
2. Hyperextend the affected digit.
3. Apply pressure to the base of the proximal phalanx until reduction is achieved.
4. Splint.

Carpometacarpal joint dislocations are comparatively rare. The joint consists of strong fibrous-osseous connections that lend a bit more protection against dislocation. When these dislocations do occur, broken bones are frequently an associated finding. Closed reduction is usually futile, and orthopedic consultation is necessary.

ANATOMICAL PITFALLS

The method of postreduction splinting of the PIP or DIP joint is generally determined by the nature of the dislocation. If the injury involves a dorsal dislodgement at the PIP joint, the joint may be splinted in slight flexion for 3 weeks or buddy taped for 3 to 6 weeks, with encouragement of early motion to prevent stiffness after healing. Similarly, lateral PIP dislocations are managed by buddy taping for 3 to 6 weeks, whereas dorsal DIP injuries are splinted to restrict movement for approximately 2 weeks.

COMPLICATIONS

Volar dislocations of any joint are often unstable and generally have a poorer prognosis. Buddy taping alone is insufficient, and orthopedic consultation with subsequent hand therapy is often required. If a patient presents to the emergency department with a dislocation of the PIP joint that was reduced outside the hospital, it is essential to determine whether the dislocation was dorsal or volar. If a volar injury is treated as a dorsal dislocation with splinting of the joint in flexion, healing occurs with the joint protruding through the torn extensor mechanism, and a boutonnière deformity may ensue.

CONCLUSIONS

Finger dislocation is a common medical emergency that presents with pain, loss of function, and occasionally tingling or numbness of the digit. Prompt radiographic imaging, appropriate anesthesia, and realignment are important in preventing permanent disability.

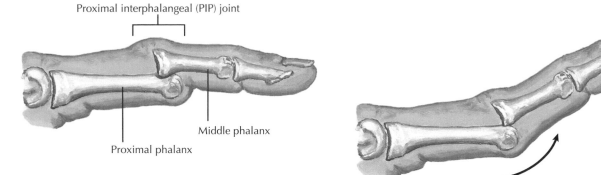

Proximal interphalangeal (PIP) joint

Middle phalanx

Proximal phalanx

1. With appropriate pain control, exaggerate the injury by hyperextending the joint while applying slight longitudinal traction until there is disctraction of the middle phalanx.

2. Apply pressure to the base of middle phalanx while flexing digit.

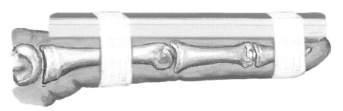

3. Splint

FIGURE 19.3 Dislocated finger reduction: reduction of proximal interphalangeal joint

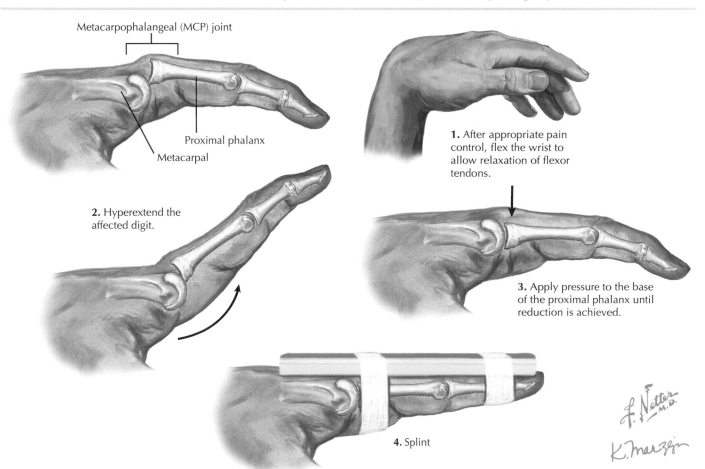

Metacarpophalangeal (MCP) joint

Proximal phalanx

Metacarpal

2. Hyperextend the affected digit.

1. After appropriate pain control, flex the wrist to allow relaxation of flexor tendons.

3. Apply pressure to the base of the proximal phalanx until reduction is achieved.

4. Splint

FIGURE 19.4 Dislocated finger reduction: metacarpophalangeal dislocations

Suggested Readings

Freiberg A. Management of proximal interphalangeal joint injuries. *Can J Plast Surg.* 2007;15:199–203.

Joyce KM, Joyce CW, Conroy F, Chan J, Buckley E, Carroll SM. Proximal interphalangeal joint dislocations and treatment: an evolutionary process. *Arch Plast Surg.* 2014;41(4):394–397.

Kannan RY, Wilmshurst AD. Unstable proximal interphalangeal joint dislocations: another cause. *EMJ.* 2006;23(10):819.

Skelley NW, McCormick JJ, Smith MV. In-game management of common joint dislocations. *Sports Health.* 2014;6(3):246–255.

Tekkis PP, Kessaris N, Enchill-Yawson M, Mani GV, Gavalas M. Palmar dislocation of the proximal interphalangeal joint—an injury not to be missed. *J Accid Emerg Med.* 1999;16(6):431–432.

Ufberg JW, McNamara RM. Management of common dislocations. In: Robert JR, Hedges JR, eds. *Clinical Procedures in Emergency Medicine*, 5th ed. Philadelphia: Elsevier; 2010:891–896.

REVIEW QUESTIONS

1. It was reported by the sports media that the outstanding 27-year-old shortstop for a New York team would miss a number of baseball games. He was hit on a fingertip while attempting to catch a ball barehanded. A tendon had been torn. The team doctor commented that the ballplayer could not straighten the last joint of the long finger of his right hand, and the finger would require surgery. From what injury did the ballplayer suffer?

   A. Claw hand deformity
   B. Boutonnière deformity
   C. Swan-neck deformity
   D. Dupuytren contracture
   E. Mallet finger

2. In a penetrating wound to the forearm of a 24-year-old man, the median nerve is injured at the entrance of the nerve into the forearm. Which of the following would most likely be apparent when the patient's hand is relaxed?

   A. The MCP and interphalangeal joints of the second and third digits will be extended.
   B. The third and fourth digits will be held in a slightly flexed position.
   C. The thumb will be flexed and slightly abducted.
   D. The first, second, and third digits will be held in a slightly flexed position.
   E. The MCP and interphalahgeal joints of the second and third digits of the hand will be flexed.

Dislocated Knee Reduction

INTRODUCTION

Knee dislocations are an underdiagnosed entity with a multifactorial etiology. The reported incidence is less than 0.02% of all musculoskeletal traumas. Many dislocations spontaneously reduce before arrival at the emergency department. Therefore emergency physicians may have little exposure to them and fail to include knee dislocation in their differential diagnosis. A high index of suspicion is required for early diagnosis and timely management to prevent a threat to the limb from occult vascular injury.

Knee dislocations are associated with high-energy injuries, with motor vehicle accidents being the most common. Other etiologies include sports-related injuries, low-energy injuries (particularly in obese patients), and accidents in which the leg is pinned under heavy objects. Knee dislocations are more common in males.

Knowledge of the anatomy of the knee is vital to a proper understanding of the development, management, and complications of a dislocated knee.

CLINICALLY RELEVANT ANATOMY

The knee, though seemingly simple, requires the interaction of bones, ligaments, tendons, muscles, and the joint capsule for proper functioning (Fig. 20.1). The medial tibiofemoral, lateral tibiofemoral, patellofemoral, and proximal tibiofibular joints together constitute the knee joint.

The many ligaments of the knee joint are classified as extracapsular or intraarticular. The extracapsular ligaments are the patellar, tibial collateral, fibular collateral, oblique popliteal, and arcuate popliteal. The ligaments within the joint capsule are the anterior cruciate, posterior cruciate, and posterior meniscofemoral.

The main movements at the knee are flexion and extension; only minimal rotational and translational movements are possible. The main muscle group responsible for extending the knee is the quadriceps femoris, composed of the vastus medialis and lateralis, rectus femoris, and vastus intermedius. Flexion is achieved by the contraction of the semimembranosus, semitendinosus, long head of the biceps femoris (together referred to as the hamstring muscles), and short head of the biceps femoris. The tensor fasciae latae is a weak extensor, and the gracilis, sartorius, gastrocnemius, and popliteus are weak flexors. Assessing the cause of an irreducible dislocation requires particular attention to these muscles because soft tissue trapped in the medial aspect of the joint can result in a failure to achieve reduction.

Adverse outcomes of knee dislocations are most commonly secondary to the injury of neurovascular structures. The arterial network around the knee has many vessels. Injury to the popliteal artery is of most concern. The popliteal artery is the continuation of the femoral artery as it passes through the adductor hiatus. It passes posterior to the knee joint and bifurcates into the anterior and posterior tibial arteries, which supply the leg and foot.

Traveling in close association with the popliteal artery is the tibial nerve, which innervates the posterior compartment of the leg. The other major nerve in the region of the knee is the common fibular, which twists its way around the head and neck of the fibula. The common fibular nerve innervates muscles of the anterior and lateral compartments of the leg via the deep and superficial fibular nerves, respectively.

INDICATIONS

In an unreduced knee, dislocation is relatively straightforward to diagnose. The possibility of a missed diagnosis arises when there is only partial displacement, spontaneous reduction has occurred, or distracting injuries are present. Signs suggesting an underlying dislocation are extensive dermabrasions and swelling of the joint, genu recurvatum (backward bending of the knee), and varus and valgus laxity.

Once a diagnosis has been made, prompt neurovascular assessment should follow. This involves palpation of the dorsalis pedis and posterior tibial pulses bilaterally to assess for symmetry. There is disagreement regarding the need for measuring the ankle-brachial index or using angiography for vascular assessment. However, computed tomographic or magnetic resonance angiography is recommended for patients with signs and symptoms of a poorly perfused limb or asymmetrical findings on physical examination.

Neurological sensation in the tibial, deep fibular, and superficial fibular distributions must be assessed. Motor function is determined by the range of motion and power of the flexor and extensor hallucis longus, tibialis anterior, and gastrocnemius. The incidence of neurovascular injury varies but is increased in open injuries.

Following a rapid but careful assessment of neurovascular function, reduction should be attempted immediately because delays may have dire consequences.

CONTRAINDICATIONS

There are no absolute contraindications to closed knee reduction. However, open reduction is preferred in some situations.

Failure of closed reduction is a possibility, albeit uncommon. It is usually suggestive of soft tissue entrapment within the medial side of the joint capsule. A skin dimple appearing between the medial femoral condyle and the medial tibial plateau as the knee is extended indicates buttonholing of the medial femoral condyle through the medial capsule. The tibial collateral ligament can also be drawn into the medial joint capsule by the traction applied to achieve reduction. Interposition of the vastus medialis has also been reported to cause irreducibility. In such cases, closed reduction should

no longer be attempted, and open reduction should be performed as quickly as possible.

Open knee dislocations require urgent surgery. Debridement and irrigation should be carried out promptly, and the injury-to-incision time must be minimized. Opinion on the timing of repair of any associated ligamentous injury varies. Open dislocations are associated with a higher incidence of neurovascular injury and therefore justify a more aggressive approach. For any patient with signs of a threatened limb, urgent surgical evaluation should be sought.

EQUIPMENT

Usually, only a skilled pair of hands is necessary to reduce a dislocated knee.

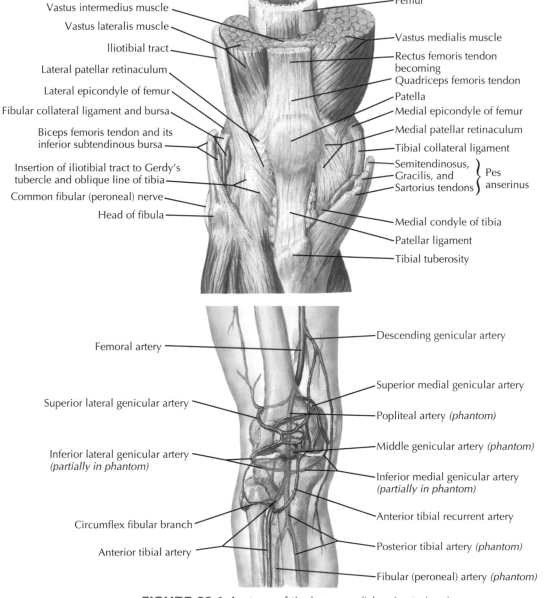

Right knee in extension

Vastus intermedius muscle
Vastus lateralis muscle
Iliotibial tract
Lateral patellar retinaculum
Lateral epicondyle of femur
Fibular collateral ligament and bursa
Biceps femoris tendon and its inferior subtendinous bursa
Insertion of iliotibial tract to Gerdy's tubercle and oblique line of tibia
Common fibular (peroneal) nerve
Head of fibula

Femur
Vastus medialis muscle
Rectus femoris tendon becoming
Quadriceps femoris tendon
Patella
Medial epicondyle of femur
Medial patellar retinaculum
Tibial collateral ligament
Semitendinosus, Gracilis, and Sartorius tendons } Pes anserinus
Medial condyle of tibia
Patellar ligament
Tibial tuberosity

Femoral artery
Superior lateral genicular artery
Inferior lateral genicular artery (partially in phantom)
Circumflex fibular branch
Anterior tibial artery

Descending genicular artery
Superior medial genicular artery
Popliteal artery (phantom)
Middle genicular artery (phantom)
Inferior medial genicular artery (partially in phantom)
Anterior tibial recurrent artery
Posterior tibial artery (phantom)
Fibular (peroneal) artery (phantom)

FIGURE 20.1 Anatomy of the knee: medial and anterior views

PROCEDURE

See Fig. 20.2.

1. Place the patient under conscious sedation.
2. After palpating anatomical landmarks, extend the knee with the aid of gentle inline traction.
3. Avoid manual pressure, especially in the popliteal area, because it can lead to iatrogenic neurovascular injury.
4. Reassessment after initial reduction is critical for detecting any missed neurovascular injury and its sequelae. The integrity of the popliteal artery and the common fibular nerve must be gauged at this time.
5. Immobilization of the limb is recommended after reassessment. This removes pressure from the soft tissues and somewhat reduces pain. It also ensures that neurovascular injury does not develop or worsen due to movement. Immobilization should be performed with the knee in approximately 20 degrees of flexion to preclude posterior slippage of the tibia. Circumferential casting or splinting should be avoided as this can hinder monitoring for compartment syndrome. Rigid casts can further restrict the leg compartment, contributing to increased intrafascial pressures.

To confirm successful reduction, radiography should follow immobilization. Imaging of the joints above and below the knee should also be obtained. The ankle-brachial index and angiography at this point are also recommended by some.

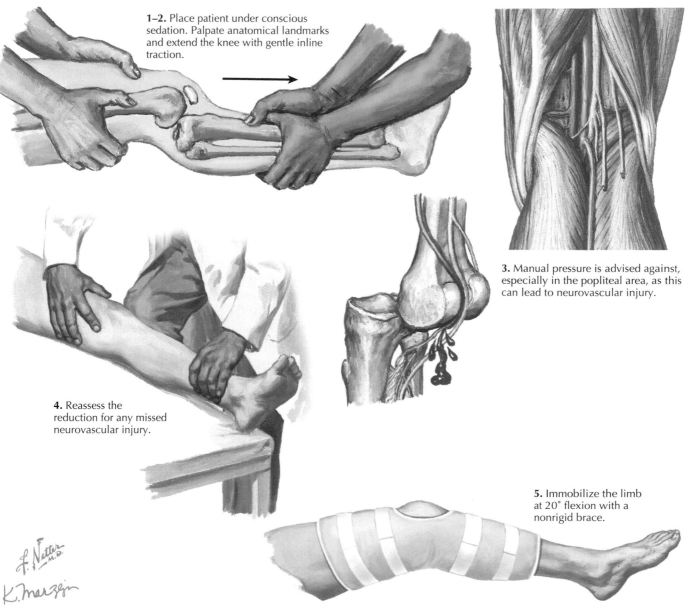

1–2. Place patient under conscious sedation. Palpate anatomical landmarks and extend the knee with gentle inline traction.

3. Manual pressure is advised against, especially in the popliteal area, as this can lead to neurovascular injury.

4. Reassess the reduction for any missed neurovascular injury.

5. Immobilize the limb at 20° flexion with a nonrigid brace.

FIGURE 20.2 Dislocated knee reduction

ANATOMICAL PITFALLS

The popliteal artery courses very close to the posterior aspect of the knee joint capsule and is separated from it by only a thin layer of fat. It is tethered both proximally and distally to the knee joint at the adductor hiatus and the arch of the soleus, respectively. These factors contribute to the risk of popliteal artery injury accompanying knee dislocation. Although the knee is surrounded by a prominent arterial network, collateral blood flow to the leg is limited. The lower leg depends almost entirely on the popliteal artery for its supply of oxygenated blood. Injury to this artery therefore entails a serious threat to the leg in knee dislocations.

COMPLICATIONS

Attempting to reduce the dislocation does not present much risk to the patient. However, forceful efforts at reduction can lead to injury to the nerves or vessels. Paresthesia, loss of sensation, or decreased or absent motor function are possible manifestations of neural injury. The most feared complication associated with knee dislocation is soft tissue injury leading to compartment syndrome and limb disability or loss. Injury to the popliteal artery can occur in the form of complete disruption, intraluminal thrombus, intimal tears, or vasospasm. Signs indicating arterial impairment include a change in skin color, asymmetric pulses, temperature changes in the limb, increasing leg pain, paresthesia, and paralysis.

CONCLUSIONS

In this uncommon orthopedic emergency, time is of the essence and the index of suspicion must be high. Closed reduction should be attempted as soon as possible once dislocation of the knee has been confirmed because delays can pose a serious threat to limb survival. Reduction should be done gently, with care taken to avoid iatrogenic injury. Reassessment is crucial to monitor for popliteal artery and common fibular nerve injuries.

Suggested Readings

Boyce RH, Singh K, Obremskey WT. Acute management of traumatic knee dislocations for the generalist. *J Am Acad Orthop Surg*. 2015;23:761–768.

Cinar M, Derincek A, Akpinar S. Irreducible dislocation of the knee joint: two-stage treatment. *Acta Othop Traumatol*. 2011;45:280–283.

Edwards GA, Sarasin SM, Davies AP. Dislocation of the knee: an epidemic in waiting? *J Emerg Med*. 2013;44:68–71.

Hirschmann MT, Müller W. Complex function of the knee joint: the current understanding of the knee. *Knee Surg Sports Traumatol Arthrosc*. 2015;23:2780–2788.

Howells NR, Brunton LR, Robinson J, Porteus AJ, Eldridge JD, Murray JR. Acute knee dislocation: an evidence based approach to the management of the multiligament injured knee. *Injury*. 2011;42:1198–1204.

Kishner S. Knee Joint Anatomy. Available at http://emedicine.medscape.com/article/1898986-overview#a2; 2015.

Lachman JR, Rehman S, Pipitone PS. Traumatic knee dislocations: evaluation, management, and surgical treatment. *Orthop Clin North Am*. 2015;46:479–493.

Paulin E, Boudabbous S, Nicodème JD, Arditi D, Becker C. Radiological assessment of irreducible posterolateral knee subluxation after dislocation due to interposition of the vastus medialis: a case report. *Skel Radiol*. 2015;44:883–888.

Peskun CJ, Levy BA, Fanelli GC, et al. Diagnosis and management of knee dislocations. *Phys Sportsmed*. 2010;38:101–111.

Skelley NW, McCormick JJ, Smith MV. In-game management of common joint dislocations. *Sports Health*. 2014;6:246–255.

Steele HL, Singh A. Vascular injury after occult knee dislocation presenting as compartment syndrome. *J Emerg Med*. 2012;42:271–274.

REVIEW QUESTIONS

1. During a football game, a 21-year-old wide receiver was illegally blocked by a linebacker, who threw himself against the posterolateral aspect of the runner's left knee. As he lay on the ground, the wide receiver grasped his knee in obvious pain. Which of the following structures is frequently subject to injury from this type of force against the knee?

   A. Fibular collateral ligament
   B. Anterior cruciate ligament
   C. Lateral meniscus and posterior cruciate ligament
   D. Fibular collateral and posterior cruciate ligament
   E. All the ligaments of the knee will be affected

2. A 34-year-old power lifter visits the outpatient clinic because he has difficulty walking. During physical examination, it is observed that the patient has a problem unlocking the knee joint to permit flexion of the leg. Which of the following muscles is most likely damaged?

   A. Biceps femoris
   B. Gastrocnemius
   C. Popliteus
   D. Semimembranosus
   E. Rectus femoris

3. A 55-year-old cowboy is admitted to the emergency department after he was knocked from his feet by a young longhorn steer. Magnetic resonance imaging reveals a large hematoma in the knee joint. Physical examination reveals that the patient suffers from the "unhappy triad" (of O'Donoghue). Which of the following structures are involved in such an injury?

   A. Tibial collateral ligament, medial meniscus, and anterior cruciate ligament
   B. Fibular collateral ligament, lateral meniscus, and posterior cruciate ligament
   C. Tibial collateral ligament, lateral meniscus, and anterior cruciate ligament
   D. Fibular collateral ligament, medial meniscus, and anterior cruciate ligament
   E. Tibial collateral ligament, medial meniscus, and posterior cruciate ligament

4. A 23-year-old man is admitted to the emergency department after injuring his knee while playing football. On physical examination, there is pain, swelling, and locking of the knee. Radiographic examination reveals a bucket-handle meniscal tear. Which of the following ligaments is most likely injured?

A. Posterior cruciate ligament
B. Tibial collateral ligament
C. Fibular collateral ligament
D. Anterior cruciate ligament
E. Coronary ligament

5. A 24-year-old woman receives a lateral blow to the knee during a tackle in a football game. Field examination reveals an "anterior drawer sign" Magnetic resonance imaging demonstrates injury to several structures of the knee, including her medial meniscus. Which structure might also have been injured by the tackle?

A. Tibial collateral ligament
B. Fibular collateral ligament
C. Lateral meniscus
D. Posterior cruciate ligament
E. Tendon of the semitendinosus

Dislocated Shoulder Joint Reduction

INTRODUCTION

The shoulder, or glenohumeral joint, is the most frequently dislocated joint in the body. The most common type of dislocation is an anterior shoulder dislocation, with posterior and inferior dislocations being much less common.

CLINICALLY RELEVANT ANATOMY

The glenohumeral joint is a diarthrotic joint with a very wide range of motion. However, this also makes it one of the more unstable joints in the body. The joint consists of the articulation of the glenoid fossa of the scapula, which is a shallow space, with the head of the humerus (Figs. 21.1 and 21.2). The glenoid labrum is a cartilaginous complex that offers additional support along the edge of the joint. Support is provided anteroinferiorly by the inferior glenohumeral ligament. This ligament is a primary deterrent to anterior dislocations.

Additional support to the glenohumeral joint is contributed by the rotator cuff muscles. The subscapularis is a thick muscle that crosses anterior to the scapulohumeral joint to attach to the humerus. It holds the head of the humerus in the glenoid cavity during movement. The supraspinatus, infraspinatus, and teres minor muscles perform a similar function posteriorly.

Shoulder dislocations are classified as anterior, posterior, or inferior. The most common type is anterior (Fig. 21.3), which is further divided according to where the head of the humerus lies, that is, subcoracoid, subglenoid, subclavicular, or intrathoracic. The latter two are uncommon.

Over 95% of dislocations of the glenohumeral joint are anterior dislocations. Typically, there is a strong blow to the arm when it is abducted, laterally rotated, and extended. This drives the humeral head out of the glenoid cavity, tearing the anterior bony and soft tissues. Tearing of the labrum is known as a Bankart lesion, which, in a small percentage of cases, includes a fracture of the glenoid. As the humeral head exits the cavity, it vigorously strikes the anteroinferior portion of the glenoid, resulting in a cortical depression or a fracture in the posterior aspect of the head of the humerus, known as a Hill-Sachs lesion.

Posterior dislocation occurs at a rate of less than 4%, and inferior glenohumeral dislocations are even less frequent, occurring in less than 1% of cases. Posterior dislocations usually occur with violent seizures or electrocution injuries, owing to severe muscle contractions that cause adduction and medial rotation of the humeral head. Inferior dislocations, also called *luxatio erecta*, occur with forceful hyperextension of the arm. This type of injury pushes the humeral head inferior to the coracoid or glenoid. It has the highest rate of complications involving neurovascular structures and bones.

INDICATIONS

Shoulder reduction is indicated for any type of acute dislocation of the humerus from the glenohumeral joint.

CONTRAINDICATIONS

Absolute Contraindications

Intrathoracic and subclavicular dislocations require surgical consultation, as do fractures involving the humerus. Standard reduction techniques place these patients at high risk for avascular necrosis of the humeral head and further neurovascular compromise of the limb.

Relative Contraindications

Nerve injuries to the brachial plexus or its branches (eg, median and axillary nerves) are a relative contraindication to closed reduction. Part of the physical examination of a dislocated shoulder includes evaluation to ensure that there are no sensory deficits, especially in the area of the deltoid muscle. Suspected arterial injury is also a relative contraindication and may require prompt arteriography. Other relative contraindications include common factures associated with shoulder dislocations such as Hill-Sachs lesions and avulsion fractures of the greater tuberosity.

EQUIPMENT

Materials used vary with the type of procedure that is selected. An assistant is needed, and equipment includes a 10- to 15-lb weight, a bed sheet, and medications.

PROCEDURE

Obtain patient consent and perform a time out.

Typical reduction methods involve traction and countertraction. When choosing a specific method, certain questions need to be taken into consideration. Is the patient able to tolerate the procedure? Does the patient require local anesthesia with lidocaine? Would conscious sedation be more appropriate? Most shoulder reductions in the emergency department are performed with local anesthesia or intravenous sedation, since the procedure is painful. Another important factor to consider is the physician's experience in performing the procedure. Physicians should be comfortable with several different reduction approaches because no single method is universally successful.

Anterior view

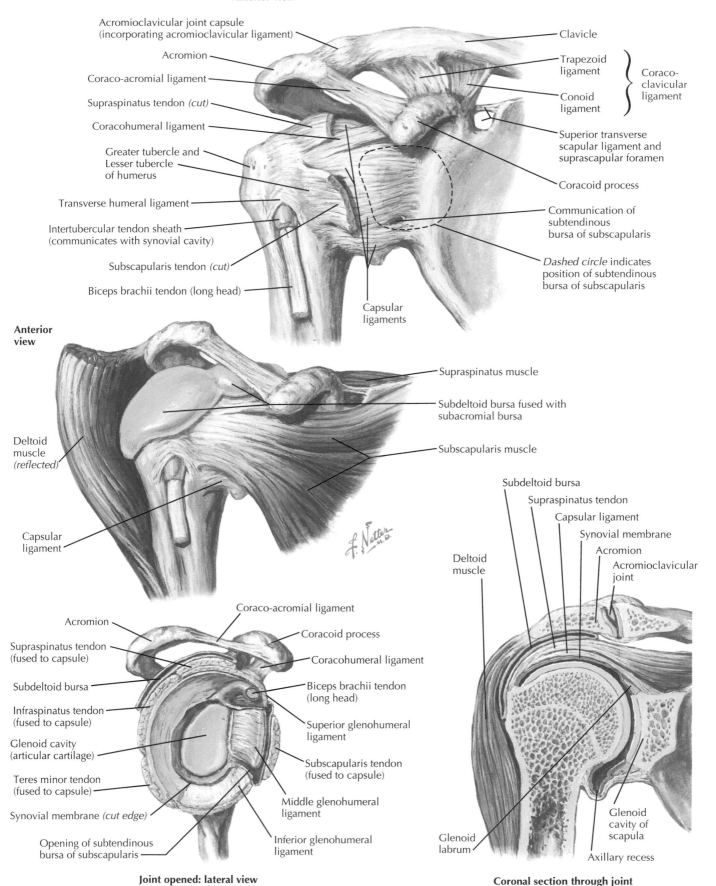

Acromioclavicular joint capsule (incorporating acromioclavicular ligament)

Acromion

Coraco-acromial ligament

Supraspinatus tendon *(cut)*

Coracohumeral ligament

Greater tubercle and Lesser tubercle of humerus

Transverse humeral ligament

Intertubercular tendon sheath (communicates with synovial cavity)

Subscapularis tendon *(cut)*

Biceps brachii tendon (long head)

Clavicle

Trapezoid ligament

Conoid ligament

} Coraco-clavicular ligament

Superior transverse scapular ligament and suprascapular foramen

Coracoid process

Communication of subtendinous bursa of subscapularis

Dashed circle indicates position of subtendinous bursa of subscapularis

Capsular ligaments

Anterior view

Deltoid muscle *(reflected)*

Capsular ligament

Supraspinatus muscle

Subdeltoid bursa fused with subacromial bursa

Subscapularis muscle

Subdeltoid bursa

Supraspinatus tendon

Capsular ligament

Synovial membrane

Acromion

Acromioclavicular joint

Deltoid muscle

Glenoid labrum

Glenoid cavity of scapula

Axillary recess

Coraco-acromial ligament

Acromion

Supraspinatus tendon (fused to capsule)

Subdeltoid bursa

Infraspinatus tendon (fused to capsule)

Glenoid cavity (articular cartilage)

Teres minor tendon (fused to capsule)

Synovial membrane *(cut edge)*

Opening of subtendinous bursa of subscapularis

Coracoid process

Coracohumeral ligament

Biceps brachii tendon (long head)

Superior glenohumeral ligament

Subscapularis tendon (fused to capsule)

Middle glenohumeral ligament

Inferior glenohumeral ligament

Joint opened: lateral view

Coronal section through joint

FIGURE 21.1 Shoulder (glenohumeral joint)

Axilla: Posterior Wall

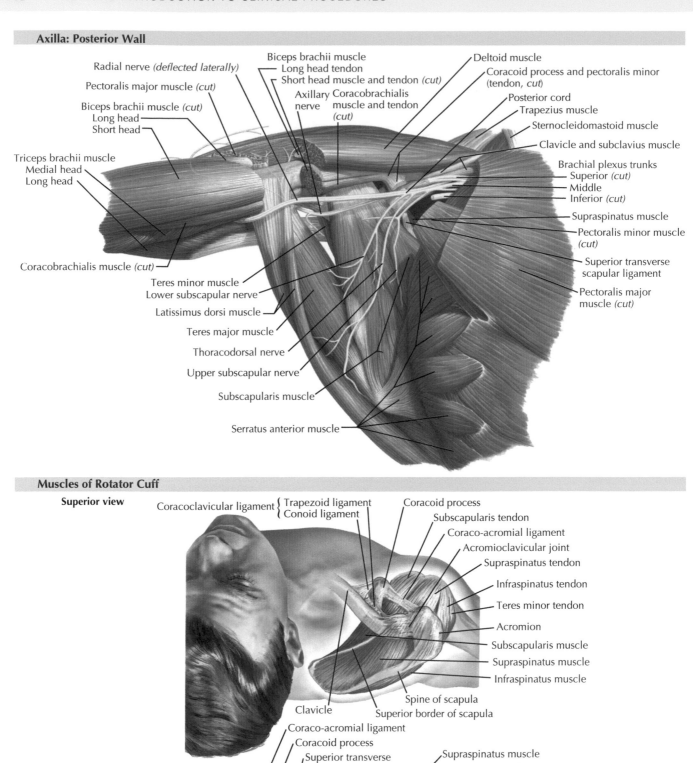

Radial nerve *(deflected laterally)*
Pectoralis major muscle *(cut)*
Biceps brachii muscle *(cut)*
Long head
Short head
Triceps brachii muscle
Medial head
Long head
Coracobrachialis muscle *(cut)*
Teres minor muscle
Lower subscapular nerve
Latissimus dorsi muscle
Teres major muscle
Thoracodorsal nerve
Upper subscapular nerve
Subscapularis muscle
Serratus anterior muscle

Biceps brachii muscle
Long head tendon
Short head muscle and tendon *(cut)*
Axillary nerve
Coracobrachialis muscle and tendon *(cut)*

Deltoid muscle
Coracoid process and pectoralis minor *(tendon, cut)*
Posterior cord
Trapezius muscle
Sternocleidomastoid muscle
Clavicle and subclavius muscle
Brachial plexus trunks
Superior *(cut)*
Middle
Inferior *(cut)*
Supraspinatus muscle
Pectoralis minor muscle *(cut)*
Superior transverse scapular ligament
Pectoralis major muscle *(cut)*

Muscles of Rotator Cuff

Superior view

Coracoclavicular ligament { Trapezoid ligament
Conoid ligament
Coracoid process
Subscapularis tendon
Coraco-acromial ligament
Acromioclavicular joint
Supraspinatus tendon
Infraspinatus tendon
Teres minor tendon
Acromion
Subscapularis muscle
Supraspinatus muscle
Infraspinatus muscle
Spine of scapula
Superior border of scapula
Clavicle

Coraco-acromial ligament
Coracoid process
Acromion
Superior transverse scapular ligament and suprascapular foramen
Supraspinatus tendon
Biceps brachii tendon (long head)
Subscapularis muscle

Supraspinatus muscle
Spine of scapula
Acromion
Supraspinatus tendon
Infraspinatus muscle
Teres minor muscle
Axillary nerve

Anterior view   **Posterior view**

FIGURE 21.2 Axilla and muscles of rotator cuff

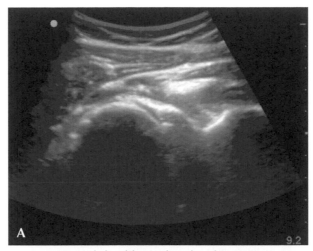

Normal shoulder (reduced in this case)

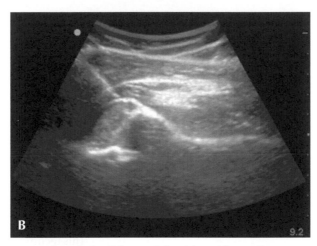

Anteriorly dislocated shoulder with needle

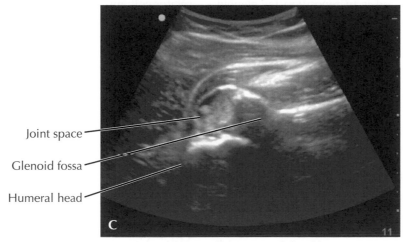

Anterior dislocation of shoulder

FIGURE 21.3 Ultrasound of normal (**A**) and anteriorly dislocated (**B** and **C**) shoulder joint

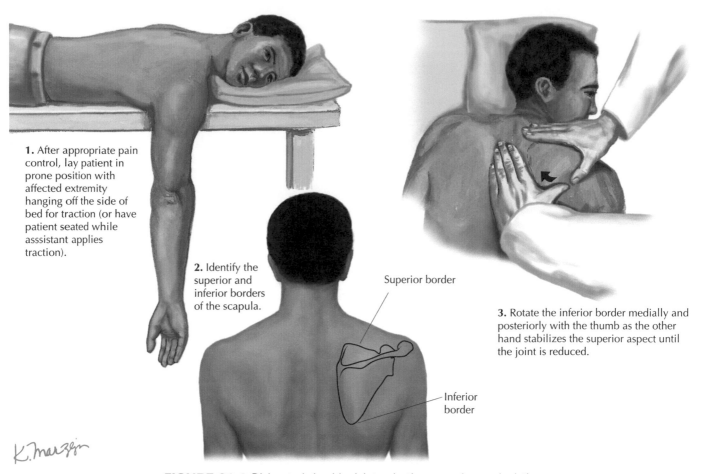

1. After appropriate pain control, lay patient in prone position with affected extremity hanging off the side of bed for traction (or have patient seated while assistant applies traction).

2. Identify the superior and inferior borders of the scapula.

Superior border

3. Rotate the inferior border medially and posteriorly with the thumb as the other hand stabilizes the superior aspect until the joint is reduced.

Inferior border

FIGURE 21.4 Dislocated shoulder joint reduction: scapular manipulation

Anterior Shoulder Dislocation Reduction Techniques

Scapular Manipulation

See Fig. 21.4.

The purpose of this method is to reposition the glenoid fossa in order to release the humeral head and allow it to reduce into the glenoid fossa.

1. The patient is seated and given appropriate pain control. An assistant gently pulls the affected arm for traction. The patient may also lie in the prone position with the arm hanging off the side of the bed for traction.
2. Identify the superior and inferior borders of the scapula.
3. Rotate the inferior border medially and posteriorly with the thumb as the other hand stabilizes the superior aspect.

Upright Best-of-Both Maneuver

This is another preferred and simple technique to perform. It is a variation of scapular manipulation and hence repositions the glenoid fossa to achieve reduction.

1. The patient is seated and given appropriate pain control. The assistant applies traction by pulling the affected arm forward and down while the clinician pushes the inferior tip of the scapula medially and the acromion downwards.
2. This causes rotation of the scapula and allows for reduction of the humeral head into the glenoid fossa.

Lateral Rotation Maneuver

See Fig. 21.5.

This technique only requires one clinician. It is safe, easy to perform, and has relatively few complications. It utilizes the rotator cuff muscles that laterally rotate the shoulder to overcome spasm of the medial rotators and reduce the humeral head back into the glenoid fossa.

1. Give appropriate pain control. The patient can either be seated or lying supine with the elbow flexed to 90 degrees and adducted.
2. Place one hand on the elbow to keep the arm adducted, and hold the patient's wrist with the opposite hand.
3. Gently and slowly laterally rotate the shoulder until the joint is reduced. This may take several attempts as the patient may experience pain or muscle spasm; with each attempt, however, the success rate increases. The reduction is very subtle, so it is easily missed, but it typically occurs when the arm is laterally rotated between 70 and 110 degrees.

Milch Maneuver

This method is easy to perform, is well tolerated, and has a very high success rate. It uses abduction and medial rotation of the shoulder with mild traction.

1. Give appropriate pain control. The patient lies supine with the affected arm close to the edge of the bed.

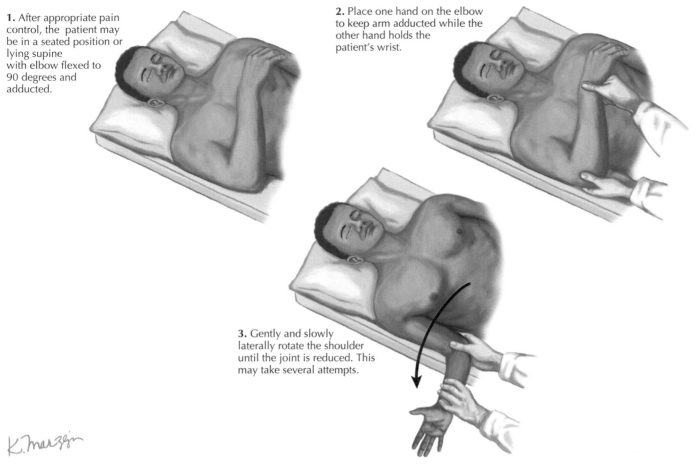

1. After appropriate pain control, the patient may be in a seated position or lying supine with elbow flexed to 90 degrees and adducted.

2. Place one hand on the elbow to keep arm adducted while the other hand holds the patient's wrist.

3. Gently and slowly laterally rotate the shoulder until the joint is reduced. This may take several attempts.

K. marzin

FIGURE 21.5 Dislocated shoulder joint reduction: lateral rotation maneuver

2. Have the patient abduct the arm while you laterally rotate it until it is over the head, applying gentle pressure in the axilla to obtain reduction.

Stimson Technique

This approach uses greater traction and is more time consuming; it should only be used if the above techniques are unsuccessful.

Give appropriate pain control. The patient lies prone with the affected arm hanging off the side of the bed with a 10- to 15-lb weight attached. Typically, reduction is achieved within 30 minutes.

Traction-Countertraction Technique

Give appropriate pain control. With the patient lying supine, wrap a bed sheet around the torso under the axilla as an assistant holds the elbow of the affected limb. Pull the sheet to apply traction to the axilla while the assistant applies countertraction to the elbow; gentle lateral rotation of the arm is used to ease the reduction. Reduction is more apparent with this technique, as an audible "clunk" is often heard as the humerus clicks back into place.

Spaso Maneuver

This technique has been reported to have a high success rate. Give appropriate pain control and have the patient lie supine. Hold the affected arm at the wrist. Lift the arm vertically toward the ceiling, simultaneously applying mild vertical traction. Maintain the traction and rotate the arm laterally. This should achieve reduction once the arm is placed back at the patient's side.

Other Techniques

Other techniques include the FARES, Cunningham, Eskimo, and Hippocrates techniques, and Kocher's method. Although these can be used, they carry greater risk to neurovascular structures.

Posterior Shoulder Dislocation Reduction Technique

Posterior shoulder dislocations are far less common than anterior dislocations. It is recommended to consult an orthopedic surgeon when dealing with such cases. Several factors must be addressed when deciding to perform a closed reduction.

Patients suffering from a posterior dislocation present with the arm medially rotated and adducted. Give appropriate pain control. Apply lateral traction to the adducted arm and countertraction with a sheet looped through the axilla. Push the humeral head anteriorly into the glenoid fossa. Once reduction is achieved, the arm should remain in neutral position in a sling.

Inferior Shoulder Dislocation Reduction Technique

Inferior shoulder dislocations are very rare but are easy to recognize when they do occur. The patient typically presents with the arm locked in abduction and the forearm flexed behind the head. In some instances, the humerus can be palpated just below the axilla. With this type of dislocation, fractures of the clavicle, acromion, and glenoid rim are possible. Neurovascular injuries are also associated with inferior dislocations. Consultation with an orthopedic surgeon is recommended if these injuries are present.

Give appropriate pain control. Apply overhead traction with gentle upward pressure on the humeral head while applying countertraction downward at the shoulder. Slowly adduct the arm, which should result in reduction. Open surgical reduction is required in cases where the head of the humerus is trapped in the inferior capsule by a tear referred to as a "buttonhole" defect.

Orthopedic Consultation

Several injuries associated with dislocation require orthopedic consultation prior to attempting reduction, regardless of the type of dislocation. These include fractures seen on prereduction imaging, articular surface defects such as a Hill-Sachs deformity affecting more than 25% of the humeral head, and dislocations older than 3 weeks. In many of these clinical situations, open reduction is advised. Surgery may also be necessary when closed reduction fails.

ANATOMICAL PITFALLS

Postreduction imaging after the procedure and follow-up are critical in preventing further complications (see Fig. 21.3). The most common complication of a shoulder dislocation is recurrent dislocation, which can occur in up to 90% of patients under 20 years of age and up to 10% of patients over 40 years of age. To prevent such an event, certain measures are advised, including immobilization with a sling, surgery, and rehabilitation.

Immobilization is traditionally used immediately after reduction. Although no specific position has been proven superior to others, the traditional and most common position places the arm in an adducted and medially rotated position. The patient is placed in a sling and swathe. Patients should be immobilized for 1 week and given a follow-up appointment with an orthopedic surgeon.

After successful closed reduction, surgery is recommended in patients who have soft tissue defects, such as bony spurs, Bankart lesions, or Hill-Sachs lesions. Repair should be performed within 10 days in order to prevent further instability and complications.

Rehabilitation is helpful in preventing recurrent dislocation. During the initial 3 weeks postreduction, patients should avoid any movement of the shoulder except while bathing or performing prescribed exercises, such as Codman's exercise (small circular movements of the affected arm). The patient should gradually strengthen the muscles of the shoulder and rotator cuff using weightless isometric exercises. The rehabilitation process can take up to 12 to 16 weeks, after which the patient can resume regular or limited sporting activities and exercises.

COMPLICATIONS

Complications of shoulder reduction include injury to neighboring nerves and vessels or a failed reduction. The most common complication is recurrent dislocation. The patient's age at the time of dislocation is inversely related to the rate of recurrence.

CONCLUSION

Knowledge of the regional anatomy and proficient technique are key to competently performing the reduction of a dislocation of the glenohumeral joint. This pathology is common, with 95% of dislocations occurring anteriorly. Thorough review of the procedural options and a methodological approach will contribute significantly to developing skill in reducing shoulder dislocations.

Suggested Readings

Cicak N. Posterior dislocation of the shoulder. *J Bone Joint Surg Br.* 2004;86:324.

Cutts S, Prempeh M, Drew S. Anterior shoulder dislocation. *Ann Royal Coll Surg Engl.* 2009;91(1):2–7.

Dodson CC, Cordasco FA. Anterior glenohumeral joint dislocations. *Orthop Clin North Am.* 2008;39(4):507–518.

Perron AD, Jones RL. Posterior shoulder dislocation: avoiding a missed diagnosis. *Am J Emerg Med.* 2000;18:189.

Robert JR, Hedges RJ. *Clinical Procedures in Emergency Medicine.* 4th ed. Philadelphia: Elsevier; 2004.

Sagarin MJ. Best of both (BOB) maneuver for rapid reduction of anterior shoulder dislocation. *J Emerg Med.* 2005;29:313.

Ufberg JW, Vilke GM, Chan TC, Harrigan RA. Anterior shoulder dislocations: beyond traction-countertraction. *J Emerg Med.* 2004;27:301.

Zacchilli MA, Owens BD. Epidemiology of shoulder dislocations presenting to emergency departments in the United States. *J Bone Joint Surg Am.* 2010;92:542.

REVIEW QUESTIONS

1. A 19-year-old man is brought to the emergency department after dislocating his shoulder while playing soccer. Following reduction of the dislocation, he has pain over the dorsal region of the shoulder and cannot abduct the arm normally. A magnetic resonance image of the shoulder shows a torn muscle. Which of the following muscles is most likely to have been damaged by this injury?

   A. Coracobrachialis
   B. Long head of the triceps brachii
   C. Pectoralis minor
   D. Supraspinatus
   E. Teres major

2. A 47-year-old female tennis professional is informed by her physician that she has a rotator cuff injury that will require surgery. Her physician explains that over the years

of play, a shoulder ligament has gradually caused severe damage to an underlying tendon. To which of the following ligaments is the physician most likely referring?

A. Acromioclavicular ligament
B. Coracohumeral ligament
C. Superior transverse scapular ligament
D. Glenohumeral ligament
E. Coracoacromial ligament

3. A 34-year-old female skier was taken by ambulance to the hospital after she struck a tree on the ski slope. Imaging demonstrates a shoulder separation. Which of the following typically occurs in this kind of injury?

A. Displacement of the head of the humerus from the glenoid cavity
B. Partial or complete tearing of the coracoclavicular ligament
C. Partial or complete tearing of the coracoacromial ligament
D. Rupture of the transverse scapular ligament
E. Disruption of the glenoid labrum

4. A 23-year-old male basketball player is admitted to the hospital after injuring his shoulder during a game. Physical and radiographic examinations reveal total separation of the shoulder. Which of the following structures has most likely been torn?

A. Glenohumeral ligament
B. Coracoacromial ligament
C. Tendon of long head of biceps brachii
D. Acromioclavicular ligament
E. Superior transverse scapular ligament

5. A 24-year-old female basketball player is admitted to the emergency department after an injury to her shoulder. Radiographic examination reveals a shoulder dislocation. What is the most commonly injured nerve in shoulder dislocations?

A. Axillary
B. Radial
C. Median
D. Ulnar
E. Musculocutaneous

Occipital Nerve Block

INTRODUCTION

Anesthetic nerve blocks have been used in many settings to alleviate pain. For the many people who suffer from occipital neuralgia or other cervicogenic headaches, an occipital nerve block can provide a diagnosis as well as therapeutic relief of pain. This chapter elucidates the relevant anatomy of the greater and lesser occipital nerves, indications for nerve block, technique, and possible complications.

CLINICALLY RELEVANT ANATOMY

The greater occipital nerve emerges as the medial branch of the C2 dorsal ramus and travels deep to the obliquus capitis inferior muscle (Figs. 22.1 and 22.2). It continues on an upward path posterior to the rectus capitis posterior major muscle before piercing the fibers of the semispinalis capitis dorsally. The nerve also passes deep to the trapezius muscle and then emerges to travel subcutaneously. In general, it courses medial to the occipital artery. The greater occipital nerve innervates the posterior scalp up to the vertex, as well as a portion of the skin of the posterior pinna.

The lesser occipital nerve arises from the ventral rami of C2 and C3. It ascends posterior to the sternocleidomastoid muscle, where it continues cephalad to pierce the deep fascia. It often communicates with the greater occipital nerve.

INDICATIONS

Occipital nerve block may provide a diagnosis of occipital neuralgia, which is confirmed by the relief of pain after performing the block. It is also done for therapeutic relief of occipital neuralgia, cervicogenic headache, and cluster headache. Observational studies report favorable results for the treatment of some migraines as well.

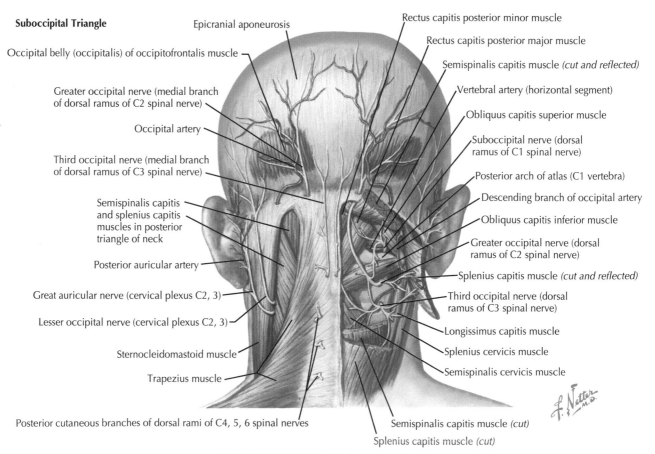

Suboccipital Triangle

Epicranial aponeurosis

Occipital belly (occipitalis) of occipitofrontalis muscle

Greater occipital nerve (medial branch of dorsal ramus of C2 spinal nerve)

Occipital artery

Third occipital nerve (medial branch of dorsal ramus of C3 spinal nerve)

Semispinalis capitis and splenius capitis muscles in posterior triangle of neck

Posterior auricular artery

Great auricular nerve (cervical plexus C2, 3)

Lesser occipital nerve (cervical plexus C2, 3)

Sternocleidomastoid muscle

Trapezius muscle

Posterior cutaneous branches of dorsal rami of C4, 5, 6 spinal nerves

Rectus capitis posterior minor muscle

Rectus capitis posterior major muscle

Semispinalis capitis muscle (cut and reflected)

Vertebral artery (horizontal segment)

Obliquus capitis superior muscle

Suboccipital nerve (dorsal ramus of C1 spinal nerve)

Posterior arch of atlas (C1 vertebra)

Descending branch of occipital artery

Obliquus capitis inferior muscle

Greater occipital nerve (dorsal ramus of C2 spinal nerve)

Splenius capitis muscle (cut and reflected)

Third occipital nerve (dorsal ramus of C3 spinal nerve)

Longissimus capitis muscle

Splenius cervicis muscle

Semispinalis cervicis muscle

Semispinalis capitis muscle (cut)

Splenius capitis muscle (cut)

FIGURE 22.1 Occipital nerve anatomy

CONTRAINDICATIONS

Occipital nerve block should not be performed in patients with a known or suspected allergy to steroids or anesthetic medications. Patients with active infection at the site of injection or a systemic infection should postpone this procedure until they are infection free. Additionally, it should not be performed for patients who are taking anticoagulants.

EQUIPMENT

- 25-gauge needle (⅝ to 1½ inch) with control-type syringe
- Local anesthetic (2% lidocaine or 0.5% bupivacaine)
- Antiseptic solution
- Alcohol prep pad
- Gloves
- Corticosteroid (2 to 4 mg betamethasone or 10 to 20 mg triamcinolone or methylprednisolone acetate injectable suspension, 40 mg/mL)
- Ultrasound machine with linear probe (optional)

PROCEDURE

Obtain patient consent and perform a time out.

The patient should be seated with the neck minimally flexed or vertically upright, with an assistant supporting the head anteriorly. The patient should be advised that locating the nerves may elicit discomfort or numbness along their distribution. To lessen the risk of intravascular injection, ultrasound guidance may be used to locate the nerves.

Locating the Greater Occipital Nerve

To locate the greater occipital nerve, palpate for the pulsation of the occipital artery; the greater occipital nerve lies immediately medial to this pulsating vessel along the superior nuchal line, approximately 2 to 3 cm lateral to the external occipital protuberance (1 to 1.5 thumb's breadth).

Ultrasound can be used to locate the nerve and the artery.

Locating the Lesser Occipital Nerve

Once the greater occipital nerve has been located, the lesser occipital nerve can be found 2 to 3 cm lateral to the greater occipital nerve, also along the superior nuchal line.

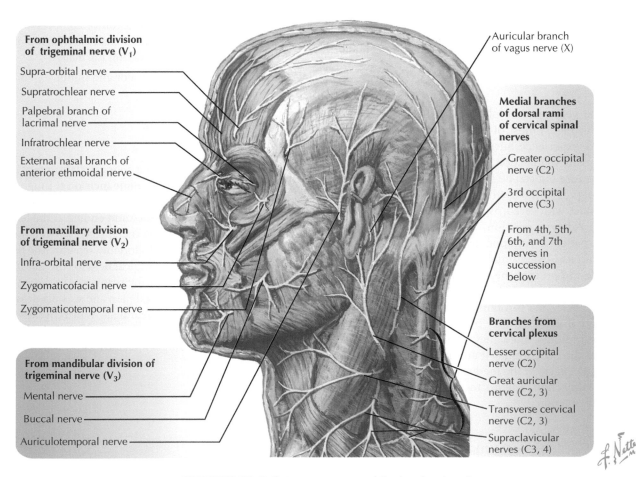

From ophthalmic division of trigeminal nerve (V₁)

Supra-orbital nerve

Supratrochlear nerve

Palpebral branch of lacrimal nerve

Infratrochlear nerve

External nasal branch of anterior ethmoidal nerve

From maxillary division of trigeminal nerve (V₂)

Infra-orbital nerve

Zygomaticofacial nerve

Zygomaticotemporal nerve

From mandibular division of trigeminal nerve (V₃)

Mental nerve

Buccal nerve

Auriculotemporal nerve

Auricular branch of vagus nerve (X)

Medial branches of dorsal rami of cervical spinal nerves

Greater occipital nerve (C2)

3rd occipital nerve (C3)

From 4th, 5th, 6th, and 7th nerves in succession below

Branches from cervical plexus

Lesser occipital nerve (C2)

Great auricular nerve (C2, 3)

Transverse cervical nerve (C2, 3)

Supraclavicular nerves (C3, 4)

FIGURE 22.2 Cutaneous nerves of the head and neck

Once the desired nerve has been located, follow these steps for occipital nerve block (Fig. 22.3):

1. Sterilize the scalp with antiseptic solution, followed by an alcohol prep pad.
2. Draw up injectate (either A or B below) into the syringe.
   a. Injectate A: 2% lidocaine with 2 to 4 mg betamethasone or 10 to 20 mg triamcinolone, for a total of 3 mL.
   b. Injectate B: 1.7 mL bupivacaine with 0.3 mL methylprednisolone acetate, for a total of 2 mL.
3. Insert the needle toward the nerve, directed perpendicularly (90 degrees) to the occiput.
4. Once the needle reaches a bony endpoint, aspirate to ensure that the needle is not in a blood vessel.
5. Inject 1 mL with the needle in this position (directly toward the nerve), and inject the remaining solution into the area around the nerve on either side.
6. Withdraw the needle and apply pressure over the injection site to achieve hemostasis.
7. Apply a sterile, dry dressing to the injection site.
8. Reevaluate the patient after 15 to 20 minutes.

NOTE: To avoid postinjection soreness, apply ice to the injection site.

ANATOMICAL PITFALLS

The skin of the occiput is innervated by several nerves. These include the greater, lesser, and third occipital nerves. These nerves have a variable course and often freely communicate with one another. The occipital artery must be avoided during injections into the occiput. This vessel usually lies about 3 cm lateral to the midline and just lateral to the greater occipital nerve.

COMPLICATIONS

There should be very few complications when performing an occipital nerve block, most of which are relatively minor. The patient may experience burning, redness, infection, or numbness at the site of injection. Intravascular injection is a risk of this procedure but can be avoided by following proper aspiration techniques to ensure that the needle tip is not in a vessel or in contact with cerebrospinal fluid in patients with cranial defects. Adverse reactions to the medication may occur in some patients. Additionally, as with any form of exogenous steroid use, overadministration of serial injections should be avoided to prevent the development of cushingoid features. It is therefore advised to perform no more than three occipital nerve blocks in a 6-month period. Patients should also be advised that although they may feel immediate relief of their pain symptoms, they may experience a rebound headache due to the injection itself around 2 days postinjection, with the true effects of the medication setting in around 3 to 5 days postinjection. Failure to respond to therapy is another possible outcome.

CONCLUSIONS

Multiple nerves can be involved in the generation of occipital neuralgia, and there are often multiple communications between these nerves. Therefore precise determination of which nerve is involved in generating the headache is very important in outlining treatment options.

Suggested Readings

International Headache Society. International Classification of Headache Disorders, 3rd edition. *Cephalagia*. 2013;33:629–808.

Jung SJ, Moon SK, Kim TY, Eom KS. A case of occipital neuralgia in the greater and lesser occipital nerves treated with neurectomy by using transcranial Doppler sonography: technical aspects. *Korean J Pain*. 2011;24(1):48–52.

Lee M, Brown M, Chepla K, et al. An anatomical study of the lesser occipital nerve and its potential compression points: implications for surgical treatment of migraine headaches. *Plast Reconstr Surg*. 2013;132(6):1551–1556.

Loukas M, El-Sedfy A, Tubbs RS, et al. Identification of greater occipital nerve landmarks for the treatment of occipital neuralgia. *Folia Morphol*. 2006;65(4):337–342.

Mosser SW, Guyuron B, Janis JE, Rohrich RJ. The anatomy of the greater occipital nerve: implications for the etiology of migraine headaches. *Plast Reconstru Surg*. 2004;113:693–697.

Ward J. Greater occipital nerve block. *Semin Neurol*. 2003;23(1):059–062.

Young WB, Marmura M, Ashkenazi A, Evans RW. Greater occipital nerve and other anesthetic injections for primary headache disorders. *Headache*. 2008;48:1122–1125.

REVIEW QUESTIONS

1. A 22-year-old man has suffered from headaches and some muscle weakness of the upper posterior deep neck muscles for the last 6 months. Magnetic resonance imaging shows a large tumor compressing the suboccipital and greater occipital nerves. Which of the following muscles will still function normally?

   A. Rectus capitis posterior major and minor
   B. Semispinalis capitis
   C. Trapezius
   D. Obliquus capitis superior
   E. Obliquus capitis inferior

2. A 48-year-old man underwent suboccipital surgery in which the surgeon made a midline incision through the ligamentum nuchae, beginning 1 cm inferior to the external occipital protuberance and ending at the level of the C2 vertebra. The surgeon then placed self-retaining retractors into the incision to forcibly separate the tissue and maintain an adequate surgical field for the duration of the 3-hour operation. During recovery, the patient complained of severe occipital pain and was diagnosed with postsurgical occipital neuralgia. Which of the following nerves was most likely directly stretched by the retractors during the surgery, resulting in this patient's postsurgical pain?

   A. Third occipital
   B. Suboccipital
   C. Greater occipital
   D. Lesser occipital
   E. Accessory

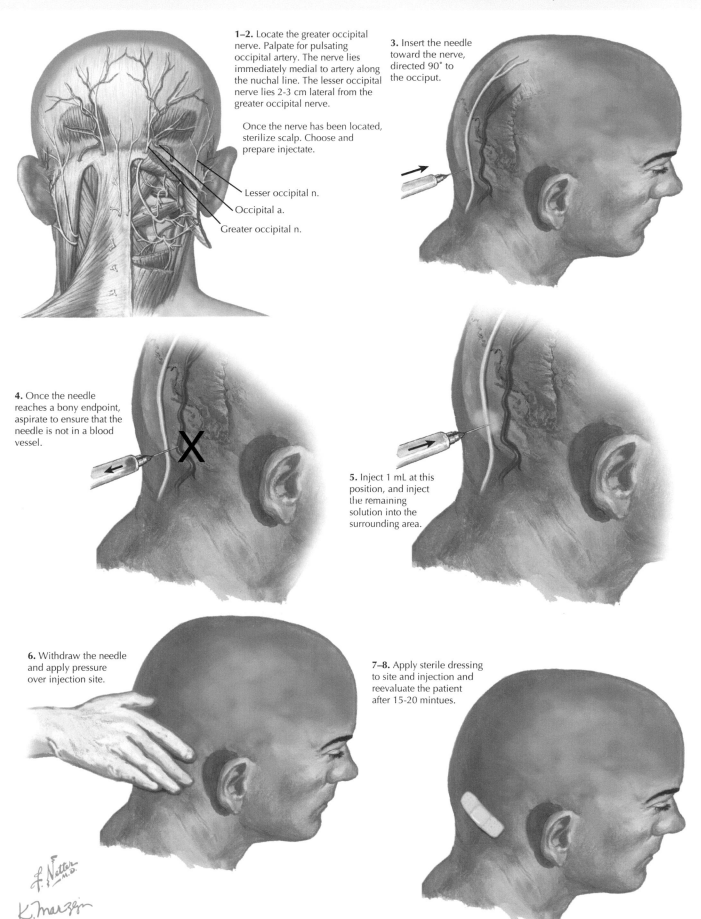

1–2. Locate the greater occipital nerve. Palpate for pulsating occipital artery. The nerve lies immediately medial to artery along the nuchal line. The lesser occipital nerve lies 2-3 cm lateral from the greater occipital nerve.

Once the nerve has been located, sterilize scalp. Choose and prepare injectate.

Lesser occipital n.

Occipital a.

Greater occipital n.

3. Insert the needle toward the nerve, directed 90° to the occiput.

4. Once the needle reaches a bony endpoint, aspirate to ensure that the needle is not in a blood vessel.

5. Inject 1 mL at this position, and inject the remaining solution into the surrounding area.

6. Withdraw the needle and apply pressure over injection site.

7–8. Apply sterile dressing to site and injection and reevaluate the patient after 15-20 mintues.

FIGURE 22.3 Occipital nerve block

Digital Nerve Block

INTRODUCTION

Digital nerve block is a commonly employed procedure performed in emergency departments to provide localized anesthesia to the skin of the middle and distal phalanges by injecting a local anesthetic. A digital nerve block allows subsequent procedures to be accomplished without causing pain.

CLINICALLY RELEVANT ANATOMY

Knowledge of the nerves to the digits is important for procedures such as incision and drainage of abscesses, debridement of regional wounds, felon treatment, ingrown nail removal, repair of nail beds, and reduction after toe fracture or dislocation. In the hand, these nerve branches arise from the ulnar, radial, and median nerves. In the palm, the median nerve divides into palmar digital branches that supply the medial and lateral aspects of the thumb, index finger, and middle finger, and the lateral aspect of the ring finger (Fig. 23.1). The palmar digital branches also provide sensation to the nail beds of these same areas. The ulnar nerve supplies both the palmar and dorsal aspects of the medial side of the ring finger and both sides of the little finger. For the dorsum of the remaining digits, the cutaneous supply is from the dorsal digital nerves of the radial nerve. Blood vessels travel with the palmar and dorsal digital nerves.

The nerves supplying the toes are branches of the fibular and tibial nerves. The medial plantar nerve supplies the plantar aspects of both sides of the first, second, and third toes and the medial aspect of the fourth toe. It also supplies the nail beds of the toes. The lateral sides of the fourth toe and both sides of the fifth toe are supplied by the lateral plantar nerve (see Fig. 23.1). The deep fibular nerve supplies the lateral side of the great toe and the medial side of the second toe dorsally. The remaining dorsal areas of the toes are supplied by the superficial fibular nerve.

INDICATIONS

Digital nerve block provides rapid analgesia, which is ideal in the acute setting and allows for treatment to be conducted comfortably. Digital nerve blocks are indicated for injuries distal to the middle phalanx, including foreign bodies, deep lacerations, paronychias with an abscess, felons, nail bed injuries, and nail avulsions.

CONTRAINDICATIONS

Digital nerve block should not be performed if there is an infection overlying the area, a history of allergy to the anesthetic, inadequate blood supply to the affected digit, prior nerve injury, or distortion of the superficial landmarks required for identification of the target nerves. The anesthetic chosen depends on the type of injury and the duration of action required. These agents may be combined with either bupivacaine or epinephrine to prolong the duration of the effect. Alternate methods of anesthesia should be considered in such cases, including topical and subcutaneous anesthetic agents. Epinephrine should be avoided in patients with an increased risk of ischemic injury, such as in those with peripheral vascular disease, due to its vasoconstrictive effect, and thus it is generally not used.

EQUIPMENT

- Local anesthetic (1% to 2% lidocaine or procaine, with or without epinephrine or bupivacaine)
- 5- to 10-mL syringe
- 18- to 22-gauge needle to draw up the anesthetic
- 25- to 30-gauge needle for injection
- Sterile gloves
- Sterile drapes
- Sterile gauze pads
- Povidone-iodine or chlorhexidine solution
- Alcohol wipes

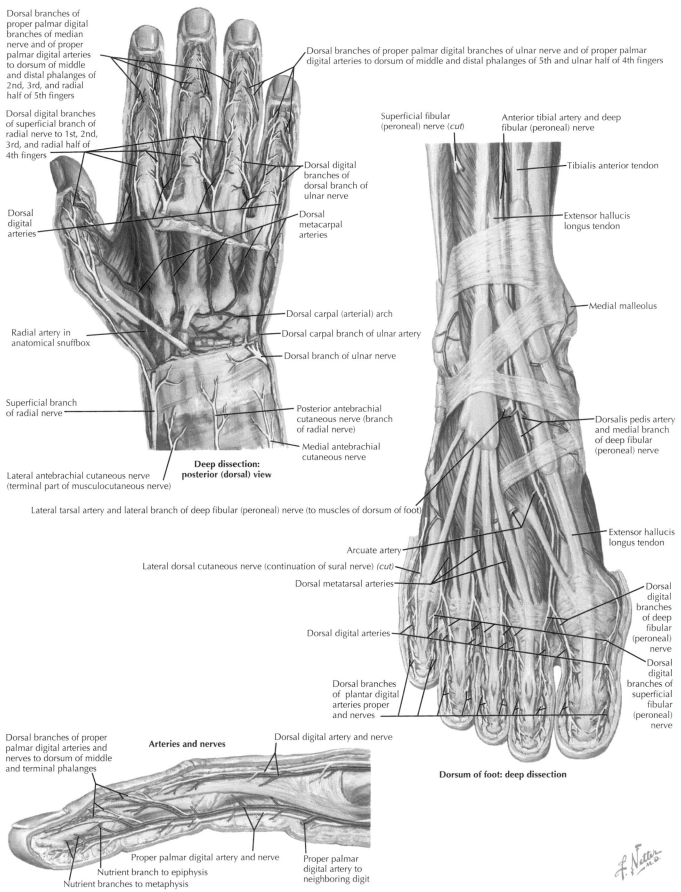

Dorsal branches of
proper palmar digital
branches of median
nerve and of proper
palmar digital arteries
to dorsum of middle
and distal phalanges of
2nd, 3rd, and radial
half of 5th fingers

Dorsal branches of proper palmar digital branches of ulnar nerve and of proper palmar
digital arteries to dorsum of middle and distal phalanges of 5th and ulnar half of 4th fingers

Dorsal digital branches
of superficial branch of
radial nerve to 1st, 2nd,
3rd, and radial half of
4th fingers

Dorsal
digital
arteries

Dorsal digital
branches of
dorsal branch of
ulnar nerve

Dorsal
metacarpal
arteries

Radial artery in
anatomical snuffbox

Dorsal carpal (arterial) arch

Dorsal carpal branch of ulnar artery

Dorsal branch of ulnar nerve

Superficial branch
of radial nerve

Posterior antebrachial
cutaneous nerve (branch
of radial nerve)

Medial antebrachial
cutaneous nerve

**Deep dissection:
posterior (dorsal) view**

Lateral antebrachial cutaneous nerve
(terminal part of musculocutaneous nerve)

Superficial fibular
(peroneal) nerve (*cut*)

Anterior tibial artery and deep
fibular (peroneal) nerve

Tibialis anterior tendon

Extensor hallucis
longus tendon

Medial malleolus

Dorsalis pedis artery
and medial branch
of deep fibular
(peroneal) nerve

Lateral tarsal artery and lateral branch of deep fibular (peroneal) nerve (to muscles of dorsum of foot)

Arcuate artery

Lateral dorsal cutaneous nerve (continuation of sural nerve) (*cut*)

Dorsal metatarsal arteries

Dorsal digital arteries

Extensor hallucis
longus tendon

Dorsal
digital
branches
of deep
fibular
(peroneal)
nerve

Dorsal
digital
branches of
superficial
fibular
(peroneal)
nerve

Dorsal branches
of plantar digital
arteries proper
and nerves

Dorsum of foot: deep dissection

Dorsal branches of proper
palmar digital arteries and
nerves to dorsum of middle
and terminal phalanges

Arteries and nerves

Dorsal digital artery and nerve

Proper palmar digital artery and nerve

Nutrient branch to epiphysis

Nutrient branches to metaphysis

Proper palmar
digital artery to
neighboring digit

FIGURE 23.1 Hand, foot, and finger dissections

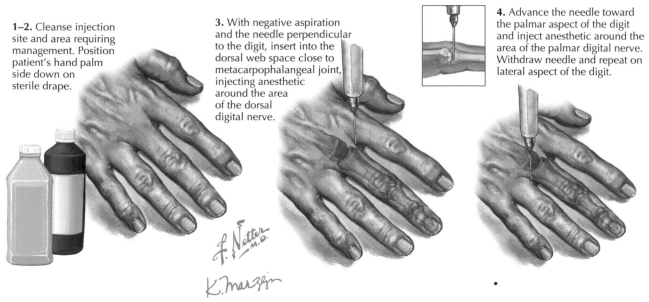

1–2. Cleanse injection site and area requiring management. Position patient's hand palm side down on sterile drape.

3. With negative aspiration and the needle perpendicular to the digit, insert into the dorsal web space close to metacarpophalangeal joint, injecting anesthetic around the area of the dorsal digital nerve.

4. Advance the needle toward the palmar aspect of the digit and inject anesthetic around the area of the palmar digital nerve. Withdraw needle and repeat on lateral aspect of the digit.

FIGURE 23.2 Finger web space block

PROCEDURE

Obtain patient consent and perform a time out. Don the proper personal protective equipment prior to performing any of the blocks listed below.

Finger Web Space Block (Traditional Digital Block) (Two-Injection Block)

The finger web space block is the most commonly employed procedure to provide anesthesia to the digit (Fig. 23.2). It can be applied to all of the fingers, including the thumb, and all of the toes except for the great toe.

1. Prepare the equipment and ensure the area is appropriately cleaned. Cleanse both the injection site and the area requiring treatment three times. If the affected digit is quite swollen or painful, a 5-minute soak in antibacterial solution can be used instead of scrubbing.
2. Position the patient's hand prone (palm side down) with the hand flat against a sterile drape.
3. Insert the needle into the dorsal aspect of the web space close to the metacarpophalangeal joint, with the needle perpendicular to the digit. Inject some anesthetic solution around the area of the dorsal digital nerve. Use a smaller-caliber needle to reduce the pain of the injection.
4. Carefully advance the needle through the palmar aspect of the digit, and inject around the area of the palmar digital nerve. After injecting a total of 1 to 3 mL of solution, withdraw the needle and repeat the same procedure on the other side of the digit.
   a. Alternatively, insert the needle from the dorsal aspect of the finger into the web space, directing it toward the metacarpophalangeal joint. Inject approximately 2 mL of anesthetic solution all at once halfway between the dorsal and palmar aspect of the digit. Withdraw the needle completely, and repeat on the other side of the digit. This modification is sometimes referred to as the metacarpal block.

Transthecal Block (Flexor Tendon Sheath Digital Block) (Volar Block)

The transthecal mode of anesthesia involves injecting anesthetic solution into the flexor tendon sheath. Although its efficacy is comparable to the subcutaneous and traditional web space blocks, the transthecal procedure is considered more painful and technically challenging to perform. This procedure can be used for all fingers and toes except for the great toe.

1. Identify the flexor tendon in the palm of the hand at the level of the distal palmar crease.
2. Ensure that the digit is adequately cleansed prior to the application of anesthesia.
3. Place the hand on a sterile drape in the supine position (palm up), with the fingers spread apart.
4. Insert the needle at a 45-degree angle toward the finger, just distal to the distal palmar crease, and push the needle into the flexor tendon sheath. Once inside the sheath, inject 1 to 2 mL of anesthetic solution. There should be a lack of resistance to the flow of fluid if the needle is properly in the sheath. If there is resistance, the needle may be against the tendon itself, which can be corrected by pulling the needle back slightly until there is a free flow of the anesthetic.

Subcutaneous Block (Volar Block) (SIMPLE: Single Subcutaneous Injection in the Midline of the Phalanx with Lidocaine and Epinephrine Block)

The subcutaneous block involves massaging the anesthetic solution into the tissues after injection just below the skin. Although several small studies have shown that the subcutaneous block is just as effective while causing lesser pain than the traditional web space and transthecal blocks, this technique may not be as effective at providing anesthesia to the dorsal aspect of the proximal digit. This procedure can be applied to all fingers and toes except for the great toe.

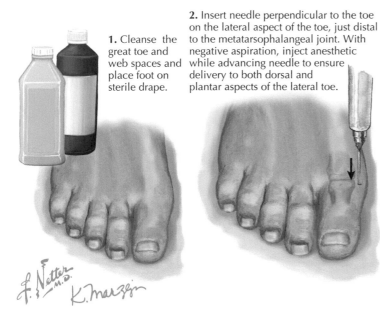

1. Cleanse the great toe and web spaces and place foot on sterile drape.

2. Insert needle perpendicular to the toe on the lateral aspect of the toe, just distal to the metatarsophalangeal joint. With negative aspiration, inject anesthetic while advancing needle to ensure delivery to both dorsal and plantar aspects of the lateral toe.

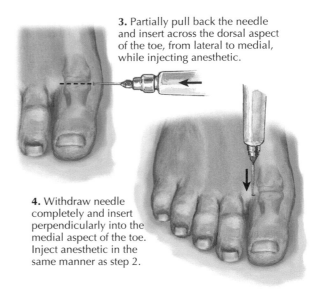

3. Partially pull back the needle and insert across the dorsal aspect of the toe, from lateral to medial, while injecting anesthetic.

4. Withdraw needle completely and insert perpendicularly into the medial aspect of the toe. Inject anesthetic in the same manner as step 2.

FIGURE 23.3 Three-sided toe block

1. Identify the proximal skin crease on the palmar aspect of the base of the affected finger.
2. Clean the skin and place the hand in the supine position with the hand open and the fingers outstretched onto a sterile drape.
3. With a sterile glove on the nondominant hand, pinch the soft tissue together just distal to the proximal skin crease to create a skin tent. With the other hand, insert the needle into this tissue tent in the middle of the skin crease just below the skin. After injecting 1 to 2 mL of anesthetic solution, massage it into the tissues.

Three-Sided Toe Block

Because the great toe and thumb have dorsal nerve branches in addition to the lateral and medial nerves, a modified block procedure must be utilized, such as the three-sided or four-sided toe block. The three-sided block is preferred over the four-sided block as it has a lesser risk of causing ischemic injury (Fig. 23.3).

1. Adequately cleanse the great toe and web spaces and then place the foot on a sterile drape with the plantar side down. Alternatively, the heel of the foot can be placed on the sterile drape and the nondominant hand used to stabilize the great toe.
2. Insert the needle perpendicular to the toe on the lateral aspect, just distal to the metatarsophalangeal joint. Once in the subcutaneous tissue, begin injecting anesthetic while advancing the needle towards the plantar aspect of the toe, ensuring that the anesthetic is delivered to both the dorsal and plantar aspects of the lateral side of the toe (approximately 1 to 2 mL of solution).
3. Partially pull back the needle and then insert it across the dorsal aspect of the toe (from the lateral to medial aspect of the dorsum of the toe) while injecting anesthetic.

4. Withdraw the needle completely and then insert it into the medial aspect of the toe, just distal to the metatarsophalangeal joint, into an area that was previously anesthetized. Inject anesthetic solution in the same manner as on the lateral side (from the dorsal to plantar aspect). With this technique, the lateral, medial, and dorsal aspects of the toe are anesthetized.

Four-Sided Ring Block

The four-sided ring block is similar to the three-sided toe block, with the addition of injection on the plantar surface of the toe as well, resulting in anesthesia in a ring-like configuration all the way around the toe.

1. Perform a three-sided ring block as above.
2. Remove the needle completely and then insert it parallel to the plane of the table into the lateral aspect of the toe on the plantar side into an area previously anesthetized, just distal to the metatarsophalangeal joint. As the needle is advanced towards the medial side of the toe, inject approximately 1 mL of anesthetic solution along the plantar aspect of the toe.

Unilateral Digital Block

A unilateral digital block is performed if there is a problem only affecting one side of the digit, such as a unilateral ingrown nail or an acute paronychia with abscess.

1. Adequately cleanse the digit and finger web space, and place the hand palmar side down on a sterile drape.
2. Place the needle on the affected side, perpendicular to the digit and parallel to the plane of the table. Insert the needle halfway between the dorsal and palmar aspects of the digit, at the base of the finger. If the needle hits bone, pull back 1 to 2 mm and then inject 0.5 mL of anesthetic solution.

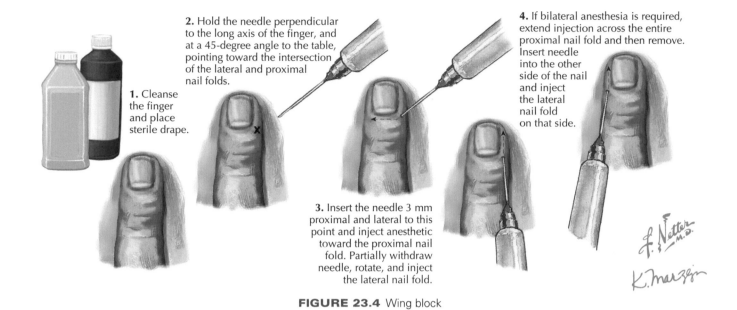

2. Hold the needle perpendicular to the long axis of the finger, and at a 45-degree angle to the table, pointing toward the intersection of the lateral and proximal nail folds.

1. Cleanse the finger and place sterile drape.

4. If bilateral anesthesia is required, extend injection across the entire proximal nail fold and then remove. Insert needle into the other side of the nail and inject the lateral nail fold on that side.

3. Insert the needle 3 mm proximal and lateral to this point and inject anesthetic toward the proximal nail fold. Partially withdraw needle, rotate, and inject the lateral nail fold.

FIGURE 23.4 Wing block

Wing Block

Sometimes a traditional digital block may not provide adequate anesthesia to the distal digit, especially if a procedure is needed on the nail plate, such as the removal of a nail. In such situations, a wing block may be performed, either in addition to another digital block procedure or on its own. The wing block may actually provide a faster onset of anesthesia compared with other digital blocks (Fig. 23.4). This procedure can be performed unilaterally or bilaterally and can be applied to the digits of either the hand or foot.

1. After adequate cleansing of the affected toe or finger, place the foot or hand with the plantar (or palmar) surface down on a sterile drape.
2. Hold the needle perpendicular to the long axis of the digit at a 45-degree angle to the table, pointing it toward the intersection of the lateral and proximal nail folds.
3. Insert the needle approximately 3 mm proximal and lateral to this intersection point and inject anesthetic solution into the deep dermis, towards the proximal nail fold. Partially withdraw the needle and then inject anesthetic solution towards the lateral nail fold. This procedure is called a wing block because the anesthetic solution blanches the skin along the lateral and proximal nail folds, creating a wing-like appearance.
4. If bilateral anesthesia is required, extend the anesthetic injection across the entire proximal nail fold and remove the needle. Insert the needle into the other side of the nail and inject across the lateral nail fold. If some sensation remains at the nail tip, inject anesthetic solution directly into that area.

ANATOMICAL PITFALLS

The close relationship between the digital nerves and accompanying blood vessels makes it possible to pierce a vessel while introducing the anesthetic needle. Prior to injecting the anesthetic solution, aspirate slowly. If there is blood return, remove the needle and reposition it.

Injection of the digital nerve itself can also occur, which can cause extreme pain. Again, the needle should be withdrawn slightly (approximately 2 mm) and then the anesthetic can be injected to bathe the nerve in the solution.

COMPLICATIONS

The most common complications of a digital nerve block are infection and bleeding. The patient may also have an allergic reaction to the anesthetic agent. More serious complications include damage to the nerve, which may result in digital paresthesia, or prolonged vasospasm or compression of vasculature, which may lead to distal digital infarction. Before the block is performed, a neurological examination should be performed in order to check for sensory deficits. If deficits are found, other methods of anesthesia should be considered.

CONCLUSION

The use of digital nerve blocks allows for the treatment of a myriad of digital injuries or infections. No one method is superior to the rest, and the decision on which one to use should be based on the practitioner's experience as well as the patient's comfort level. With proper technique, these procedures cause minimal discomfort and carry minimal risks.

Suggested Readings

Bashir MM, Khan FA, Khan BA. Comparison of traditional two injections dorsal digital block with volar block. *J Coll Physicians Surg Pak.* 2008;18:768–770.

Chowdry S, Seidenstricker L, Cooney D, et al. Do not use epinephrine in digital blocks: myth or truth? Part II. A retrospective review of 1111 cases. *Plast Reconstr Surg.* 2010;126:2031–2034.

Summers A. Use of digital nerve blocks to provide anaesthetic relief. *Emerg Nurse.* 2011;19:25–28.

Vinycomb TI, Sahhar LJ. Comparison of local anesthetics for digital nerve blocks: a systematic review. *Hand Surg [Am]*. 2014;39:744–751.

Wheelock ME, et al. Is it true that injecting palmar finger skin hurts more than dorsal skin? New level 1 evidence. *Hand*. 2011;6:47–49.

REVIEW QUESTIONS

1. A 35-year-old patient has a small but painful tumor under the nail of the little finger. Which of the following nerves would have to be anesthetized for painless removal of the tumor?

    A. Superficial radial nerve
    B. Common palmar digital of the median nerve
    C. Common palmar digital of the ulnar nerve
    D. Deep radial nerve
    E. Recurrent branch of the median nerve

2. A 48-year-old female piano player visited the outpatient clinic with numbness and tingling in her left hand. A diagnosis was made of nerve compression in the carpal tunnel, and the patient underwent an endoscopic nerve release. Two weeks postoperatively the patient com-plained of profound weakness in the thumb with loss of thumb opposition. The sensation to the hand, however, was unaffected. Which of the following nerves was injured during the operation?

    A. The first common digital branch of the median nerve
    B. The second common digital branch of the median nerve
    C. Recurrent branch of the median nerve
    D. Deep branch of the ulnar nerve
    E. Anterior interosseous nerve

3. A 16-year-old boy presents to the emergency department with a fracture of the first and second toes of his right foot. He receives an anesthetic injection in the first web space of his foot to permit easy manipulation and correction. Which nerve is blocked by the anesthesia?

    A. Saphenous nerve
    B. Cutaneous branch of deep fibular nerve
    C. Cutaneous branch of superficial fibular nerve
    D. Sural nerve
    E. Common fibular nerve

Dental Nerve Blocks

INTRODUCTION

Dental pathologies are not usually treated in the emergency department. However, dental-related emergency room visits are increasingly common. This can be partially attributed to underexamined or unnoticed dental disease and the lack of appropriate short- and long-term patient follow-up, as well as to the lack of access to dental care. Although, many dental pathologies are not inherently life threatening, if left untreated, there is a risk of spread of infection, foreign body aspiration, and airway compromise. Dental emergencies involving trauma may also present to the emergency department, where dental nerve blocks are necessary for pain management. All dental-related emergency department visits require clear and complete documentation of the patient's dental history and a thorough oral examination.

The medical interview should elicit information regarding the etiology or mechanism of injury, the frequency and duration of any symptoms, any aggravating and alleviating factors, details regarding the patient's self-management of the condition, and recent dental procedures. It is also important to determine whether the patient is experiencing any difficulty breathing, speaking, or swallowing because airway compromise can occur suddenly and warrants urgent medical management. In addition, any relevant medical history, such as diabetes or other immunocompromised status, bleeding or clotting disorders, tetanus immunization status, and allergies should be documented.

Oral examination should begin by recording the patient's vital signs. The gingiva of a healthy oral cavity should be moist, firm, and pink. It is important to check for malocclusion, tooth mobility, soft tissue lesions, or difficulty in opening the mouth. Percussion should be performed by tapping the crown of the tooth, which may elicit sensitivity secondary to infection. The maxilla and mandible should be assessed for tenderness and step-off or malocclusion, which may indicate an underlying bone fracture. The zygoma should be assessed for deformity and pain. The oral examination is not complete until the head and neck are assessed for any obvious trauma, facial asymmetry, swelling, decreased neck mobility, or lymphadenopathy. Dental radiography should be requested if there is any doubt regarding dental trauma or infection.

Dental emergencies may be trauma related or involve infections that range from a simple cavity or abscess to deeper life-threatening infections such as Ludwig angina. Dental blocks are used to provide adequate pain relief to allow full examination or to temporize until a dentist or oral surgeon can provide definitive dental treatment.

Dental emergencies include odontogenic infections, orofacial pain, and bleeding. Traumatic injury to the teeth, alveolar portions of the maxilla or mandible, and the surrounding soft tissue structures are common and can result in cracked, misaligned, or avulsed teeth. Management depends on the severity of the injury. Sometimes immediate intervention is required, but most patients need pain management, tetanus vaccination, and follow-up care by a dentist within 24 hours. Bleeding from the gums occurs secondary to surgery, trauma, or systemic or local disease. If a patient presents with excessive bleeding following a recent dental procedure, an underlying bleeding disorder should be ruled out.

Odontogenic infections refer to a range of pathologies that are initially limited to the tooth enamel (dental cavities) but which, if left untreated, may eventually penetrate into the dentin and pulp cavity (pulpitis), with the potential of spreading to the head and neck structures. Patients with odontogenic infections may present with pain, tooth mobility, cervical lymphadenopathy, fever, and malaise. Patients with chronic periodontal infections present late with intraoral drainage or chronic fistula. Facial cellulitis requires urgent treatment due to the risk of infection spreading to the brain and meninges. Ludwig angina refers to a particularly aggressive type of cellulitis that involves the sublingual, submandibular, and submental spaces bilaterally. The patient presents with fever, drooling, and difficulty in breathing and swallowing. Bilateral swelling may expand down the neck and mediastinum, compromising the airway. This warrants immediate airway management and intravenous antibiotic administration.

Orofacial pain is a frequent presenting complaint in the emergency department. Pain originating from the dental pulp is usually dull, pulsating, poorly localized, and extremely sensitive to thermal stimuli. However, tooth pain can also be referred from nonodontogenic sources such as the temporomandibular joint, neuralgias, intracranial pathologies, cervical spine, psychogenic conditions, and other contiguous anatomical structures. When indicated, the administration of local anesthesia may be performed to ensure patient compliance and comfort during emergency management. Anesthetic failure can be minimized with an appropriate understanding of the anatomy of the oral cavity.

CLINICALLY RELEVANT ANATOMY

The oral cavity consists of the oral vestibule, which lies between the teeth and cheeks, and the oral cavity proper, which is bordered by the dental arches, the hard and soft palates, the tongue and the floor of the month, and the oropharynx (Fig. 24.1). A tooth is made up of a crown and one or more root portions. The crown portion is visible above the gingiva, the soft tissue that surrounds the base of the tooth, and is composed of enamel, dentin, and pulp. The cementum is the outermost layer of the root portion, which is anchored to the alveolar bone of the maxilla or mandible by the periodontal ligament (Fig. 24.2). The maxilla is a bone of the midface that houses the upper teeth. The mandible is a mobile horseshoe-shaped bone made up of a body, ramus, and processes that provide attachment for the muscles of mastication and support for the mandibular teeth (see Fig. 24.2).

Clinically important nearby structures are the potential spaces and fascial planes that offer paths of minimal resistance to the spread of odontogenic infections. The sublingual space resides between the mucosa of the floor of the oral cavity and the mylohyoid muscle. It is bounded by the mandible and hyoid and communicates with the submandibular spaces posteriorly. The submandibular space lies inferior to the mylohyoid muscle and is bordered by the hyoglossus, styloglossus, and platysma muscles, the anterior and posterior bellies of the digastric muscle, and the adjacent mandible. The submental space is located anterior to the submandibular space (see Fig. 24.2). The superficial and deep cervical fasciae surround the muscles of the neck and provide potential pathways to the pharynx and face.

INDICATIONS

Indications for a dental nerve block include a dental abscess, pulpitis, orofacial injury and its repair, orofacial pain, and dental trauma.

CONTRAINDICATIONS

There are no absolute contraindications to the procedure except for an allergy to the anesthetic solution, for which there may be alternatives. Relative contraindications include bleeding or clotting disorders, anticoagulant therapy, or an inability of the patient to cooperate.

EQUIPMENT

* Nonsterile gloves
* Tongue depressor
* Anesthetic agent (local and topical)
* Sterile 3-mL syringe
* 25- to 27-gauge needle
* 4 × 4 gauze

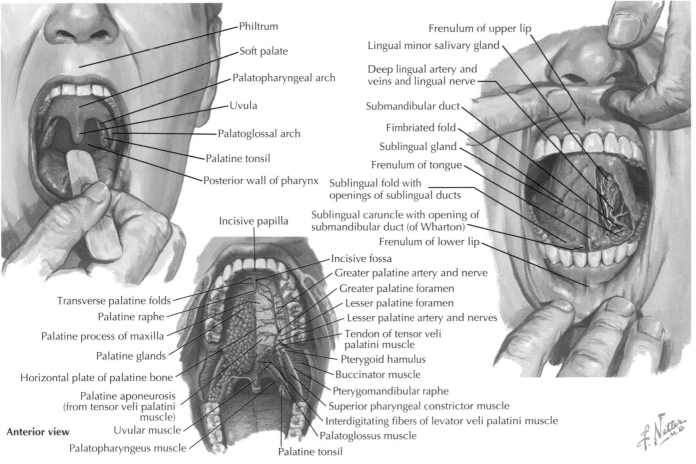

FIGURE 24.1 Oral cavity

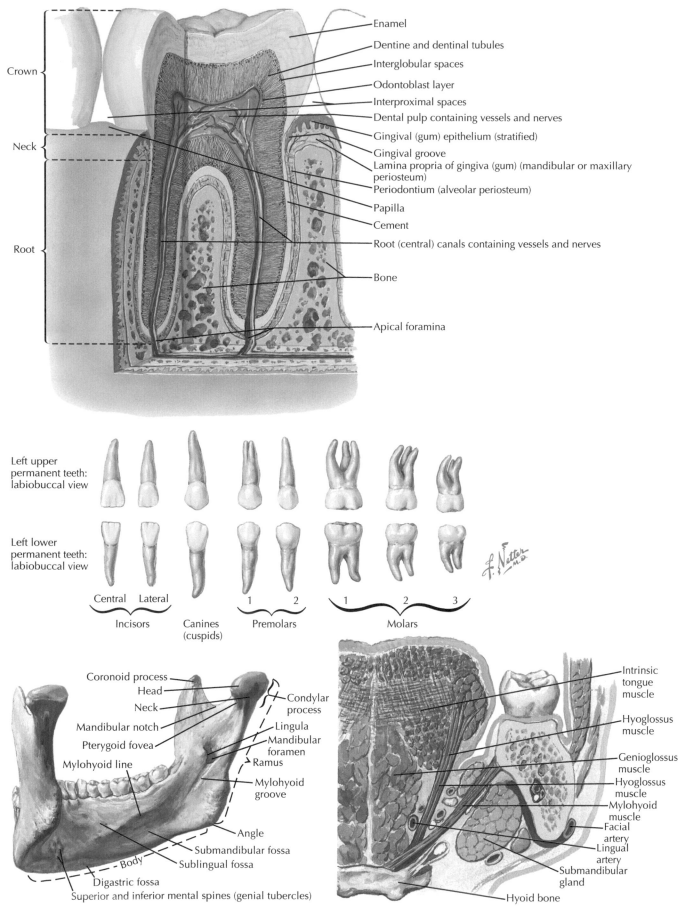

Crown

Neck

Root

Enamel
Dentine and dentinal tubules
Interglobular spaces
Odontoblast layer
Interproximal spaces
Dental pulp containing vessels and nerves
Gingival (gum) epithelium (stratified)
Gingival groove
Lamina propria of gingiva (gum) (mandibular or maxillary periosteum)
Periodontium (alveolar periosteum)
Papilla
Cement
Root (central) canals containing vessels and nerves
Bone
Apical foramina

Left upper permanent teeth: labiobuccal view

Left lower permanent teeth: labiobuccal view

Central   Lateral

Incisors

Canines (cuspids)

1   2
Premolars

1   2   3
Molars

Coronoid process
Head
Neck
Mandibular notch
Pterygoid fovea
Mylohyoid line

Condylar process
Lingula
Mandibular foramen
Ramus
Mylohyoid groove

Angle
Submandibular fossa
Sublingual fossa

Body
Digastric fossa
Superior and inferior mental spines (genial tubercles)

Intrinsic tongue muscle
Hyoglossus muscle
Genioglossus muscle
Hyoglossus muscle
Mylohyoid muscle
Facial artery
Lingual artery
Submandibular gland
Hyoid bone

FIGURE 24.2 Teeth and mandible

- Cotton-tipped applicators
- Light source

PROCEDURE

Before any dental nerve block is attempted, the procedure should be explained to the patient. Obtain consent and perform a time out. Don proper personal protective equipment.

SUPERIOR ALVEOLAR NERVE BLOCK

Superior alveolar nerve blocks anesthetize the maxillary teeth (Fig. 24.3).

1. Place the patient supine with the mouth open and the body of the mandible parallel to the floor.

2. Locate the mucobuccal fold above the tooth to be anesthetized by pulling the upper lip out and upward with the gauze.
3. Apply topical anesthetic to the injection site.
4. Advance a 25- to 27-gauge needle attached to a syringe containing the anesthetic approximately 2 cm at a 45-degree angle to the tooth into the mucobuccal fold toward the maxilla.
5. When the maxilla is contacted, withdraw the needle 1 to 2 mm and aspirate.
6. If the aspirate is free of blood, gradually inject 1 to 2 mL of local anesthetic solution at the apex of the root tip.
7. Withdraw the needle and discard in the sharps bin.

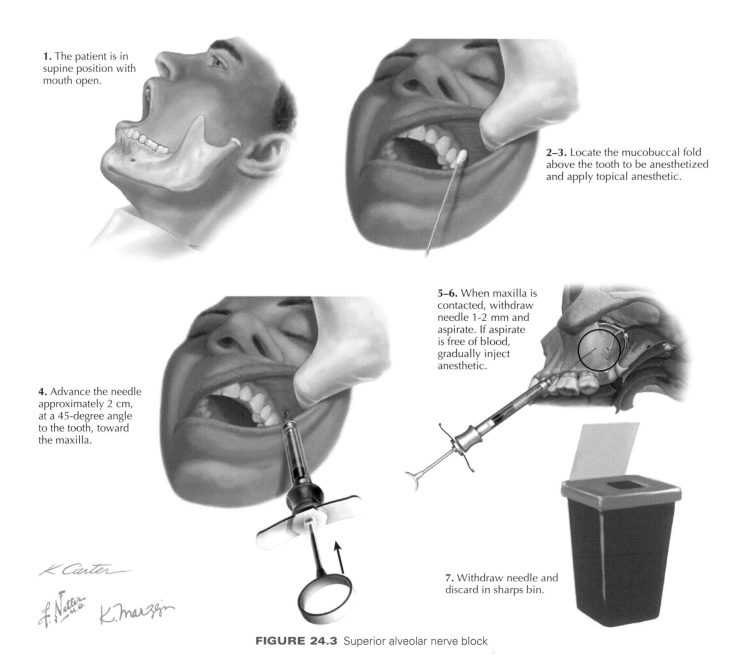

1. The patient is in supine position with mouth open.

2–3. Locate the mucobuccal fold above the tooth to be anesthetized and apply topical anesthetic.

4. Advance the needle approximately 2 cm, at a 45-degree angle to the tooth, toward the maxilla.

5–6. When maxilla is contacted, withdraw needle 1-2 mm and aspirate. If aspirate is free of blood, gradually inject anesthetic.

7. Withdraw needle and discard in sharps bin.

FIGURE 24.3 Superior alveolar nerve block

Inferior Alveolar Nerve Block

Inferior alveolar nerve blocks anesthetize the mandibular teeth but are more difficult to administer than superior alveolar nerve blocks (Fig. 24.4).

1. Place the patient supine with the mouth open and the body of the mandible parallel to the floor.
2. Pull at the angle of the mouth with the thumb of the nondominant hand. The mandibular foramen is located at about one-quarter of the distance between the deepest part of the pterygomandibular raphe and coronoid notch and above the biting surface of the mandibular teeth.
3. Apply topical anesthetic.
4. Position the syringe parallel to the surface of the teeth, with the barrel of the syringe angled toward the opposite corner of the mouth.
5. Advance the 25- to 27-gauge needle about 1.5 cm until the mandible is contacted.
6. Withdraw the needle 1 to 2 mm and aspirate.

7. If the aspirate is void of blood, gradually inject 1 to 2 mL of local anesthetic solution.
8. Withdraw the needle and discard in the sharps bin.

ANATOMICAL PITFALLS

The diffusion of the anesthetic is generally sufficient to overcome variations in the location of the mandibular foramen and other bony or neural anatomical variations. Anesthetic success is primarily dependent upon operator technique.

COMPLICATIONS
Anesthetic Access

One of the more common complications is anesthesia failure, which has implications for patient compliance and comfort during dental treatment. Needle insertion though infected tissues can result in the spread of infection. Toxicity can occur if the anesthetic solution is inadvertently injected intravascularly, which can be minimized by aspirating prior to injection

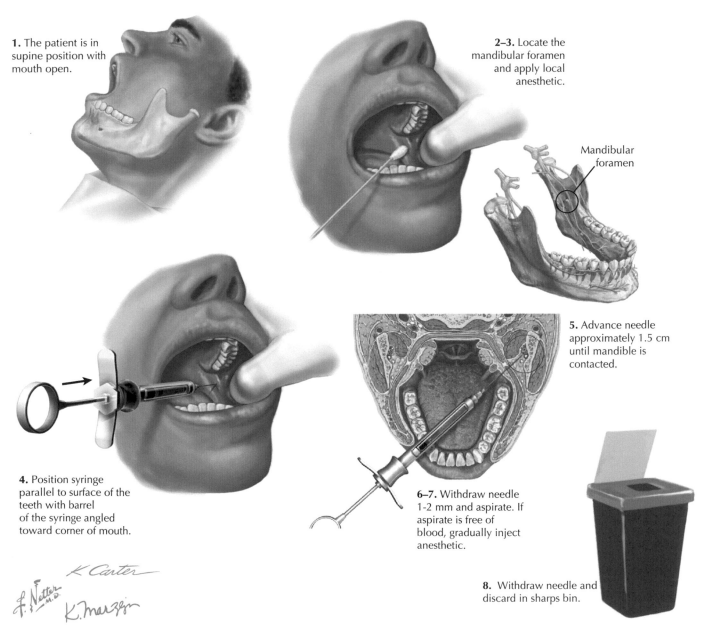

1. The patient is in supine position with mouth open.

2–3. Locate the mandibular foramen and apply local anesthetic.

Mandibular foramen

5. Advance needle approximately 1.5 cm until mandible is contacted.

4. Position syringe parallel to surface of the teeth with barrel of the syringe angled toward corner of mouth.

6–7. Withdraw needle 1-2 mm and aspirate. If aspirate is free of blood, gradually inject anesthetic.

8. Withdraw needle and discard in sharps bin.

FIGURE 24.4 Inferior alveolar nerve block

to ensure that there is no blood return. Bleeding and neuropathies may occur secondary to neurovascular damage.

Dental Trauma

A child's underlying permanent teeth can be damaged if there is an attempt to reinsert an avulsed primary tooth. Also, there is a risk for tooth fragment aspiration, especially in patients with an altered mental status. The proper handling and prompt transportation of any avulsed teeth except a primary tooth is important for maintaining tooth viability.

Odontogenic Infections

Odontogenic infections have the potential to spread in any direction within the head or neck. Typically, a tract starts at the root apex and continues through the marrow cavity of the mandible or maxilla before gaining access to the superficial tissues of the oral cavity. The infection may also travel within the sublingual, submental, or submandibular spaces or along the deeper fascial planes of the neck. Once the infection gains access to these potential spaces, resolution can only be accelerated by incision and drainage or spontaneous rupture, along with appropriate antibiotic cover. Extensive swelling can compromise a patient's airway or affect vision if there is spread to the eye. Facial cellulitis must be treated aggressively due to the risk of cavernous sinus thrombosis and meningitis.

CONCLUSION

The prompt diagnosis and management of dental emergencies is crucial to minimizing morbidity. Pain management through a dental nerve blocks plays a vital role in treatment. However, effective management of these pathologies relies on the physician's tactful alleviation of dental phobia, pain management, and prompt triage to a dental professional for definitive management.

Suggested Readings

Douglass AB, Douglass JM. Common dental emergencies. *Am Fam Physician.* 2003;67:511–516.

Hodgdon A. Dental and related infections. *Emerg Med Clin North Am.* 2013;31:465–480.

Khalil H. A basic review on the inferior alveolar nerve block techniques. *Anesth Essays Res.* 2014;8:3–8.

Klokkevold P. Common dental emergencies: evaluation and management for emergency physicians. *Emerg Med Clin North Am.* 1989;7:29–63.

Kumar A, Brennan MT. Differential diagnosis of orofacial pain and temporomandibular disorder. *Dent Clin North Am.* 2013;57:419–428.

Murray JM. Mandible fractures and dental trauma. *Emerg Med Clin North Am.* 2013;31:553–573.

Nixdorf DR, Law AS, John MT, Sobieh RM, Kohli R, Nguyen RH, National Dental PBRN Collaborative Group. Differential diagnoses for persistent pain after root canal treatment: a study in the national dental practice-based research network. *J Endod.* 2015;41:457–463.

Pynn BR, Sands T, Pharoah MJ. Odontogenic infections: part one. Anatomy and radiology. *Oral Health.* 1995;85:7–10. 13-4, 17–8.

Tellez M, Kinner DG, Heimberg RG, Lim S, Ismail AI. Prevalence and correlates of dental anxiety in patients seeking dental care. *Community Dent Oral Epidemiol.* 2015;43:135–142.

Turkistani J, Hanno A. Recent trends in the management of dentoalveolar traumatic injuries to primary and young permanent teeth. *Dent Traumatol.* 2011;27:46–54.

REVIEW QUESTIONS

1. A 24-year-old man had a third molar (wisdom tooth) extracted from his lower jaw. This resulted in the loss of general sense and taste sensation from the anterior two-thirds of the tongue. This loss was most likely due to injury of which of the following nerves?

    A. Auriculotemporal
    B. Chorda tympani
    C. Lingual
    D. Mental
    E. Inferior alveolar

2. A 38-year-old patient is admitted to the dental clinic with acute dental pain. The attending dentist found penetrating dental caries (tooth decay) affecting one of the mandibular molar teeth. Which of the following nerves would the dentist need to anesthetize to remove the caries in that tooth?

    A. Lingual
    B. Inferior alveolar
    C. Buccal
    D. Mental
    E. Nerve to mylohyoid

3. A 45-year-old man is admitted to the emergency department with severe dyspnea. On physical examination, there is swelling in the floor of his mouth and pharynx so that his airway is nearly totally occluded. In addition, there is a swelling in his lower jaw and upper neck. His history indicates that one of his lower molars was extracted a week ago, and he had been feeling worse every day since that event. Which of the following conditions is the most likely diagnosis?

    A. Quinsy
    B. Torus palatinus
    C. Ankyloglossia
    D. Ranula
    E. Ludwig angina

4. A 5-year-old boy playing soccer was kicked in the mouth, and his primary central incisor was knocked out. The boy was brought to the emergency department. Which of the following actions should be advised by the physician?

    A. Place the tooth in milk and send to the dentist as soon as possible.
    B. Scrub the tooth in betadine, put it on ice, and send the patient to the dentist as soon as possible.
    C. Give it back to the boy and tell him to put it under his pillow for the tooth fairy.
    D. Insert the tooth promptly back in place and wire it to the teeth next to it.

Abdominal Paracentesis

INTRODUCTION

The term *paracentesis* (Greek *para*, "beside," and *kentesis*, "puncture") translates to "pierce the side." Abdominal paracentesis ("abdominal tap") involves the surgical advancement of a needle or cannula through the abdominal wall to evacuate ascitic fluid from the peritoneal cavity.

Abdominal paracentesis is a clinically useful procedure for both diagnostic and therapeutic purposes. In diagnostic paracentesis, a small amount of ascitic fluid is removed for analysis to determine the cause of the ascites. Therapeutic paracentesis involves the removal of much larger quantities of fluid to relieve the symptoms of ascites, such as abdominal pain or shortness of breath. This procedure may be performed on an outpatient or inpatient basis. Adequate anatomical and procedural knowledge will enable the successful performance of abdominal paracentesis by physicians of any specialty, especially with the aid of ultrasound. This chapter describes the most current technique used when performing abdominal paracentesis.

CLINICALLY RELEVANT ANATOMY

If ultrasound is used to locate the ascetic fluid, the anatomic location for the procedure would be the general posterior-inferior area that is clear of structures. if ultrasound is not available, then abdominal paracentesis is performed at two locations: the infraumbilical midline (ML) and the left lower quadrant (LLQ) (Figs. 25.1 and 25.2). The advantages of these locations are the thinness of the abdominal wall in the LLQ and the relative avascularity of the ML location. The LLQ site is two fingerbreadths medial and two fingerbreadths cranial to the left anterior superior iliac spine. The ML location is midway between the umbilicus and pubis. Of the two locations, the LLQ is preferred over the ML because of the growing prevalence of abdominal obesity, which increases the ML wall thickness. In addition, more fluid can be removed from the LLQ because it is the point of maximum pooling. The clinician should keep in mind that the inferior epigastric artery courses from a point lateral to the pubic tubercle and runs cranially between the rectus abdominis and the posterior lamellae of its sheath. Puncture of this artery can result in significant hemorrhage. In pregnancy, a supraumbilical approach can be used with the aid of ultrasound.

Note that the right lower quadrant can also be used but is usually avoided because of the gaseous distention of the cecum in patients taking lactulose and the frequent presence of an appendectomy scar.

CAUSES AND COMPLICATIONS OF ASCITES

Ascites is defined as an unusual collection of fluid (greater than 25 mL) in the peritoneal cavity, which can be caused by several conditions (Fig. 25.3A). The most common cause of ascites is a liver parenchymal disease such as cirrhosis. In fact, ascites is the most common complication of cirrhosis. Cancer is the second most common cause of ascites, including peritoneal carcinomatosis, ovarian cancer, and lymphoma. Heart failure is the third most common cause. Other less-frequent etiologies are tuberculosis, pancreatic diseases, nephrogenous causes (such as peritoneal dialysis ascites and nephritic or nephrotic conditions), chlamydial infection, surgical peritonitis, and trauma to the lymphatic system or ureters. A serum-to-ascites albumin gradient of 1.1 g/dL or greater indicates that the cause of the ascites is portal hypertension, whereas a gradient of less than 1.1 g/dL may suggest peritoneal causes such as neoplasm or infection.

The most common complications associated with ascites are spontaneous bacterial peritonitis, congestive heart failure, and renal failure.

CLINICAL PRESENTATION AND PHYSICAL EXAMINATION

Ascites can manifest differently depending on the degree of fluid accumulation. If it is minimal, patients may be asymptomatic. However, large collections of fluid may result in abdominal fullness, anorexia, early satiety, nausea, or abdominal pain. In some cases, lung capacity may be restricted by a large fluid volume, resulting in dyspnea and respiratory compromise. Patients with chronic ascites have a characteristic appearance. The patient will be emaciated, have multiple spider nevi (if ascites is secondary to liver disease), and a caput medusae. There may be marked distension from the accumulation of the ascetic fluid.

On physical examination, the abdomen is distended, and percussion of the flanks with the patient lying supine reveals dullness because the fluid collects in the most dependent areas. Approximately 1500 mL of fluid must accumulate for dullness to be present in the flanks. Testing for shifting dullness has a sensitivity and specificity of approximately 83% and 56%, respectively.

Other findings, such as shifting dullness, a "puddle sign," or a "fluid wave" (Fig. 25.3B), are not sensitive or specific enough. When there is doubt regarding the location and presence of ascitic fluid, ultrasound should be used for clarification, if available.

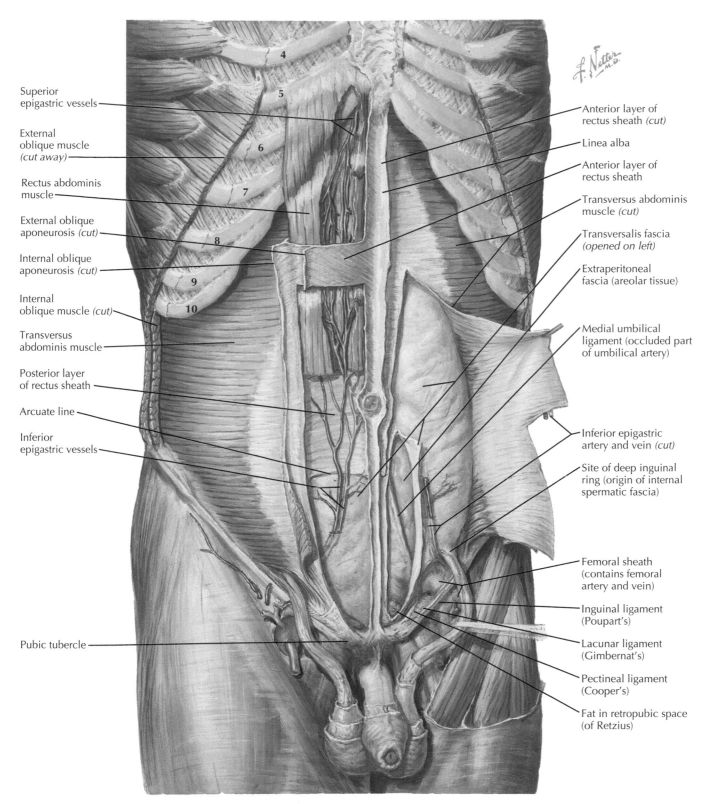

Superior
epigastric vessels

External
oblique muscle
(cut away)

Rectus abdominis
muscle

External oblique
aponeurosis (cut)

Internal oblique
aponeurosis (cut)

Internal
oblique muscle (cut)

Transversus
abdominis muscle

Posterior layer
of rectus sheath

Arcuate line

Inferior
epigastric vessels

Pubic tubercle

Anterior layer of
rectus sheath (cut)

Linea alba

Anterior layer of
rectus sheath

Transversus abdominis
muscle (cut)

Transversalis fascia
(opened on left)

Extraperitoneal
fascia (areolar tissue)

Medial umbilical
ligament (occluded part
of umbilical artery)

Inferior epigastric
artery and vein (cut)

Site of deep inguinal
ring (origin of internal
spermatic fascia)

Femoral sheath
(contains femoral
artery and vein)

Inguinal ligament
(Poupart's)

Lacunar ligament
(Gimbernat's)

Pectineal ligament
(Cooper's)

Fat in retropubic space
(of Retzius)

FIGURE 25.1 Anterior abdominal wall: deep dissection

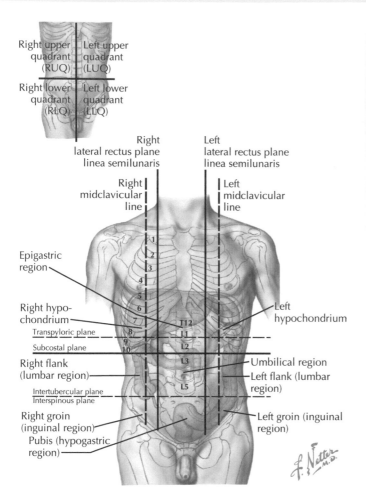

Right upper quadrant (RUQ) | Left upper quadrant (LUQ)
Right lower quadrant (RLQ) | Left lower quadrant (LLQ)

Right lateral rectus plane linea semilunaris

Left lateral rectus plane linea semilunaris

Right midclavicular line

Left midclavicular line

Epigastric region

Right hypo-chondrium

Transpyloric plane

Subcostal plane

Right flank (lumbar region)

Intertubercular plane
Interspinous plane

Right groin (inguinal region)

Pubis (hypogastric region)

Left hypochondrium

Umbilical region

Left flank (lumbar region)

Left groin (inguinal region)

T12
L1
L2
L3
L5

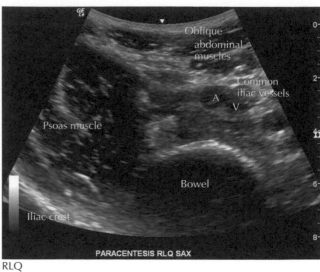

Oblique abdominal muscles

Common iliac vessels

Psoas muscle

Bowel

Iliac crest

PARACENTESIS RLQ SAX

RLQ

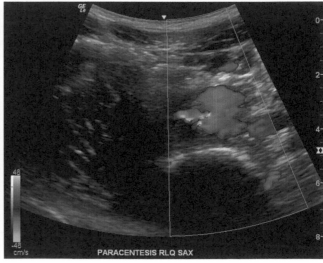

Obliques

A

V

Psoas

Bowel

Iliac crest

PARACENTESIS LLQ SAX

LLQ

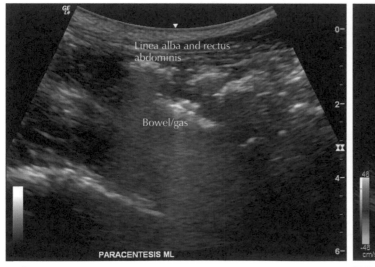

Linea alba and rectus abdominis

Bowel/gas

PARACENTESIS ML

Midline

PARACENTESIS RLQ SAX

RLQ

FIGURE 25.2 Regions and planes of the abdomen

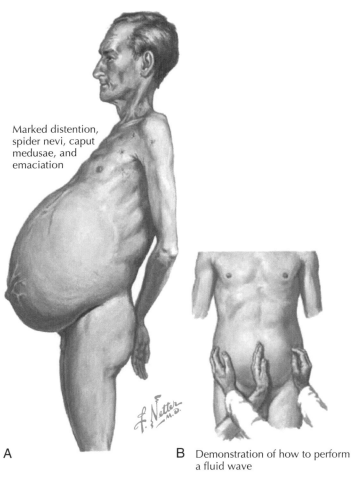

Marked distention, spider nevi, caput medusae, and emaciation

A

B Demonstration of how to perform a fluid wave

FIGURE 25.3 Ascites

INDICATIONS

New-onset ascites, the development of ascites in a previously admitted patient regardless of the reason for admission, and deterioration in the clinical condition are all indications for abdominal paracentesis. Signs of deterioration include abdominal pain or tenderness, fever, peripheral leukocytosis, hepatic encephalopathy, metabolic acidosis, and worsening renal function. However, the most common reasons for performing paracentesis is for the detection of spontaneous bacterial peritonitis and the therapeutic alleviation of symptoms caused by the ascites.

CONTRAINDICATIONS

Abdominal paracentesis is regarded as a relatively safe procedure with minimal complications. The only absolute contraindications are clinically evident fibrinolysis or disseminated intravascular coagulation. Other contraindications include significant bowel distention or ileus unless the procedure is performed with ultrasound guidance, since the risk of perforating the bowel is higher without it. Surgical scars may be present close to the entry site, suggesting the possibility of adhesions, which also increase the risk of bowel perforation during paracentesis. Infected skin may contaminate the entry site and should be avoided. Pregnancy is a relative contraindication, and paracentesis in this case should always be performed under ultrasound guidance, if available.

Moderate to severe coagulopathy from liver disease is also a relative contraindication that may need correction before the procedure. These patients are at higher risk of bleeding complications.

EQUIPMENT

The following materials are necessary when doing abdominal paracentesis:

Consent form
Personal protective equipment (sterile gloves, gown, and face shield)
Sterile drape
Multiple sterile gauze sponges
Antiseptic solution: chlorhexidine-alcohol or povidone-iodine for skin preparation
Ultrasound machine (should always be used if available)
Local anesthetic (1% lidocaine with epinephrine)
Needles
    1- or 1.5-inch, 22-gauge needle for diagnostic paracentesis
    3.5-inch, 22-gauge needle possibly needed for obese patients
    15- or 16-gauge needle for therapeutic paracentesis
    Over-the-needle cannula
    18-gauge needle for drawing up the local anesthetic
    1.5-inch, 25- or 27-gauge needle for injecting anesthetic
Syringes: 5, 20, and 50 mL
High-pressure drainage tubing and vacuum containers (for large-volume therapeutic paracentesis)
Culture bottles: anaerobic and aerobic
Hematology, chemistry, and microbiology sample tubes

PROCEDURE

Before beginning the procedure, obtain informed consent and perform a time out. Don appropriate personal protection equipment and follow sterile technique, including washing the hands before and after the procedure. The patient's urinary bladder should be empty. Use ultrasound guidance if available, especially in pregnant patients, to visualize the pockets of fluid that have become loculated secondary to mesenteric attachments, surgery, or adhesions (Fig. 25.4).

Place the patient in a supine position with the head raised 30 to 45 degrees to allow fluid to accumulate in the lower abdomen (Fig. 25.5, Video 25.1). The left lateral decubitus position may be used for smaller volumes of ascites.

1. Choose the best puncture site by percussion and mark it with an X. Four other points at 12, 3, 6, and 9 o'clock positions to the X should be marked outside the area to be cleansed. The fluid is usually drained lateral to the rectus abdominis muscle in the LLQ, carefully avoiding the inferior epigastric vessels.
2. Sterilize the skin with circular motions starting from the central X, which is erased in the process. The other four points act as a marker for the puncture site in the center.
3. Drape the site using sterile technique.

Loops of bowel Ascites fluid

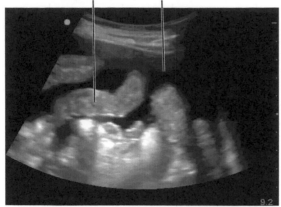

Abdominal ascites - no needle

Needle tip

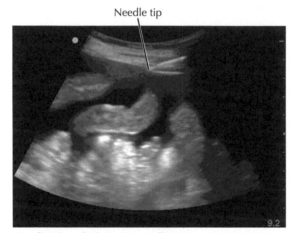

Visualization of advancing needle

Needle tip

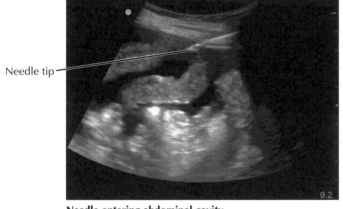

Needle entering abdominal cavity

FIGURE 25.4 Imaging of abdominal paracentesis

4. Draw up lidocaine using an 18-gauge needle, and anesthetize the site using the 25- or 27-gauge needle, aspirating as the needle is advanced into the soft tissue.
5. Attach the appropriate paracentesis needle to a large syringe. Advance the needle using the Z-track technique (see next section).
6. A small "give" will be felt as the needle penetrates the peritoneal cavity, and fluid can be aspirated into the syringe. A small incision using a #11 scalpel blade should

be made at the site if a larger-diameter needle or cannula is needed for therapeutic paracentesis.
7. For diagnostic paracentesis, enough fluid should be aspirated for analysis and the needle removed swiftly while aspirating, releasing skin tension only when the needle is completely removed. Apply pressure to the site, and dress the wound.
8. For therapeutic purposes, after advancing the needle with the cannula, hold the cannula in place while the needle is withdrawn, blocking the opening of the cannula with a finger or a stopcock. Attach the hub of the high-pressure drainage tube to the cannula. Attach the opposite end of the tube to a vacuum container bottle. Many patients have more than 1 to 2 L of fluid drained. After removal of the desired volume, withdraw the cannula and dress the site.

Z-Track Technique

The Z-track technique for needle advancement reduces the risk of persistent leakage and infection by producing a discontinuous entry path (see Fig. 25.5). This is achieved by using the nondominant hand to apply caudal tension on the skin while the dominant hand advances the needle and intermittently attempts aspiration. The nondominant hand is not released until the needle is fully withdrawn after aspiration. As the needle advances through the skin, muscle, and fascia, the puncture holes will not overlap, thus decreasing postprocedural leakage.

ANATOMICAL PITFALLS

A thorough understanding of abdominal anatomy is important for avoiding inadvertent injury during abdominal paracentesis. The operator should be aware of the position of major organs in this cavity, such as the liver and colon, as well as large blood vessels such as the aorta and inferior vena cava. When entering the lower quadrants, the inferior epigastric vessels must be avoided. A distended urinary bladder must also be avoided. Paracentesis in a pregnant patient requires particular caution.

COMPLICATIONS

The most common complication of abdominal paracentesis is ascitic fluid leakage, which most often occurs if the Z-track technique is not used, the paracentesis needle is very large, or the incision is wide. Fluid leakage is usually self-limited, but if it persists, a purse-string suture can be placed over the site or adhesive glue can be used.

Bleeding is also another common complication and usually presents in the form of an abdominal wall hematoma or hemoperitoneum secondary to the puncture of the inferior epigastric vessels. Patients with renal failure, liver disease, and severe coagulopathy are at an increased risk of bleeding, although mild-to-moderate coagulopathy does not appear to pose a major risk. A figure-of-eight suture can be placed over the needle entry site to curtail bleeding if it occurs. Laparotomy may be needed only if these measures fail, which is rare. Bowel or bladder perforation is also rare but may occur if the procedure is performed in the presence of a full urinary bladder or close to a surgical scar with adherent bowel. Treatment is not usually required unless signs

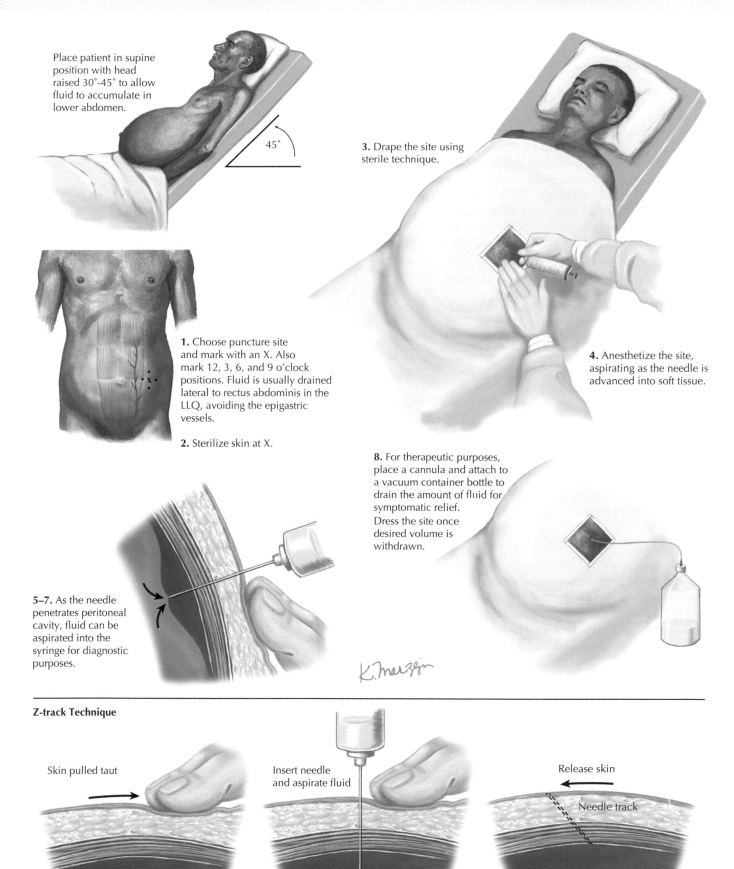

Place patient in supine position with head raised 30°-45° to allow fluid to accumulate in lower abdomen.

45°

3. Drape the site using sterile technique.

1. Choose puncture site and mark with an X. Also mark 12, 3, 6, and 9 o'clock positions. Fluid is usually drained lateral to rectus abdominis in the LLQ, avoiding the epigastric vessels.

2. Sterilize skin at X.

4. Anesthetize the site, aspirating as the needle is advanced into soft tissue.

8. For therapeutic purposes, place a cannula and attach to a vacuum container bottle to drain the amount of fluid for symptomatic relief. Dress the site once desired volume is withdrawn.

5–7. As the needle penetrates peritoneal cavity, fluid can be aspirated into the syringe for diagnostic purposes.

K. Marzejon

Z-track Technique

Skin pulled taut

Insert needle and aspirate fluid

Release skin

Needle track

FIGURE 25.5 Abdominal paracentesis

of infection such as fever and abdominal tenderness develop. The risk of introducing infection into the peritoneal cavity is minimal, particularly if sterile precautions are undertaken.

CONCLUSION

Abdominal paracentesis is a clinically valuable procedure used to remove ascitic fluid for diagnostic and therapeutic purposes. This procedure has been found to reduce mortality rates in hospitalized patients. It should be performed in any patient with new-onset ascites, malignant ascites, or a suspicion of spontaneous bacterial peritonitis. The indications in hospitalized patients also include new-onset ascites, tense or diuretic-resistant ascites, and clinical deterioration in a patient with ascites. Special care should be taken to avoid vascular and visceral structures. Ultrasound should always be used, if available.

Suggested Readings

Hou W, Sanyal AJ. Ascites: diagnosis and management. *Med Clin North Am.* 2009;93(4):801–817.

McGibbon A, Chen GI, Peltekian KM, van Zanten SV. An evidence-based manual for abdominal paracentesis. *Dig Dis Sci.* 2007;52(12): 3307–3315.

Rosen P, Chan TC, Vilke GM, Sternbach G. Paracentesis. In: *Atlas of emergency procedures.* St Louis: Mosby; 2001.

Runyon BA. Paracentesis of ascitic fluid: a safe procedure. *Arch Intern Med.* 1986;146(11):2259–2261.

Runyon MS, Marx JA. Peritoneal procedures. In: Custalow CB, Chanmugam AS, Chudnofsky CR, McManus LT, eds. *Roberts and Hedges' clinical procedures in emergency medicine.* 5th ed. Philadelphia: Saunders-Elsevier; 2010.

Wong CL, Holroyd-Leduc J, Thorpe KE, Straus SE. Does this patient have bacterial peritonitis or portal hypertension? How do I perform a paracentesis and analyze the results? *JAMA.* 2008;299(10):1166–1178.

REVIEW QUESTIONS

1. The decision is made by emergency department surgeons to perform an exploratory laparotomy on a 32-year-old woman with severe abdominal pain. Bleeding occurs during the dissection of the lower quadrant and superficially with manipulation of the rectus abdominis muscle. Which of the following arteries is most likely injured?

   A. Superior epigastric artery
   B. Thoracoepigastric artery
   C. Intercostal artery
   D. Aorta
   E. Inferior epigastric artery

2. A 65-year-old man is admitted to the emergency department with abdominal fullness, anorexia, early satiety, and nausea or abdominal pain. On physical examination, the abdomen is distended, and percussion of the flanks in the supine position reveals dullness because fluid will collect mostly in the most dependent areas in this position. Testing for shifting dullness, the puddle sign, and fluid wave is positive. An LLQ paracentesis is performed. Which of the following is the most appropriate directional landmark for identifying the inferior epigastric artery during this procedure?

   A. Lateral to the pubic tubercle
   B. Medial to the pubic tubercle
   C. Medial to the rectus abdominis muscle
   D. Medial to the triangle of Hesselbach
   E. Lateral to the transversus abdominis muscle

3. Which of the following is a contraindication to performing an abdominal paracentesis?

   A. Disseminated intravascular coagulation
   B. Pregnancy
   C. Acute tubular necrosis
   D. Sepsis
   E. Children less than 10 years old

Auricular Hematoma Drainage

INTRODUCTION

An auricular hematoma is a common injury that occurs during contact sports such as wrestling, boxing, and mixed martial arts. Motor vehicle accidents, falls, and assaults may also cause an auricular hematoma. The overwhelming majority of auricular hematomas are trauma related, but they can occur spontaneously.

The main goal of treatment is to drain the accumulated blood and prevent deformities such as a cauliflower ear. The traditional treatment is incision and drainage, followed by the application of a compressive dressing. A silicone putty mold, fibrin glue, an absorbable mattress suture, or a Silastic sheet can also be used.

CLINICALLY RELEVANT ANATOMY

The external ear is composed of the auricle (pinna) and the external acoustic meatus. The auricle consists of the lobule, tragus, antitragus, concha, antihelix, and helix. The external acoustic meatus runs from the deepest part of the concha to the tympanic membrane (eardrum) (Figs. 26.1 and 26.2). The arterial supply of the auricle arises from the posterior auricular, superficial temporal, and occipital arteries. The great auricular nerve innervates the skin of the anterior and posterior inferior portions of the auricle, the lesser occipital nerve innervates the posterior superior portion, and the auriculotemporal nerve innervates the anterior superior portion of the auricle. The deeper parts of the external ear are innervated by the vagus nerve (Fig. 26.3).

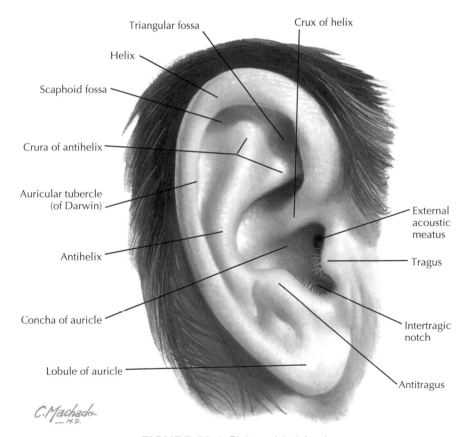

Triangular fossa

Crux of helix

Helix

Scaphoid fossa

Crura of antihelix

Auricular tubercle (of Darwin)

External acoustic meatus

Antihelix

Tragus

Concha of auricle

Intertragic notch

Lobule of auricle

Antitragus

FIGURE 26.1 Right auricle (pinna)

Coronal oblique section of external acoustic meatus and middle ear (tympanic cavity)

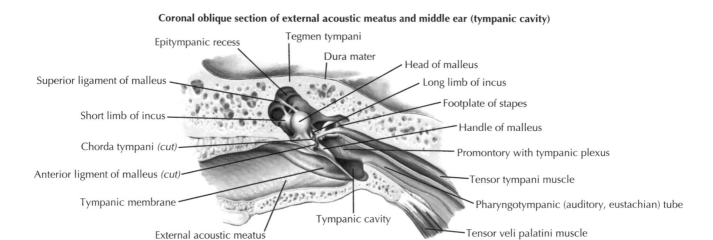

Epitympanic recess

Tegmen tympani

Dura mater

Head of malleus

Long limb of incus

Footplate of stapes

Superior ligament of malleus

Short limb of incus

Handle of malleus

Chorda tympani *(cut)*

Promontory with tympanic plexus

Anterior ligment of malleus *(cut)*

Tensor tympani muscle

Tympanic membrane

Pharyngotympanic (auditory, eustachian) tube

Tympanic cavity

Tensor veli palatini muscle

External acoustic meatus

Right tympanic cavity after removal of tympanic membrane (lateral view)

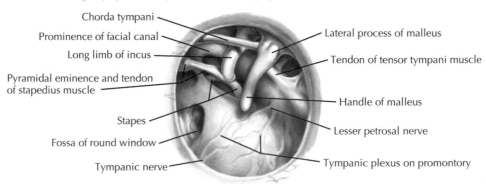

Chorda tympani

Prominence of facial canal

Long limb of incus

Lateral process of malleus

Tendon of tensor tympani muscle

Pyramidal eminence and tendon of stapedius muscle

Handle of malleus

Stapes

Lesser petrosal nerve

Fossa of round window

Tympanic nerve

Tympanic plexus on promontory

C. Machado M.D.

FIGURE 26.2 Tympanic membrane

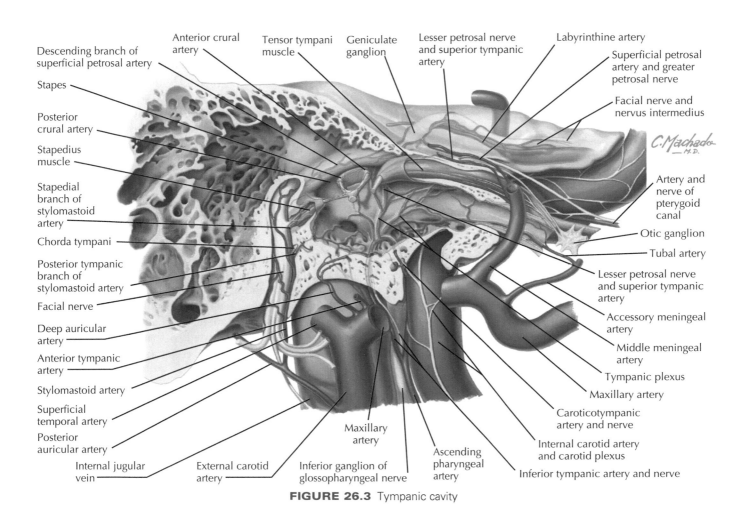

Descending branch of superficial petrosal artery

Stapes

Posterior crural artery

Stapedius muscle

Stapedial branch of stylomastoid artery

Chorda tympani

Posterior tympanic branch of stylomastoid artery

Facial nerve

Deep auricular artery

Anterior tympanic artery

Stylomastoid artery

Superficial temporal artery

Posterior auricular artery

Internal jugular vein

External carotid artery

Inferior ganglion of glossopharyngeal nerve

Maxillary artery

Ascending pharyngeal artery

Anterior crural artery

Tensor tympani muscle

Geniculate ganglion

Lesser petrosal nerve and superior tympanic artery

Labyrinthine artery

Superficial petrosal artery and greater petrosal nerve

Facial nerve and nervus intermedius

Artery and nerve of pterygoid canal

Otic ganglion

Tubal artery

Lesser petrosal nerve and superior tympanic artery

Accessory meningeal artery

Middle meningeal artery

Tympanic plexus

Maxillary artery

Caroticotympanic artery and nerve

Internal carotid artery and carotid plexus

Inferior tympanic artery and nerve

FIGURE 26.3 Tympanic cavity

INDICATIONS

Once an auricular hematoma is diagnosed, incision and drainage followed by a compressive dressing should be performed as soon as possible. Patients with an auricular hematoma should be evaluated thoroughly to rule out serious injuries such as skull fractures, as well as for tympanic membrane rupture and hearing loss.

CONTRAINDICATIONS

There are no contraindications to this procedure.

EQUIPMENT

Antiseptic solution
Ear drape
No. 15 scalpel
Local anesthetic (2% lidocaine)
Compressive dressing (eg, cotton bolster, silicone putty mold, Silastic sheet)
Suture kit including 3-0 silk suture
Antibiotic ointment

PROCEDURE

Explain the procedure to the patient and obtain consent; don the appropriate personal protective equipment, and perform a time out. See Fig. 26.4.

1. Drape the ear.
2. Cleanse the auricle with antiseptic solution.
3. Inject a local anesthetic in the area of the auricular hematoma where the scalpel will be used as well as in the posterior surface of the auricle for complete anesthesia during suturing. Alternatively, a periauricular nerve block can be performed.
4. Make a 4- to 5-mm incision with a No. 15 scalpel over the hematoma and drain the blood.
5. Apply antibiotic ointment to a compressive dressing.
6. Place the compressive dressing on the anterior surface of the auricle. Using 3-0 silk, suture the dressing to the auricle, passing the suture through the superior portion of the auricle and back through the inferior portion, and then tie it over the dressing.

ANATOMICAL PITFALLS

When applying a local anesthetic, isolated nerve blocks should be avoided because the sensory innervation of the auricle is very complex, with multiple nerves innervating it. For instance, attempting a great auricular nerve block might accidentally result in Horner's syndrome (ipsilateral partial ptosis, miosis, and facial anhidrosis) if the sympathetic trunk is blocked.

COMPLICATIONS

Adequate cleansing of the ear is important for preventing infection. The patient should be advised to seek help immediately if signs of infection appear. Drainage of all accumulated blood and the correct use of a compressive dressing are critical for preventing a cauliflower ear deformity.

Competitive athletes such as wrestlers and boxers may need to resume their careers before full healing occurs. In these patients, mattress sutures should be considered instead of traditional compressive dressings to allow a return to training as soon as possible.

CONCLUSION

A hematoma is a common traumatic injury to the auricle of the ear. It is important to perform incision and drainage and apply a compressive dressing as soon as possible. Although the procedure is straightforward, physicians need to make sure that all the blood is drained so that a cauliflower ear deformity is avoided. In addition, patients with an auricular hematoma should be thoroughly evaluated so that any life-threatening injury such as a skull fracture is recognized and managed.

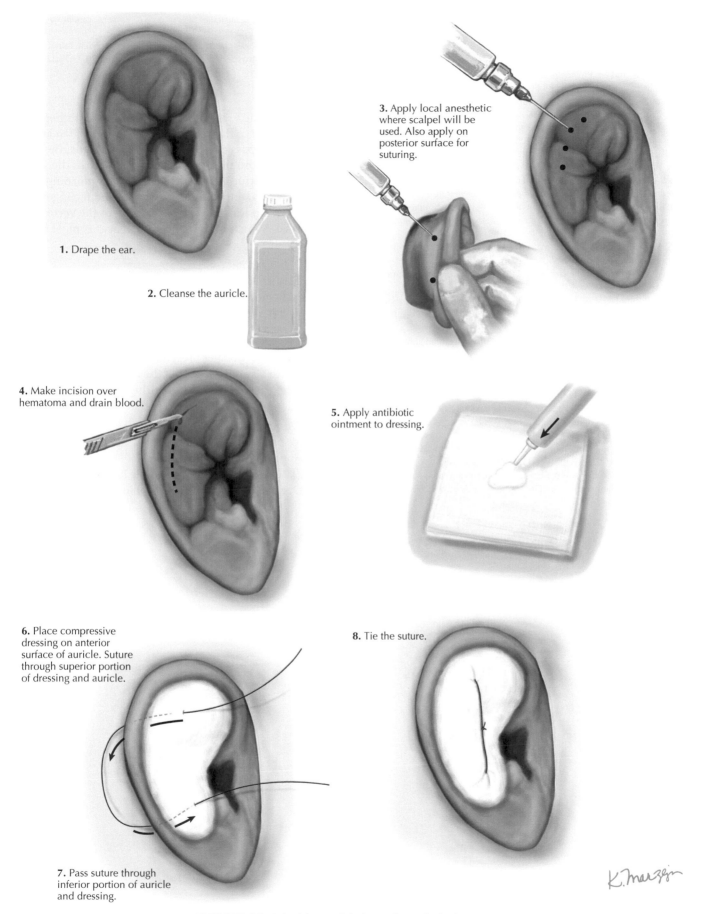

1. Drape the ear.

2. Cleanse the auricle.

3. Apply local anesthetic where scalpel will be used. Also apply on posterior surface for suturing.

4. Make incision over hematoma and drain blood.

5. Apply antibiotic ointment to dressing.

6. Place compressive dressing on anterior surface of auricle. Suture through superior portion of dressing and auricle.

7. Pass suture through inferior portion of auricle and dressing.

8. Tie the suture.

FIGURE 26.4 Incision and drainage for auricular hematoma

Suggested Readings

Cassaday K, Vazquez G, Wright JM. Ear problems and injuries in athletes. *Curr Sports Med Rep.* 2014;13:22–26.

Drake RL, Vogl AW, Mitchell AWM. Head and neck. In: *Gray's Anatomy for Students.* 2nd ed. Philadelphia: Elsevier; 2010:902–919.

Giles WC, Iverson KC, King JD, Hill FC, Woody EA, Bouknight AL. Incision and drainage followed by mattress suture repair of auricular hematoma. *Laryngoscope.* 2007;117:2097–2099.

Kakarala K, Kieff DA. Bolsterless management for recurrent auricular hematomata. *Laryngoscope.* 2012;122:1235–1237.

Martin RJ, Carey VM, Philbert RF, Carter JB. Prevention of haematomas after auricular injuries. *Br J Oral Maxillofac Surg.* 2000;38:238–240.

Mathur S, Clarke R, John CM. "Spontaneous" auricular haematoma: a rare differential diagnosis of NAI. *Acta Paediatr.* 2009;98:928.

Mohamad SH, Barnes M, Jones S, Mahendran S. A new technique using fibrin glue in the management of auricular hematoma. *Clin J Sport Med.* 2014;24:e65–e67.

Nahl SS, Kent SE, Curry AR. Treatment of auricular haematoma by silicone rubber splints. *J Laryngol Otol.* 1989;103:1146–1149.

O'Donnell BP, Eliezri YD. The surgical treatment of traumatic hematoma of the auricle. *Dermatol Surg.* 1999;25:803–805.

Quine SM, Roblin DG, Cuddihy PJ, Tomkinson A. Short communications: treatment of acute auricular haematoma. *J Laryngol Otol.* 1996;110:862–863.

Rah YC, Park MH. Use of Silastic sheets with mattress-fashion sutures for the treatment of auricular hematoma. *Laryngoscope.* 2015;125:730–732.

Ross MH, Pawlina W. Cartilage. In: *Histology: A Text and Atlas: With Correlated Cell and Molecular Biology.* 6th ed. Philadelphia: Lippincott Williams & Wilkins; 2011.

Roy S, Smith LP. A novel technique for treating auricular hematomas in mixed martial artists (ultimate fighters). *Am J Otolaryngol.* 2008;31:21–24.

Schuller DE, Dankle SD, Strauss RH. A technique to treat wrestlers' auricular hematoma without interrupting training or competition. *Arch Otolaryngol Head Neck Surg.* 1989;115:202–206.

Starck WJ, Kaltman SI. Current concepts in the surgical management of traumatic auricular hematoma. *J Oral Maxillofac Surg.* 1992;50:800–802.

Summers A. Managing auricular haematoma to prevent "cauliflower ear." *Emerg Nurse.* 2012;20:28–30.

Zohn S. In response to: acute management of auricular haematoma: a novel approach and retrospective review. *Clin J Sport Med.* 2013;23:329.

REVIEW QUESTIONS

1. While at a party, an intoxicated teenager asks her friend to pierce the tragus of her left ear. When attempting to pass a needle through the tragus, the friend slips and the needle deeply punctures the skin directly anterior to the tragus. The next morning the teenager awakens to find that she has no feeling on the left temporal side of her scalp up to the vertex of her head. Which of the following nerves is most likely damaged?

   A. Lesser occipital
   B. Greater occipital
   C. Auriculotemporal
   D. Zygomaticotemporal
   E. Great auricular

2. A 20-year-old wrestler presents to the emergency department with a swollen tragus of the left ear after being kicked in the side of his head during a match. Which of the following is the most appropriate treatment?

   A. Warm soaks
   B. Ice packs
   C. Apply a compression dressing
   D. Explore and evacuate a possible hematoma
   E. Obtain a computed tomographic scan

Cerumen Removal

INTRODUCTION

Cerumen is a yellow, waxy mixture of secretory products from both sebaceous and modified apocrine glands in the external acoustic meatus. It serves a protective function and can inhibit infection by trapping foreign substances in the meatus. Lipid content derived from the sebaceous gland lubricates the meatus, preventing itching and burning. The external acoustic meatus possesses unique anatomy and physiology that permit an efficient self-cleaning system. Under normal conditions, cerumen is naturally swept away with dirt and debris by ear cilia and jaw movement. When this self-cleaning mechanism fails, cerumen can become impacted and generate a tough plug, blocking the meatus.

A cerumen plug can cause dizziness, pain, itching, ringing or decreased hearing. Among the elderly, cerumen impaction may be secondary to the stiffening of ear cilia or the placement of hearing aids.

CLINICALLY RELEVANT ANATOMY

The accumulation of cerumen is limited to the external acoustic meatus, which begins at the meatus of the auricle and ends at the tympanic membrane (Figs. 27.1 and 27.2). The outer one-third of the meatus consists of hair and gland-bearing skin on top of fibrocartilaginous tissue. Secretions from the sebaceous and ceruminous glands within the skin are responsible for the components of cerumen. The inner two-thirds of the external acoustic meatus consist of thin skin adherent to the periosteum of the temporal bone. The meatus narrows in most individuals at the isthmus, which is located at the junction of the bony and fibrocartilaginous portions of the meatus. The isthmus is a frequent site of cerumen impaction because it is the narrowest cerumen-containing portion. Cerumen trapped medial to the isthmus tends to become impacted and cause hearing loss. At the innermost end of the external meatus is the tympanic membrane. The lateral layer of the tympanic membrane consists of keratinizing squamous epithelium in continuity with the epithelium of the external acoustic meatus.

INDICATIONS

A clinician must assess patients with a complaint of cerumen accumulation. Removal is frequently indicated in patients who present with symptoms such as hearing loss, earache, ear fullness, itchiness, reflex cough, dizziness, and tinnitus. The use of an otoscope can confirm the diagnosis on physical examination.

CONTRAINDICATIONS

Syringing or irrigation should be avoided for patients with tympanic membrane damage as there is a risk of introducing infection. In cases when a patient is unaware of a ruptured tympanic membrane and an aural lavage has been performed, a prophylactic antibiotic should be administered. Patients with otitis externa should not undergo irrigation because aberrations in temperature worsen symptoms. Self-cleaning of the external acoustic meatus should be avoided as it may lead to damage.

EQUIPMENT

Otoscope and microscope, if available
Syringe with a tapered tip, filled with water at body temperature
Blunt ear curettes

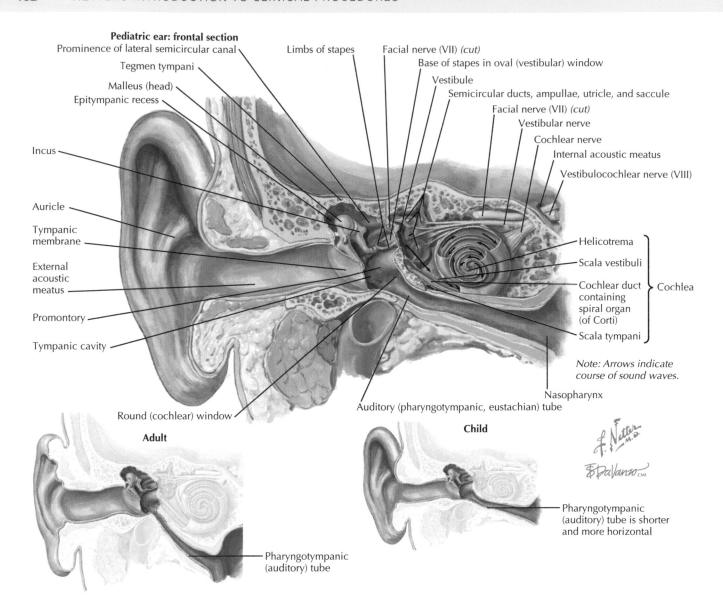

Pediatric ear: frontal section

Prominence of lateral semicircular canal

Tegmen tympani

Malleus (head)

Epitympanic recess

Limbs of stapes

Facial nerve (VII) *(cut)*

Base of stapes in oval (vestibular) window

Vestibule

Semicircular ducts, ampullae, utricle, and saccule

Facial nerve (VII) *(cut)*

Vestibular nerve

Cochlear nerve

Internal acoustic meatus

Vestibulocochlear nerve (VIII)

Incus

Auricle

Tympanic membrane

External acoustic meatus

Promontory

Tympanic cavity

Helicotrema

Scala vestibuli

Cochlear duct containing spiral organ (of Corti)

Scala tympani

} Cochlea

Note: Arrows indicate course of sound waves.

Round (cochlear) window

Auditory (pharyngotympanic, eustachian) tube

Nasopharynx

Adult

Child

Pharyngotympanic (auditory) tube

Pharyngotympanic (auditory) tube is shorter and more horizontal

FIGURE 27.1 Anatomy of the ear

PROCEDURE

Obtain patient consent and perform a time out.

Ear Irrigation

See Fig. 27.3.

1. Straighten the meatus by pulling the pinna up and back in an adult or down and back in an infant.
2. Place a syringe full of water at body temperature just inside the external acoustic meatus so that the tip is visible.
3. Irrigate the fluid toward the posterior wall of the meatus at a steady rate until the cerumen is removed.

    a. Slow the stream of water if it is painful.

    b. The flow of water from the syringe should be slower for children.

Irrigation of the external acoustic meatus to remove cerumen is becoming less popular in primary care facilities because it is executed blindly, substantially increasing the likelihood of serious complications such as perforation of the tympanic membrane. Earwax in the elderly tends to contain more keratin, which can make irrigation more challenging. Some otic solutions contain glycerin, which softens cerumen and facilitates the ease of cleaning via lavage or irrigation.

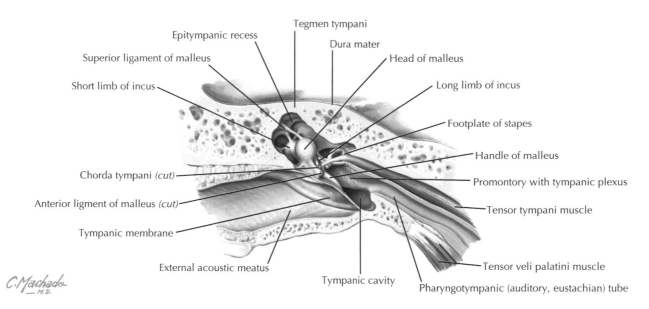

FIGURE 27.2 Coronal oblique section of external acoustic meatus and middle ear (tympanic cavity)

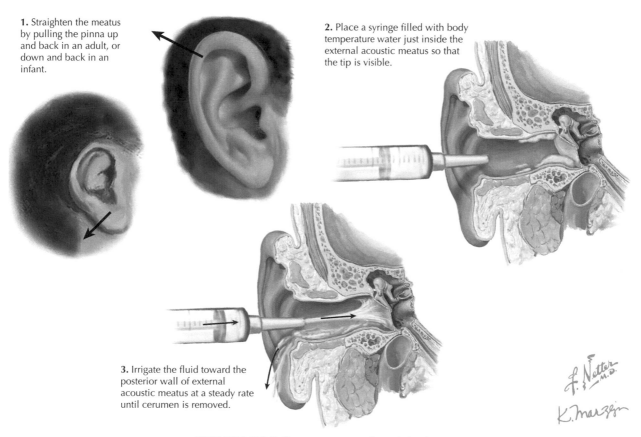

1. Straighten the meatus by pulling the pinna up and back in an adult, or down and back in an infant.

2. Place a syringe filled with body temperature water just inside the external acoustic meatus so that the tip is visible.

3. Irrigate the fluid toward the posterior wall of external acoustic meatus at a steady rate until cerumen is removed.

FIGURE 27.3 Cerumen removal: ear irrigation

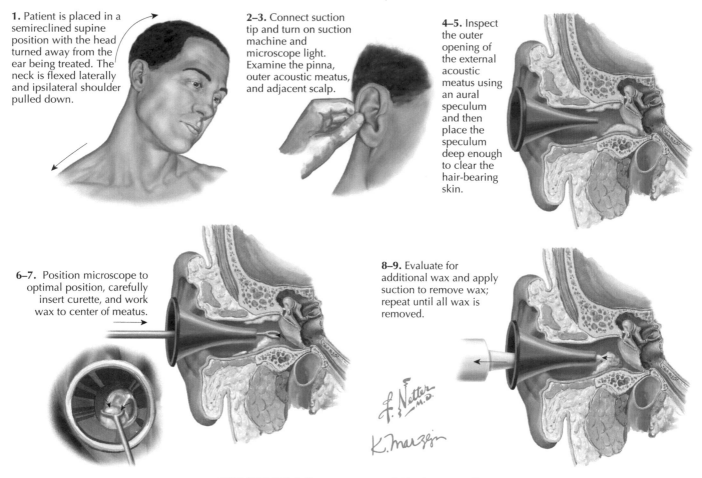

1. Patient is placed in a semireclined supine position with the head turned away from the ear being treated. The neck is flexed laterally and ipsilateral shoulder pulled down.

2–3. Connect suction tip and turn on suction machine and microscope light. Examine the pinna, outer acoustic meatus, and adjacent scalp.

4–5. Inspect the outer opening of the external acoustic meatus using an aural speculum and then place the speculum deep enough to clear the hair-bearing skin.

6–7. Position microscope to optimal position, carefully insert curette, and work wax to center of meatus.

8–9. Evaluate for additional wax and apply suction to remove wax; repeat until all wax is removed.

FIGURE 27.4 Cerumen removal: blunt ear curettes

Blunt Ear Curettes

See Fig. 27.4.

1. Place the patient in a semireclined supine position with the head turned away from the ear being entered. The neck is flexed laterally and the ipsilateral shoulder pulled down.
2. Connect a suction tip and turn on the suction machine and microscope light.
3. Examine the pinna, outer portions of the external acoustic meatus, and the adjacent scalp for any evidence of previous surgery incisions.
4. Inspect the outer opening of the external acoustic meatus using the appropriate aural speculum.
5. Place the speculum deep enough to clear the hair-bearing skin.
6. Position the microscope for an optimal view.
7. Carefully insert the curette and work the wax to the center of the meatus.
8. Apply suction to remove the wax.
9. Repeat the procedure until all wax is removed, then reposition the microscope to evaluate for additional wax.

Placement of the curette is critical for successful removal as well as preventing posterior displacement of the wax further down the acoustic meatus toward the tympanic membrane. If cerumen is still difficult to remove, a patient may be sent home with eardrops and a follow-up appointment scheduled within 4 days. The patient should anticipate a small amount of pain and loss of hearing when using the drops because cerumenolytics cause the wax to expand in the ear meatus. The patient should also be advised to avoid getting shampoo, soap, or alcohol in the ear. At follow-up, ear lavage or irrigation should be performed to remove the wax.

Endoscopy

Although a microscope is used more commonly, a rigid endoscope coupled to a Jobson-Horne probe and St. Bartholomew's wax hook is relatively inexpensive and easier to use for primary care physicians and otolaryngologists.

Of the many treatments available for the removal of impacted cerumen, no technique has proven more effective than any other. The recommended procedure calls for taking a careful history, examining the patient for prior pathology, and using sterile instruments, good lighting, and accepted methods of cerumen removal. Knowing when to stop irrigation and use cerumenolytic drops or refer to a specialist is key to maximizing patient comfort and minimizing complications.

ANATOMICAL PITFALLS

The external acoustic meatus is longer and more angulated in adults than in children. The meatus is exquisitely sensitive to touch and is highly innervated. One known consequence of irritation of the meatus, especially its posterior wall, is bradycardia resulting from stimulation of the cutaneous branch of the vagus nerve.

COMPLICATIONS

Tympanic membrane perforation occurs in 1% of patients undergoing earwax removal. Perforation is more likely to occur in children due to the shorter length of their ear meatus. Damage to the external acoustic meatus epithelium may lead to bacterial infection, resulting in external otitis. The irrigating fluid should be maintained at body temperature to avoid nausea, vomiting, and vertigo. Perforation of the tympanic membrane and permanent hearing loss are also possible, as are secondary infections from traumatic cerumen removal.

Partial removal of cerumen by irrigation can result in the accumulation of water behind the cerumen, potentially leading to maceration and infection. Immunosuppressed patients must be managed with caution because they have an increased risk of developing malignant otitis externa as a complication of cerumen removal.

CONCLUSION

In reasonable amounts, cerumen provides protection to the external acoustic meatus. Pathological accumulation, however, can result in symptomatic complaints, requiring its removal. Treatment should be reserved for individuals who experience symptoms associated with cerumen accumulation. The current literature suggests irrigation with saline and cerumenolytics as the first-line treatment in most primary care settings. In the event of treatment failure with the above two modalities, manual removal with direct visualization may be performed by otolaryngologists or other trained individuals.

Suggested Readings

Afolabi AO, et al. Attitude of self ear cleaning in black Africans: any benefit? *East Afr J Public Health*. 2009;6(1):43–46.

Almeyda R, Babar-Craig H. A comparison of endoscopic and microscopic removal of wax: a randomised clinical trial. *Clin Otolaryngol*. 2007;32(1):73–74.

Bortz JT, Wertz PW, Downing DT. Composition of cerumen lipids. *J Am Acad Dermatol*. 1990;23(5 Pt 1):845–849.

Burton MJ, Doree C. Ear drops for the removal of ear wax. *Cochrane Database Syst Rev*. 2009;(1):CD004326.

Grossan M. Cerumen removal–current challenges. *Ear Nose Throat J*. 1998;77(7):541–546, 548.

Grossan M. Safe, effective techniques for cerumen removal. *Geriatrics*. 2000;55(1):80, 83–86.

Ijaz A, Lee WC, Binnington JD. External auditory canal measurements: localization of the isthmus. *Otorhinolaryngol Nova*. 1996;10:183–186.

Jabor MA, Amedee RG. Cerumen impaction. *J La State Med Soc*. 1997;149(10):358–362.

Kelly KE, Mohs DC. The external auditory canal: anatomy and physiology. *Otolaryngol Clin North Am*. 1996;29:725.

Lum CL, Jeyanthi S, Prepageran N, et al. Antibacterial and antifungal properties of human cerumen. *J Laryngol Otol*. 2009;123:375–378.

REVIEW QUESTIONS

1. A 3-year-old girl ruptured her eardrum when she inserted a pencil into her external ear canal. She was urgently admitted to the emergency department. Physical examination revealed pain in her ear and a few drops of blood in the external auditory meatus. There was concern that there might have been an injury to the nerve that principally innervates the external surface of the tympanic membrane. Which of the following tests is most likely to be performed during physical examination to check for injury to this nerve?

   A. Check the taste in the anterior two-thirds of the tongue
   B. Check the sensation of the pharynx and palate
   C. Check for paresthesia at the temporomandibular joint
   D. Check for sensation in the larynx
   E. Check for sensation in the nasal cavity

2. A 55-year-old man with severe ear pain visits an otolaryngologist. On otoscopic examination, the tympanic membrane is found to be ruptured. Which of the following nerves is responsible for sensory innervation of the inner surface of the tympanic membrane?

   A. Glossopharyngeal
   B. Auricular branch of facial
   C. Auricular branch of vagus
   D. Great auricular
   E. Lingual

3. A 70-year-old man presents to his otologist for the evaluation of his sudden hearing loss. Upon examination, the physician sees a large amount of cerumen in the external auditory meatus and removes it to fully evaluate the tympanic membrane. During this process, the patient begins to cough. The cough results from stimulation of an area of the meatus that is innervated by which nerve?

   A. Vestibulocochlear
   B. Vagus
   C. Trigeminal
   D. Facial
   E. Accessory

Ear and Nose Foreign Body Removal

INTRODUCTION

Patients presenting with foreign bodies in the nose or ear are most commonly between the ages of 2 and 8 years. The anatomical structure of the ear canal and nasal cavity allows foreign bodies to occlude them. Patients with foreign bodies in the ear are typically asymptomatic, although some may present with pain, symptoms of otitis media, hearing loss, or a sense of ear fullness. The most common foreign bodies found in the ear include beads, plastic toys, pebbles, and popcorn kernels. In patients over the age of 10 years, insects are a more common foreign body in the ear.

In order to properly treat a patient with a foreign body, it is important to classify the object into three categories: animal, vegetable, or mineral. This classification helps to determine which type of treatment should be used based on the composition of the foreign body. Animals, such as ants or flies, are commonly found in adults and require urgent attention because of the irritation and pain they cause. Vegetables such as beans and peas as well as paper matter can lead to inflammation if left inside the ear or nose over an extended period because of swelling from exposure to moisture. Mineral foreign bodies include objects such as beads, parts of toys, lead from pencils, and erasers.

One of the main reasons for the use of anesthesia in young patients is that they may be uncooperative or frightened. Only 30% of patients younger than the age of 7 years require general anesthesia to facilitate the removal of a foreign body in the ear. Graspable objects such as foam rubber, paper, and vegetable material have higher rates of successful removal under direct visualization.

CLINICALLY RELEVANT ANATOMY
Nose

The nose consists of two nasal fossae separated by a vertical septum and subdivided into three passages by the superior, middle, and inferior turbinates. Nasal foreign bodies tend to be located on the floor of the nasal passage, just below the inferior turbinate or in the upper nasal fossa anterior to the middle turbinate (Fig. 28.1). Small foreign bodies can be further aspirated through the nasal cavity into either the esophagus or trachea after passing the soft palate and epiglottis.

Ear

The external acoustic meatus is a narrow passage consisting of bone and cartilage lined with a thin layer of periosteum and skin. The canal narrows further toward the tympanic membrane, which can be a site of foreign body impaction (Fig. 28.2).

INDICATIONS
Nose

In some cases, the patient may not realize that a foreign body is in the nasal cavity until experiencing mucopurulent discharge and a foul odor. These two symptoms, especially if unilateral in children, suggest that a foreign body is present. Nasal obstruction and epistaxis, as well as unexplained pain or sneezing, snoring, or mouth breathing, may also occur when a foreign body is lodged in the nose. Anterior rhinoscopy can confirm the diagnosis.

Ear

If a foreign body has caused injury to the external acoustic meatus, tympanic membrane, or middle ear, or if vestibular symptoms such as nausea, vomiting, and nystagmus are present, the patient must be referred to an otolaryngologist. This is also the case if the object is not successfully removed on the first attempt.

Timing

Many foreign bodies are removed within 24 hours of being embedded in the ear or nose. It is critical to recognize the urgency required based on the characteristics of the object. For example, button batteries and magnets require urgent care in comparison with food items, paper, or foam.

CONTRAINDICATIONS

Referral to an otolaryngologist is necessary if the foreign body is a button battery because urgent removal is required to avoid chemical irritation and damage to surrounding tissues. If the foreign body cannot be removed on the first attempt because of bleeding or lack of proper instrumentation or if the foreign body has been pushed posteriorly into the cavity, a specialist should be consulted.

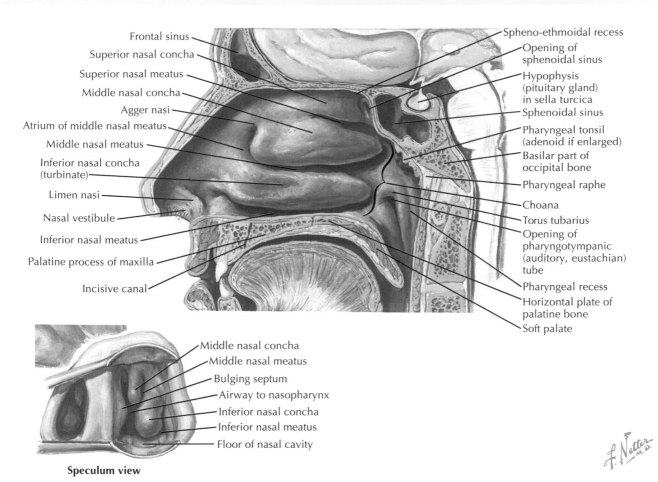

Speculum view

FIGURE 28.1 Lateral wall of nasal cavity

EQUIPMENT

Nose

The removal of nasal foreign bodies can be performed with various instruments, depending on the composition of the object. Proper visualization is necessary before removal is attempted. Use of instruments to remove foreign bodies in the anterior nasal cavity is preferred over positive pressure. The proper equipment required for removal includes the following:

Topical anesthesia and vasoconstrictor nose drops (if necessary)
Otoscope
Headlight

Blunt hooks
Itard probes
Bayonet forceps
Hartmann-type forceps
Right-angle hook, wire loop or curette

Ear

Forceps
Cerumen loop
Right-angle ball hook
Suction catheter
Angled wire loop
Angled cerumen curette

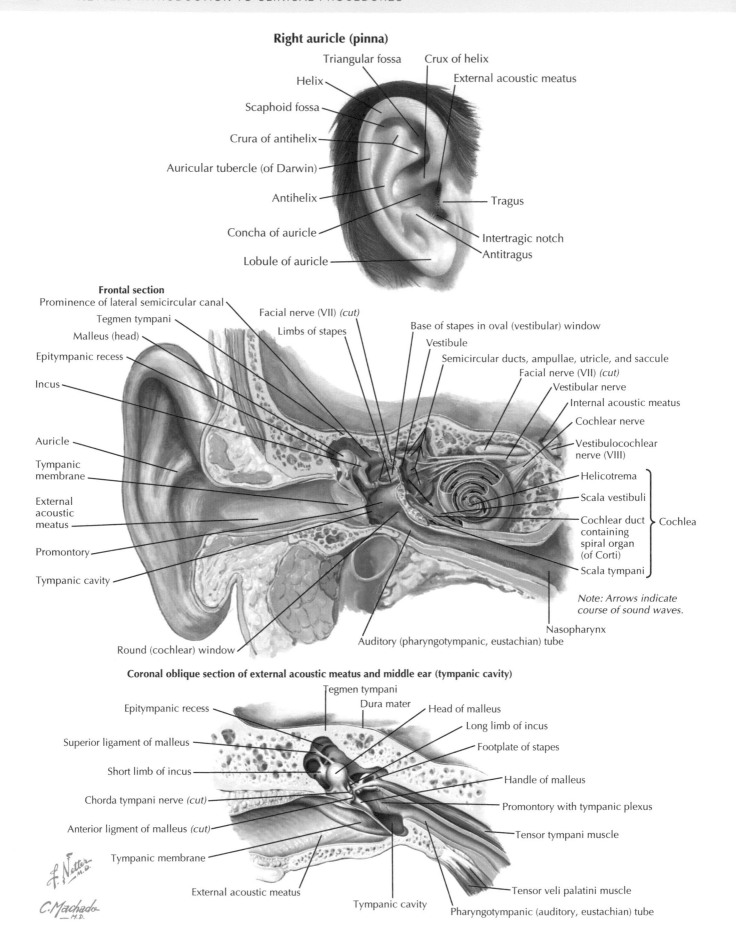

Right auricle (pinna)

Triangular fossa

Crux of helix

Helix

External acoustic meatus

Scaphoid fossa

Crura of antihelix

Auricular tubercle (of Darwin)

Antihelix

Tragus

Concha of auricle

Intertragic notch

Lobule of auricle

Antitragus

Frontal section

Prominence of lateral semicircular canal

Tegmen tympani

Malleus (head)

Epitympanic recess

Incus

Auricle

Tympanic membrane

External acoustic meatus

Promontory

Tympanic cavity

Round (cochlear) window

Facial nerve (VII) (cut)

Limbs of stapes

Base of stapes in oval (vestibular) window

Vestibule

Semicircular ducts, ampullae, utricle, and saccule

Facial nerve (VII) (cut)

Vestibular nerve

Internal acoustic meatus

Cochlear nerve

Vestibulocochlear nerve (VIII)

Helicotrema

Scala vestibuli

Cochlear duct containing spiral organ (of Corti)

Cochlea

Scala tympani

Note: Arrows indicate course of sound waves.

Nasopharynx

Auditory (pharyngotympanic, eustachian) tube

Coronal oblique section of external acoustic meatus and middle ear (tympanic cavity)

Tegmen tympani

Dura mater

Head of malleus

Epitympanic recess

Long limb of incus

Superior ligament of malleus

Footplate of stapes

Short limb of incus

Handle of malleus

Chorda tympani nerve (cut)

Promontory with tympanic plexus

Anterior ligment of malleus (cut)

Tensor tympani muscle

Tympanic membrane

External acoustic meatus

Tympanic cavity

Tensor veli palatini muscle

Pharyngotympanic (auditory, eustachian) tube

FIGURE 28.2 Anatomy of the ear

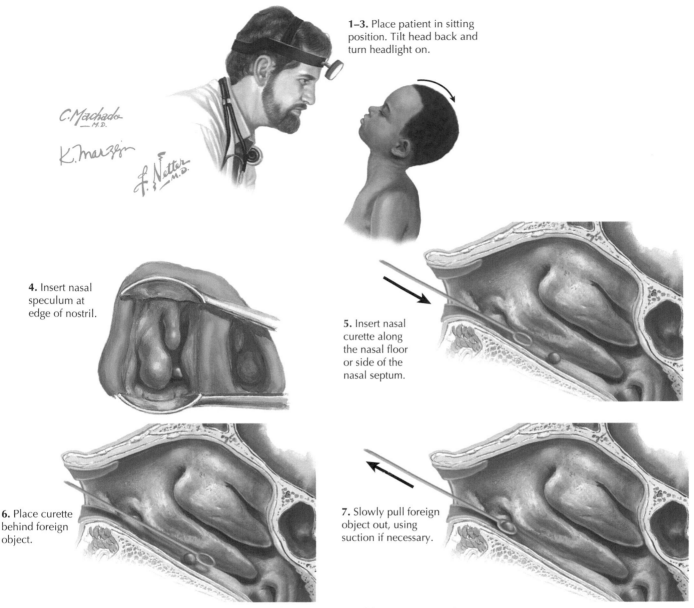

1–3. Place patient in sitting position. Tilt head back and turn headlight on.

4. Insert nasal speculum at edge of nostril.

5. Insert nasal curette along the nasal floor or side of the nasal septum.

6. Place curette behind foreign object.

7. Slowly pull foreign object out, using suction if necessary.

FIGURE 28.3 Direct removal of foreign body in the nose

PROCEDURE

Obtain patient consent and perform a time out.

Direct Removal from the Nose

See Fig. 28.3.

1. Have the patient seated.
2. Tilt the head back.
3. Turn the headlight on.
4. Insert the nasal speculum at the edge of the nostril.
5. Insert the nasal curette along the nasal floor or the side of the nasal septum.
6. Place the curette behind the foreign object.
7. Slowly pull the foreign object out, using suction if necessary.

Direct Removal from the Ear

1. Perform otoscopy to ensure that the tympanic membrane is intact.
2. Place the patient in the supine position with the affected ear up. Use restraints if needed. Cooperative patients can remain in a chair or on the stretcher with the head upright and stable.
3. If removing an insect, instill mineral oil, 95% ethanol, or 1% lidocaine to kill it prior to irrigation.
4. A butterfly cannula with the needle cut off is soft, flexible, nontraumatic, and easily available in the emergency department. It can be attached to a syringe for the irrigation of the ear canal.
5. The flow of the fluid (tap water at body temperature or normal saline in a 20- to 50-mL syringe) should be brisk and aimed at the superior part of the ear canal.

Alternative Treatment Methods

Nose

An alternative to direct removal, especially in children, is the use of increased upper airway pressure in order to propel the foreign body out of the nostril.

1. Have a caregiver hold the patient.
2. The patient's parent then occludes the contralateral nostril.
3. The parent gives mouth-to-mouth puffs of air to cause increased air pressure in the ipsilateral nostril.
4. If unsuccessful, the direct removal method can be used.

Ear

The cyanoacrylate method provides an alternative approach with few complications to removing foreign bodies from the external acoustic meatus. This method requires the use of cyanoacrylate glue on the tip of a cotton bud, straightened paper clip, or camel-hair paintbrush.

1. Place less than 0.25 mL of cyanoacrylate glue directly on the tip of a cotton bud.
2. Place the tip onto the foreign body in the external acoustic meatus.
3. Allow the glue to dry for a minimum of 25 seconds before removal.

ANATOMICAL PITFALLS

The osseous component of the external acoustic meatus is sensitive to pain and is protected only by the overlying skin, with potential for pain during the removal of foreign bodies. Narrowing of the external acoustic meatus toward the tympanic membrane also poses the risk of foreign objects being pushed further in during removal and becoming more firmly lodged in the canal. Foreign bodies remaining in the ear can cause dermatitis, inflammation, local swelling, and skin ischemia.

COMPLICATIONS

Nasal Complications

The most serious complications can occur with intranasal button batteries, including septal perforation with saddle nose deformity, nasal meatus stenosis, inferior turbinate necrosis, and collapse of the alar cartilage.

The first attempt to remove an object is likely to be the most successful. Multiple unsuccessful tries cause further swelling and bleeding and compromise patient cooperation. One of the main risks in removing a foreign body from the nose is aspiration, especially in young children who may cry and inhale the object into the airway.

Rhinolithiasis is a rare entity caused by a foreign body remaining in the nose over time. Long-standing foreign bodies can adhere to the inferior turbinate, causing local inflammation. Chronic foreign bodies may occlude the inferior or middle meatus and lead to sinusitis. In certain cases, patients can experience bilateral purulent rhinorrhea due to foreign bodies. It is recommended that a careful examination be performed before prescribing antibiotics for sinusitis because missing a foreign body may cause severe damage.

Instrumentation in the nose may cause trauma to the nasal cavity and epistaxis. This is typically temporary and can be controlled with direct pressure. The patient should be examined again before discharge to ensure that all pieces of the foreign body have been removed.

Auditory Complications

The anatomical structure of the external acoustic meatus makes it susceptible to abrasion or laceration during foreign body removal in up to 50% of patients. The risk of complications is increased with multiple attempts. Treatment consists of topical antibiotic eardrops. Tympanic membrane perforation and middle ear damage are possible but not as common as the lacerations of the external acoustic meatus. Serious complications are associated with button batteries and require urgent consultation with an otolaryngologist.

CONCLUSION

Proper and timely removal of foreign bodies in the external acoustic meatus and nasal passages will avoid complications in the impacted area, which include traumatic damage and eventual infection. Patients presenting with foreign bodies are typically children in the toddler age group, and they are frequently asymptomatic. A caregiver may have witnessed the insertion of a foreign object into the nares or ear canal or the patient may present with otorrhea, rhinorrhea, or bleeding. Diagnosis can be confirmed upon visual inspection with rhinoscopy or otoscopy. Occasionally, a foreign body may be an incidental finding.

The choice of extraction method lies with the practitioner, and the decision to use irrigation versus manual extraction in the ear is a clinical judgment based on the anatomical location of impaction, shape, and type of the object. Urgent referral to an otolaryngologist should be considered with any evidence of trauma to surrounding tissues, sharp objects, or suspicion of button batteries.

Suggested Readings

Antonelli PJ, Ahmadi A, Prevatt A. Insecticidal activity of common reagents for insect foreign bodies of the ear. *Laryngoscope.* 2001;111:15.

Backlin SA. Positive-pressure technique for nasal foreign body removal in children. *Ann Emerg Med.* 1995;25:554.

Balbani AP, Tanit GS, Ossamu B, Márcia AK, et al. Ear and nose foreign body removal in children. *Int J of Pediatric Otorhinol.* 1998;46.1-2:37–42.

Botma M, Bader R, Kubba H. "A parent's kiss": evaluating an unusual method for removing nasal foreign bodies in children. *J Laryngol Otol.* 2000;114:598.

Bressler K, Clough S. Ear foreign-body removal: a review of 98 consecutive cases. *The Laryngoscope.* 1993;103.4:367–370.

Davies PH. Foreign bodies in the nose and ear: a review of techniques for removal in the emergency department. *Emerg Med J.* 2000;17.2:91–94.

Figueiredo RR, Azevedo AA, Kós AO, Tomita S. Nasal foreign bodies: description of types and complications in 420 cases. *Braz J Otorhinol.* 2006;72:18.

François M, Hamrioui R, Narcy P. Nasal foreign bodies in children. *Eur Arch Otorhinol.* 1998;255:132.

Guidera AK, Stegehuis HR. Button batteries: the worst case scenario in nasal foreign bodies. *N Z Med.* 2010;123:68.

Heim SW, Maughan KL. Foreign bodies in the ear, nose, and throat. *Am Fam Physician.* 2007;76:1185.

McLaughlin R, Ullah R, Heylings D. Comparative prospective study of foreign body removal from external acoustic meatus of cadavers with right angle hook or cyanoacrylate glue. *Emerg Med J.* 2002;19:43.

Schulze SL, Kerschner J, Beste D. Pediatric external acoustic meatus foreign bodies: a review of 698 cases. *Otolaryngol Head Neck Surg.* 2002;127:73.

Votey S, Dudley JP. Emergency ear, nose, and throat procedures. *Emerg Med Clin North Am.* 1989;7:117–154.

REVIEW QUESTIONS

1. A 5-year-old boy is admitted to the hospital with otitis media. Otoscopic examination reveals a bulging and inflamed eardrum. It is decided to incise the tympanic membrane to relieve the painful pressure and allow drainage of the infection associated with otitis media. Which of the following is the best location for making an opening (myringotomy) for drainage?

   A. The anterior superior quadrant of the eardrum
   B. The posterior superior quadrant of the eardrum
   C. Directly through the site of the umbo
   D. The posterior inferior quadrant of the eardrum
   E. A vertical incision should be made in the eardrum, from the 12 o'clock to the 6 o'clock position of the rim of the eardrum

2. A 55-year-old man with severe ear pain visits an otorhinolaryngologist. On otoscopic examination, the tympanic membrane is seen to be ruptured. Which of the following nerves is responsible for the sensory innervation of the inner surface of the tympanic membrane?

   A. Glossopharyngeal nerve
   B. Auricular branch of the facial nerve
   C. Auricular branch of the vagus nerve
   D. Great auricular nerve
   E. Lingual nerve

3. A 15-year-old boy was brought to the emergency department complaining of pain in the right ear. While attempting to clean his itchy ear with a swab, his little brother bumped his elbow, causing the stick to penetrate deeply into the ear. On examination with the otoscope, the tympanic membrane was pearly white and there was no cone of light visible. There was clotted blood in the external auditory meatus. The Rinne test was positive (bone conduction was better than air conduction). Which of the following best describes the nerves responsible for the perception of pain from the injured area?

   A. Auriculotemporal and great auricular nerves
   B. Facial, glossopharyngeal, and vagus nerves
   C. Lesser occipital and great auricular nerve
   D. Chorda tympani and glossopharyngeal nerve
   E. Tympanic plexus and lesser petrosal nerve

Burr Hole Craniotomy

INTRODUCTION

Traumatic injuries to the head can result in extensive damage to the brain and may be life threatening in the event of bleeding within the cranial cavity. Blunt trauma or acceleration injuries can cause the rupture and tearing of arteries or veins, leading to blood pooling in distinct intracranial compartments. A rise in intracranial pressure and the resultant mass effect on the brain can cause a variety of complications such as uncal herniation, brain stem compression, and ischemia. If untreated, the result may be a loss of neurologic function, coma, or death. Treatment for such hemorrhages is usually performed by trained neurosurgeons, but if a surgeon is unavailable, the emergency physician may need to perform a burr hole craniotomy as a life-saving procedure.

Burr hole craniotomy is performed for the management of cranial trauma when a patient has a suspected or confirmed acute epidural hematoma (EDH) or subdural hematoma (SDH). It is a temporizing procedure, but it may be life-saving until a definitive neurosurgical operation can be performed. The goal is to drill a small hole into the patient's skull and expand the opening, so that blood clots can be removed from the intracranial space to relieve pressure. An SDH occurs below the dura mater, requiring further penetration through the dura in order to evacuate pooled blood.

Burr hole craniotomy may not be as effective for treating SDH as it is for treating EDH. The literature shows that the critical time factor for treating SDH is not the interval from injury to surgical treatment but rather the time between clinical deterioration and treatment. This emphasizes the need for careful evaluation by a clinician other than a neurosurgeon when deciding whether to perform an emergency burr hole craniotomy for SDH. The time needed for the procedure from the decision to operate to the opening of the dura mater is usually less than 20 minutes, so it can be performed quickly in a patient who is deteriorating.

CLINICALLY RELEVANT ANATOMY
Epidural Hematoma

EDH occurs between the periosteal layer of the dura and the bones of the skull where the meningeal arteries (particularly the middle meningeal artery) reside (Figs. 29.1, 29.2, and 29.3). When these arteries are ruptured by a skull fracture from blunt trauma, they bleed into the tight space, forming an EDH. A common location for this is in the temporal region, with the EDH resulting from trauma to the pterion, an area of the lateral skull that is thin and beneath which lie the branches of the middle meningeal artery. A distinguishing feature of EDH on computed tomography (CT) is a visible biconvex hematoma that does not cross suture lines.

A lucid interval, also called "talk and deteriorate," may occur when the patient is initially rendered unconscious, regains consciousness, and then deteriorates a short time later, sometimes after having left the medical facility. Although some consider this to be the rule, it actually occurs in only 12% to 32% of patients who become comatose after head trauma and in less than 50% of those with EDH. A study of 211 patients who had a lucid interval found that 71% deteriorated within the first 24 hours after injury. Mortality from EDH is nearly 20%, but early intervention may improve outcomes.

Subdural Hematoma

SDH occurs in the space between the meningeal layer of the dura mater and the arachnoid mater (see Figs. 29.1, 29.2, and 29.3). This is normally a potential space, but in SDH the layers become separated by venous blood from the rupture of the bridging veins crossing the dura mater or from the intracranial dural venous sinuses. Because of the low pressure of the venous vessels, it may take days to weeks for noticeable symptoms to occur. By that time, the patient may not associate the problem with previous trauma. On CT imaging, SDH appears as a "crescent" shape that crosses suture lines (Fig. 29.4). Although mortality rates from acute SDH have historically been reported to be nearly 60%, more recent studies report a mortality rate of 22% to 40% after definitive surgery.

INDICATIONS

The primary indication for an emergency burr hole craniotomy is if the time required for transfer to a facility for definitive neurosurgical treatment is deemed too long to wait. This judgment must be made based on factors such as the distance to the nearest neurosurgical unit and the severity of injury. A Glasgow Coma Scale score of 8 or less or other signs of intracranial hypertension such as anisocoria or hemiparesis indicate the need for emergency intervention, as does the failure of first-line procedures such as intravenous (IV) mannitol and hyperventilation.

CONTRAINDICATIONS

Emergency burr hole craniotomy is contraindicated when the condition does not meet the criteria noted above. In cases where there is a nearby neurosurgical unit, a Glasgow Coma Scale score greater than 8, and no signs of intracranial

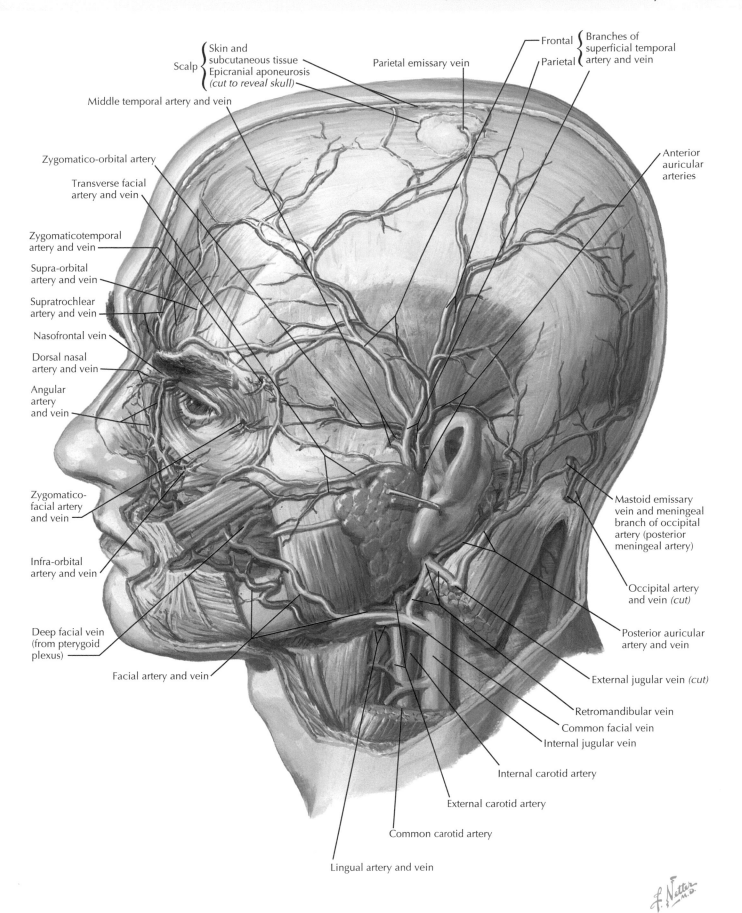

FIGURE 29.1 Superficial arteries and veins of face and scalp

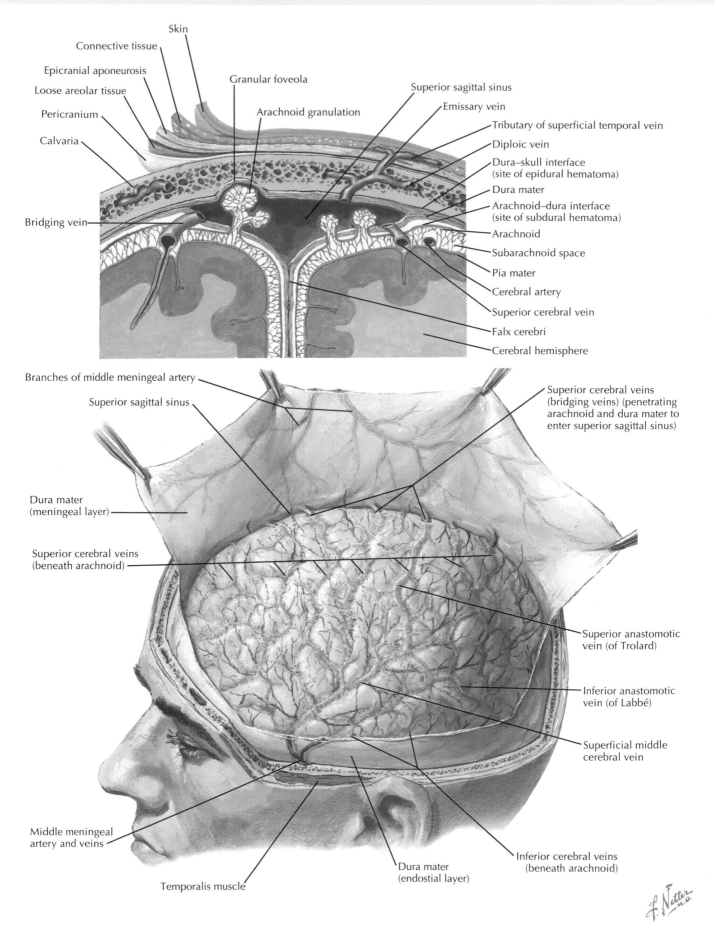

Skin

Connective tissue

Epicranial aponeurosis

Loose areolar tissue

Pericranium

Calvaria

Granular foveola

Arachnoid granulation

Superior sagittal sinus

Emissary vein

Tributary of superficial temporal vein

Diploic vein

Dura–skull interface (site of epidural hematoma)

Dura mater

Arachnoid–dura interface (site of subdural hematoma)

Arachnoid

Subarachnoid space

Pia mater

Cerebral artery

Superior cerebral vein

Falx cerebri

Cerebral hemisphere

Bridging vein

Branches of middle meningeal artery

Superior sagittal sinus

Dura mater (meningeal layer)

Superior cerebral veins (beneath arachnoid)

Middle meningeal artery and veins

Temporalis muscle

Dura mater (endostial layer)

Superior cerebral veins (bridging veins) (penetrating arachnoid and dura mater to enter superior sagittal sinus)

Superior anastomotic vein (of Trolard)

Inferior anastomotic vein (of Labbé)

Superficial middle cerebral vein

Inferior cerebral veins (beneath arachnoid)

FIGURE 29.2 Meninges and superficial cerebral veins

Temporal Fossa Hematoma

Shift of normal midline structures

Compression of posterior cerebral artery

Skull fracture crossing middle meningeal artery

Shift of brain stem to opposite side may reverse lateralization of signs by tentorial pressure on contralateral pathways

Herniation of temporal lobe under tentorium cerebelli

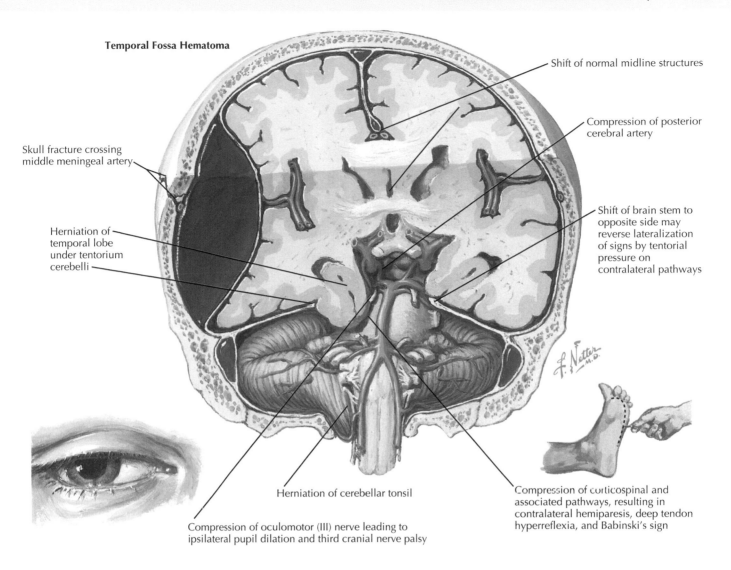

Herniation of cerebellar tonsil

Compression of corticospinal and associated pathways, resulting in contralateral hemiparesis, deep tendon hyperreflexia, and Babinski's sign

Compression of oculomotor (III) nerve leading to ipsilateral pupil dilation and third cranial nerve palsy

Subfrontal Hematoma
Frontal trauma: headache, poor cerebration, intermittent disorientation, anisocoria

Acute Subdural Hematoma

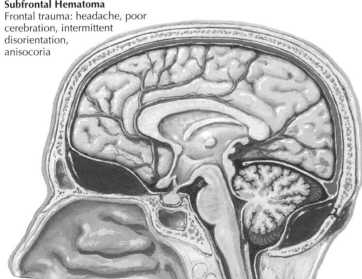

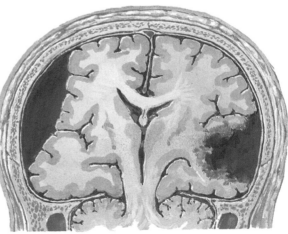

Posterior Fossa Hematoma
Occipital trauma and/or fracture: headache, meningismus, cerebellar and cranial nerve signs, Cushing's triad

Section showing acute subdural hematoma on right side and subdural hematoma associated with temporal lobe intracerebral hematoma ("burst" temporal lobe) on left

FIGURE 29.3 Hematomas

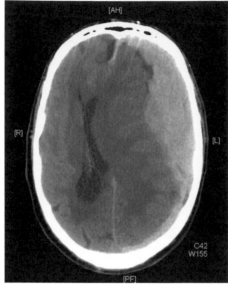
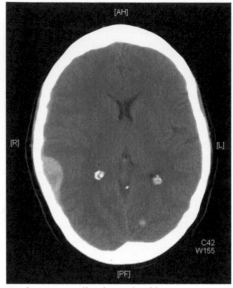

CT showing left subdural hematoma　　　　CT showing small right epidural hematoma

FIGURE 29.4 General features of hemorrhage

herniation, an emergency burr hole craniotomy should not be performed. If the volume of an EDH is less than 30 cm³, other less-invasive maneuvers should be considered first. If imaging such as CT is not available to localize the bleed, a burr hole craniotomy should not be attempted.

EQUIPMENT

Hudson brace or twist drill or trephinator or motorized drill
Perforator drill bit and burr bit (make sure they fit the equipment being used)
Saline
Suction catheter
Sterile drapes
Antiseptic prep
Scalpel, No. 15 or 11
Self-retaining retractors
Dural hook
Periosteal elevator
Bone rongeur
Bone wax
Needle driver
Suture scissors
Head support
Absorbable suture
Monofilament suture
Forceps, toothed
0.5% lidocaine with 1:200,000 epinephrine (optional)

PROCEDURE

Obtain patient consent and perform a time out. See Fig. 29.5.

Patient Preparation

1. Contact the nearest neurosurgeon for consultation and advice for the procedure, as there may be individual variables that determine the best course of action.

2. Intubate the patient and hyperventilate to a PCO_2 of 25 to 28 mm Hg. Use IV lidocaine (100 mg) or anesthesia to prevent hypertension due to intubation, if deemed necessary. Administer 20% mannitol 1 g/kg IV over 20 minutes.

3. Angle the bed between 15 and 30 degrees, with the head rotated as needed for a temporal, frontal, or parietal burr hole. The head should be supported by a headrest, and padding should be put underneath the ipsilateral shoulder for support. For a posterior fossa or occipital burr hole, the patient should be placed prone with the head flexed.

4. Shave a 5-cm area where the incision will be made.

5. Sterilize the area and apply a drape.

Scalp Incision

6. Since the area of blood collection is readily visualized with CT, it is possible to ascertain the precise location of the hemorrhage. Scalp infiltration with 0.5% lidocaine and 1:200,000 epinephrine can be used to prevent bleeding at the incision.

   a. Temporal: Center a 4-cm vertical incision about 2 cm anterior to the tragus and 2 cm above the zygomatic arch. The incision should penetrate the temporalis muscle. Palpate the superficial temporal artery to prevent injury to this vessel. Use the back of the scalpel to scrape the temporalis muscle off the underlying bone.

   b. Parietal: Make a vertical incision 3 cm posterior to the external acoustic meatus and 5 cm lateral to the midline.

   c. Frontal: Make a horizontal incision anterior to the coronal suture and at least 3 cm lateral to the midline at approximately the mid-pupillary line. The burr hole should be placed anterior to the coronal suture to help avoid any damage to the motor cortex.

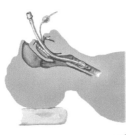

1–3. Contact nearest neurosurgeon. Intubate and ventilate patient. Place patient in proper position, rotating head and supporting ipsilateral shoulder.

4–6. Shave 5 cm area where incision will be made. Sterilize incision area and drape. Make a vertical incision 3 cm posterior to external acoustic meatus and 5 cm lateral to midline.

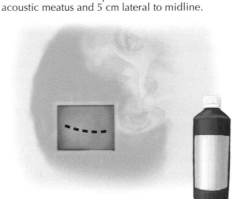

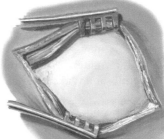

7. Retract any muscle and incision with self-retaining retractor for maximum exposure.

8–9. Drill into the skull until bit traverses the inner table of the bone. Use saline and suction to irrigate field and clear off bone dust.

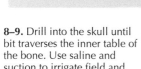

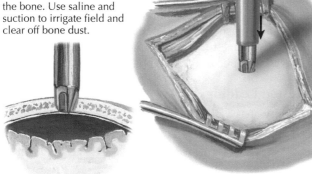

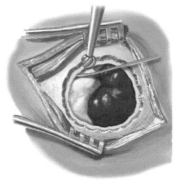

10. Switch to burr bit and make a cylindrical hole, leaving a thin fine rim of inner table at edges. Use an elevator to separate the rim from dura mater if necessary.

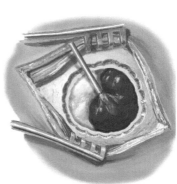

11. Suction the hematoma.

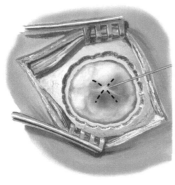

12–13. Dark blue color is visible in the case of a subdural hematoma. Use dural hook to lift dura and carefully make two incisions, forming a cross, with scalpel. Take care not to suction brain while suctioning hematoma.

14. Close wound in two layers.

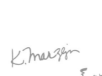

K. Marzin
F. Netter M.D.

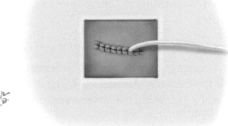

FIGURE 29.5 Emergent craniotomy for intracranial hematoma

d. Posterior cranial fossa or occipital: Make a vertical incision 3 cm medial to the mastoid process. When the burr hole is made, care must be taken not to make it too high or it may penetrate the transverse sinus.

Drilling and Evacuation

7. After the incision is made and the muscle overlying the bone is scraped off, insert a self-retaining retractor to hold the incision open for maximal exposure. Retractors are also useful for partial hemostasis.

8. Use the triangular perforator drill bit in the Hudson brace at the midpoint of the calculated location of the hematoma, angled perpendicularly to the skull. Drill into the skull until the perforating bit traverses the inner table.

9. Use saline and suction to irrigate the field, clearing off bone debris.

10. Switch the perforator drill bit for the burr bit to expand the hole and make it cylindrical while leaving a thin, fine rim of inner table at the edges. An elevator should be used to separate the rim from the dura mater. The rim is removed with a bone rongeur. Use bone wax to control bone bleeding.

11. An EDH should be amenable to evacuation by suction; however, if extensive clotting has occurred, it may be

necessary to further expand the hole. Use a rongeur to expand the hole to a 4-cm diameter, taking care not to damage the dura mater.

12. An SDH may appear as a dark blue area seen through the dura mater. Use a dural hook to hold up the dura carefully and make two incisions forming a "cross" with a No. 15 or No. 11 scalpel blade.

13. When using suction for an SDH, use lower suction pressures and take extra care not to apply suction directly to the brain. If necessary to fully evacuate the clot, expand the burr hole with a rongeur, as indicated in step 5.

14. Close the wound in two layers. Absorbable sutures are used for the galeal layer and staples or monofilament sutures for the skin.

ANATOMICAL PITFALLS
Brain and Motor Cortex

Possible mechanical injury to the brain is a cause for concern when attempting to perform a burr hole craniotomy. Although the brain is covered by the meningeal layers, uncontrolled drilling may cause either blunt or sharp injury to the cortex, if a "plunging" motion occurs. Use of a variable depth stop or a clutched drill can prevent this. In addition, positioning the burr hole over the area of blood collection provides an extra barrier. As stated above, frontal burr holes should be placed anterior to the coronal suture to prevent accidental injury to the motor cortex.

Superior Sagittal Sinus

The superior sagittal sinus lies in the midline of the skull and travels back to the confluence of sinuses. It is formed by the dural folds that come together to form the falx cerebri. Always avoid drilling in the midline to prevent damage to this structure.

Superficial Temporal Artery

With a temporal burr hole, the superficial temporal artery is at risk for damage. Accidental incision of this artery can be avoided by palpating the artery and positioning the incision accordingly.

Transverse Sinus

The transverse sinus is formed by the dura of the tentorium cerebelli against the posterior aspect of the occipital bone where it meets at the confluence of sinuses in the midline. In the rare case a posterior fossa or occipital burr hole is required, care must be taken not to make the hole too far superior so as to avoid bleeding from the sinus.

COMPLICATIONS

Bleeding from the scalp and skull may occur, although this is infrequent. Performing a burr hole craniotomy typically does not allow for the localization and treatment of the source of the intracranial bleed, which is why this procedure is not the primary operation of choice. The burr hole craniotomy may cause an additional hematoma, particularly when performed for chronic SDH. Accidental penetration of the superior sagittal sinus may cause life-threatening bleeding, which is why it is imperative to drill well away from the midline.

Plunging of the drill bit into the cavity may cause a penetrating injury to the dura, blood vessels, or the brain itself, possibly causing intracerebral hematoma, cortical lacerations, and subdural, extradural, and interventricular hematomas. However, proper equipment and placement of the burr hole may help reduce the chance of plunging, as noted above.

There is a risk of wound infection, meningitis, and encephalitis following burr hole craniotomy. Although it is preferred that the procedure be performed in the operating room, proper sterile technique should minimize the risk of infection, even if it must be performed in the emergency department.

CONCLUSION

Burr hole craniotomy performed by an emergency physician is a potentially life-saving procedure that requires careful judgment as to whether it is required. By rapidly relieving building pressure within the cranial cavity, a burr hole is a temporizing measure that may reduce the chance of severe neurologic damage to the brain and brainstem until further treatment by a neurosurgeon is possible.

Suggested Readings

Bullock MR, Chesnut R, Ghajar J, et al. Surgical management of acute subdural hematomas. *Neurosurgery*. 2006;58:S16–S24.

Donovan DJ, Moquin RR, Ecklund JM. Cranial burr holes and emergency craniotomy: review of indications and technique. *Mil Med*. 2006;171: 12–19.

Liu JT, Tyan YS, Lee YK, Wang JT. Emergency management of epidural haematoma through burr hole evacuation and drainage. A preliminary report. *Acta Neurochir (Wien)*. 2006;148:313–317.

Rohde V, Graf G, Hassler W. Complications of burr-hole craniostomy and closed-system drainage for chronic subdural hematomas: a retrospective analysis of 376 patients. *Neurosurg Rev*. 2002;25:89–94.

Smith SW, Clark M, Nelson J, Heegaard W, Lufkin KC, Ruiz E. Emergency department skull trephination for epidural hematoma in patients who are awake but deteriorate rapidly. *J Emerg Med*. 2010;39:377–383.

Springer MFB, Baker FJ. Cranial burr hole decompression in the emergency department. *Am J Emerg Med*. 1988;6:640–646.

Tian H, Chen S, Xu T, et al. Risk factors related to hospital mortality in patients with isolated traumatic acute subdural haematoma: analysis of 308 patients undergone surgery. *Chin Med J*. 2008;121:1080–1084.

Tien HCN, Jung V, Pinto R, Mainprize T, Scales DC, Rizoli SB. Reducing time-to-treatment decreases mortality of trauma patients with acute subdural hematoma. *Ann Surg*. 2011;253:1178–1183.

Yoshino Y, Aoki N, Oikawa A, Ohno K. Acute epidural hematoma developing during twist-drill craniostomy: a complication of percutaneous subdural tapping for the treatment of chronic subdural hematoma. *Surg Neurol*. 2000;53:601–604.

REVIEW QUESTIONS

1. A 40-year-old unconscious man is admitted to the emergency department after being hit in the head with a baseball. CT reveals a fractured pterion and an epidural hematoma. Branches of which of the following arteries are most likely to be injured?

   A. External carotid

   B. Superficial temporal

C. Maxillary
D. Deep temporal
E. Middle meningeal

2. A 65-year-old man is admitted to the hospital 3 weeks after what he reported to be a "small bump of his head" sustained from hitting a low-hanging branch while driving his tractor through the apple orchard. On physical examination, the patient displays mental confusion and poor physical coordination. CT reveals an intracranial thrombus probably due to leakage from a cerebral vein over the right cerebral hemisphere. From what condition is the patient most likely suffering?

A. Subarachnoid hemorrhage
B. Epidural hematoma
C. Intracerebral bleeding into the brain parenchyma
D. Subdural hematoma
E. Bleeding into the cerebral ventricular system

Elbow Joint Aspiration

INTRODUCTION

Joint aspiration, also known as *arthrocentesis*, is a safe and minimally invasive clinical procedure in which a needle and syringe are used to collect synovial fluid from the joint capsule. This procedure can be used to establish a diagnosis, alleviate discomfort, drain infected fluid or blood, or inject medication into the joint space. As a diagnostic aid, arthrocentesis helps distinguish inflammatory arthropathies from osteoarthritis or crystal-induced arthritides. This chapter focuses on elbow joint arthrocentesis.

If available, ultrasonography should be used as an adjunct. Recent studies suggest that ultrasound-guided arthrocentesis is superior to the classic anatomical landmark- and palpation-guided procedure. The use of ultrasonography greatly minimizes procedural pain, improves arthrocentesis success, yields more synovial fluid, allows greater joint decompression, and improves clinical outcomes. Ultrasonography can be used to guide needle insertion under direct visualization. Alternatively, it can be used indirectly, visualizing and marking the site targeted for needle insertion and estimating the depth and direction of needle placement.

If ultrasonography is not readily available, the procedure must be performed by palpation-guided arthrocentesis. When using anatomical landmarks, the risk of injury can be minimized by following the procedural approach outlined below. In either case, it is important to have a fundamental understanding of the clinically relevant anatomy to avoid injury to tendons, ligaments, muscles, and neurovascular structures when performing arthrocentesis of the elbow.

CLINICALLY RELEVANT ANATOMY

The elbow joint is a complex synovial hinge joint that consists of three joints within one joint capsule: the humeroradial, humeroulnar, and radioulnar joints. The humeroradial and humeroulnar joints are responsible for flexion and extension of the elbow, whereas the radioulnar joint is responsible for pronation and supination of the forearm and wrist at the elbow (Fig. 30.1).

The humeroradial joint is a ball-and-socket joint with articulation between the capitulum of the humeral condyle and the head of the radius. The humeroulnar joint is a synovial hinge joint with articulation between the trochlea of the humeral condyle and the trochlear notch of the ulna. The radioulnar joint is a pivot-type synovial joint with articulation between the head of the radius and the radial notch of the ulna.

The joint capsule is continuous over all three joints. The inner portion of the joint capsule is lined by synovium (also known as synovial membrane), which produces the synovial fluid responsible for lubricating the joint (Fig. 30.2). Anteriorly, the joint capsule extends from the distal humerus to the coronoid process, annular ligament, and radial head. Posteriorly, the capsule extends from the distal humerus to the olecranon process and annular ligament. Fat pads near the olecranon, coronoid fossa, and radial notch lie between the synovium and joint capsule (Fig. 30.3). When the synovial sac is distended with fluid, the fat pads are displaced away from the humerus. On lateral elbow radiographs, this finding helps establish the diagnosis of joint effusion.

The ulnar and radial collateral ligaments are triangular bands that blend with and reinforce the surrounding joint capsule. Functionally, these ligaments help the articular surfaces to remain in contact with each other and serve to limit lateral movement. The ulnar collateral ligament has its apex on the medial epicondyle and has three main bands. The anterior band, the most important component, runs from the medial epicondyle to the coronoid process. The middle band is oriented toward the coronoid process, and the posterior band is directed toward the olecranon. The radial collateral ligament extends from the lateral epicondyle and blends distally into the annular ligament of the radius. This ligament wraps around the head of the radius and attaches to the ulna anteriorly and posteriorly. The surface of the annular ligament is lined with synovial membrane and allows the head of the radius to rotate during supination and pronation while maintaining the stability of the radioulnar joint.

There are many bursae in the elbow, with the most clinically significant being the subcutaneous, subtendinous, and intratendinous. The subcutaneous olecranon bursa is found in the connective tissue over the olecranon. The subtendinous bursa, located between the olecranon and the tendon of the triceps brachii, helps to reduce the friction between the two structures during flexion and extension of the arm. The intratendinous bursa is found within the distal tendon of the triceps brachii.

Several vital structures share a close anatomical relationship with the elbow joint capsule. Structures such as ligaments, nerves, muscles, and vessels are at risk of injury during joint aspiration. Hence, it is important to have a sound knowledge of the regional anatomy.

INDICATIONS

Before arthrocentesis is performed, periarticular entities, such as bursitis, cellulitis, contusion, and tendonitis, must be differentiated from articular processes. Typically, periarticular

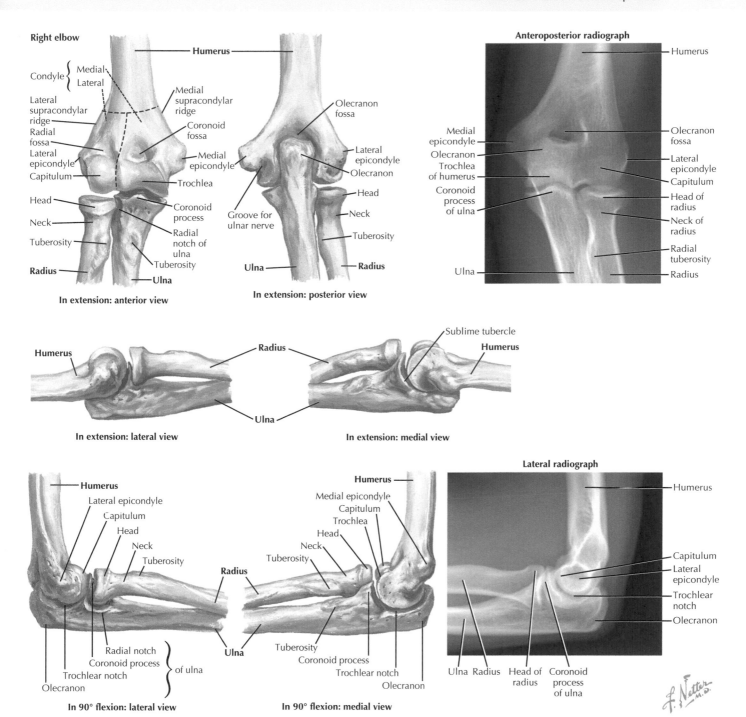

FIGURE 30.1 Bones of the elbow

processes restrict the active range of motion more than the passive range and are localized to a specific area, whereas articular processes restrict both active and passive ranges of motion and often produce circumferential pain and swelling.

Elbow joint aspiration can be used for both diagnostic and therapeutic purposes.

Diagnostic Elbow Joint Aspiration

Diagnostic elbow joint aspiration is indicated when evaluating for chronic arthritis (rheumatoid arthritis, osteoarthritis), crystal-induced arthritis (gout, pseudogout), septic arthritis,

articular inflammation of unknown origin, joint effusion, and hemarthrosis (Fig. 30.4).

Aspirated synovial fluid is of high diagnostic value and can be analyzed for viscosity, glucose, total protein, uric acid, lactate, cell count, rheumatoid factor, mucin clots, and crystals. The fluid sample can also undergo polymerase chain reaction studies, Gram stain, and culture for bacteria, mycobacteria, and fungi.

Therapeutic Elbow Joint Aspiration

Therapeutically, elbow joint aspiration is used to aspirate effusion or blood to relieve pain; improve mobilization of the

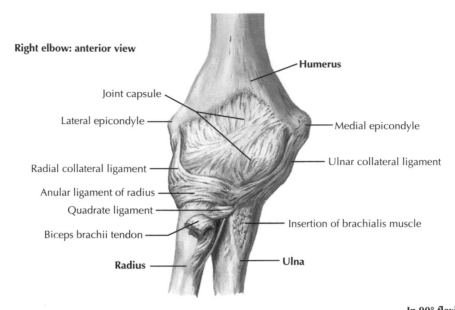

Right elbow: anterior view

Humerus

Joint capsule

Lateral epicondyle

Medial epicondyle

Radial collateral ligament

Ulnar collateral ligament

Anular ligament of radius

Quadrate ligament

Insertion of brachialis muscle

Biceps brachii tendon

Radius

Ulna

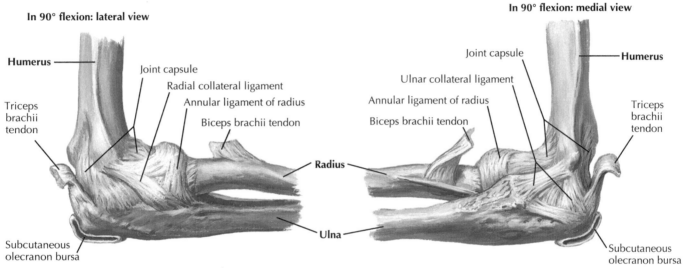

In 90° flexion: lateral view

In 90° flexion: medial view

Humerus

Joint capsule

Radial collateral ligament

Annular ligament of radius

Biceps brachii tendon

Triceps
brachii
tendon

Radius

Ulna

Subcutaneous
olecranon bursa

Joint capsule

Ulnar collateral ligament

Annular ligament of radius

Biceps brachii tendon

Humerus

Triceps
brachii
tendon

Subcutaneous
olecranon bursa

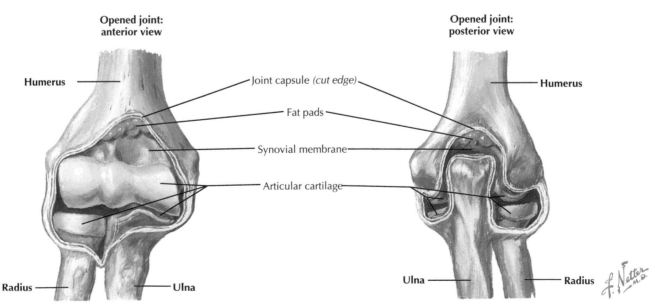

**Opened joint:
anterior view**

**Opened joint:
posterior view**

Humerus

Joint capsule (*cut edge*)

Humerus

Fat pads

Synovial membrane

Articular cartilage

Radius

Ulna

Ulna

Radius

FIGURE 30.2 Ligaments of the elbow

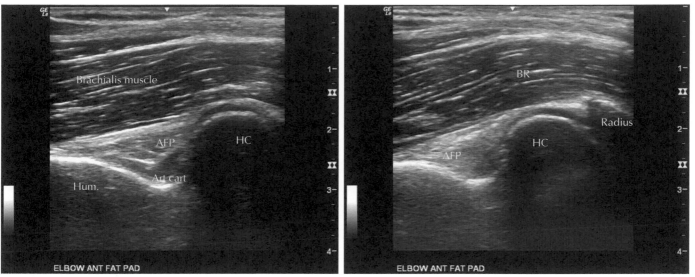

FIGURE 30.3 Ultrasound imaging of the elbow joint. AFP, anterior fat pad; Art cart, articular cartilage; BR, brachialis; HC, Humerus capitulum; Hum., humerus.

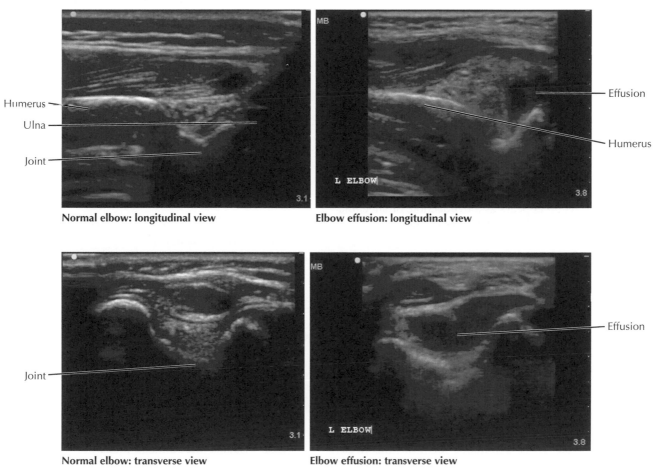

FIGURE 30.4 Ultrasound imaging of normal elbow joint and elbow joint effusion

joint; inject medications such as corticosteroids, antibiotics, or anesthetics; and drain septic effusions.

CONTRAINDICATIONS

There are few contraindications to elbow joint aspiration. Relative contraindications include cellulitis, dermatitis, or skin infection overlying the site of needle entry; adjacent osteomyelitis; uncontrolled coagulopathy; and joint prosthesis. Suspected bacteremia is a relative contraindication, but arthrocentesis should still be performed if septic arthritis is suspected.

EQUIPMENT

Sterile gloves and drapes
Sterile gauze squares
Sterile hemostat
Sterile bandage
Tray table
Skin antiseptic solution: povidone-iodine or chlorhexidine
Syringes
One small syringe (5 or 10 mL) for anesthetic
Three large syringes (30 mL) for aspiration
Selection of needles: 18, 20, and 25 gauge
Local anesthetic (1% lidocaine)
Specimen tubes
Ultrasound, if available

PROCEDURE

Obtain patient consent and perform a time out.

Traditionally, elbow joint aspiration has been performed using external anatomical landmarks. A medial approach is generally advised against, so a needle is advanced into the joint space via a lateral approach, using the center of the anconeus triangle as a landmark. However, if available, ultrasonography can facilitate a lateral, posterior, or medial approach. The lateral approach is preferred for arthrocentesis. On ultrasound, a joint capsule effusion appears as a hypoechoic or anechoic fluid collection that superficially displaces the fat pad.

Traditional Lateral Approach for Elbow Joint Arthrocentesis

See Fig. 30.5.

Explain the procedure and reassure the patient that the procedure has very few risks. Inform the patient that there may be some pain during the injection of local anesthetic and when the synovial cavity is entered.

1. Position the patient sitting up with the affected arm abducted, resting at the patient's side, and pronated and flexed to 90 degrees.
2. Carefully examine, palpate, and identify the lateral olecranon process, lateral epicondyle of the humerus, and radial head. These landmarks form the anconeus triangle, with its center as the site of needle insertion.
3. Mark the site with a plastic needle sheath or sterile marker.
4. Don the appropriate personal protective equipment. Wearing sterile gloves, sterilize the skin with antiseptic

solution, starting from the marked site and working outward in concentric circles. Allow the application to dry. If the patient is allergic to iodine, 70% alcohol can be used. Sterile drapes may be used but are not required.

5. Anesthetize the region with 1% lidocaine in a 5-mL syringe with a 25-gauge needle. Make a small wheal to anesthetize the skin and subcutaneous tissue at the insertion site. Insert the needle deeper, anesthetizing along the anticipated track of the arthrocentesis needle.
6. Place an 18- or 20-gauge needle on a 5- or 10-mL syringe, and use the nondominant hand to stretch the patient's skin.
7. Insert the needle at a 90-degree angle to the skin in the depression between the olecranon and lateral epicondyle.
8. Slowly advance the needle medially, directed toward the medial epicondyle. Gently pull back on the syringe plunger to check for the return of synovial fluid.
9. If aspiration is unsuccessful, draw the needle back, reidentify the landmarks, and correct the needle position. If the needle hits bone, it should be pulled back and redirected at a slightly different angle.
10. Once the syringe has filled, place a hemostat on the hub of the needle. With the needle stabilized, disconnect the syringe. A new syringe can be attached to drain more fluid or to deliver medicine, such as a corticosteroid, into the joint space.
11. Slowly withdraw the needle and syringe from the joint space. Once withdrawn, place the safety cap over the needle and ensure proper disposal.
12. Apply pressure over the procedure site with gauze for a few minutes until the site is clear of fluid or blood. Dress with a sterile bandage and elastic wrap.
13. The synovial fluid should be placed in properly labeled specimen tubes and sent promptly for analysis.

Ultrasound-Guided Lateral Approach for Elbow Joint Arthrocentesis

1. Follow sterile procedures.
2. Position the patient sitting up with the affected arm abducted, resting at the patient's side, and pronated and flexed to 90 degrees.
3. Place towels or sheets under the elbow to elevate the joint. This makes the procedure easier to perform.
4. First, examine the nonaffected elbow with ultrasound, then compare it with the examination of the joint capsule of the affected elbow. The goal is to find the landmarks that form the anconeus triangle.
5. Place the linear, transducer (10-5 MHz) longitudinally along the proximal forearm, parallel to the shaft of the radius, and with the probe marker toward the patient's head. Visualize the rounded radial head, lateral epicondyle, and capitulum. The lateral radiocapitellar joint space can be assessed for effusion.
6. The common extensor tendon is superficial to the radiocapitellar joint space and can be easily identified and avoided when seen on ultrasound.

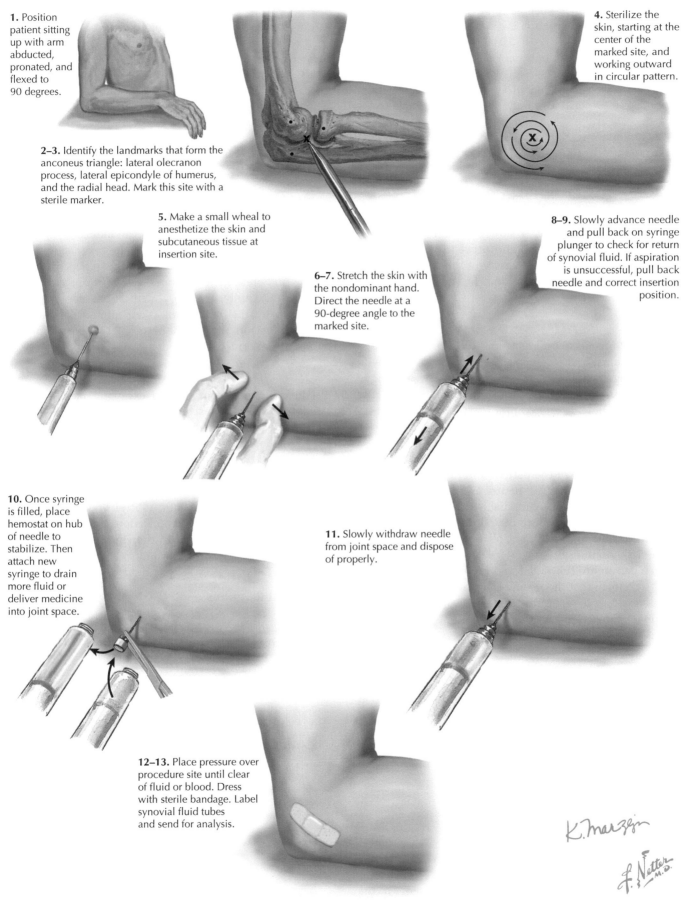

1. Position patient sitting up with arm abducted, pronated, and flexed to 90 degrees.

2–3. Identify the landmarks that form the anconeus triangle: lateral olecranon process, lateral epicondyle of humerus, and the radial head. Mark this site with a sterile marker.

4. Sterilize the skin, starting at the center of the marked site, and working outward in circular pattern.

5. Make a small wheal to anesthetize the skin and subcutaneous tissue at insertion site.

6–7. Stretch the skin with the nondominant hand. Direct the needle at a 90-degree angle to the marked site.

8–9. Slowly advance needle and pull back on syringe plunger to check for return of synovial fluid. If aspiration is unsuccessful, pull back needle and correct insertion position.

10. Once syringe is filled, place hemostat on hub of needle to stabilize. Then attach new syringe to drain more fluid or deliver medicine into joint space.

11. Slowly withdraw needle from joint space and dispose of properly.

12–13. Place pressure over procedure site until clear of fluid or blood. Dress with sterile bandage. Label synovial fluid tubes and send for analysis.

FIGURE 30.5 Elbow joint aspiration

7. Once the effusion has been clearly visualized, ensure that the center of the probe is located at the middle of the effusion.

8. Inject 5 mL of local anesthetic just below the center of the transducer.

9. Use a 5- or 10-mL syringe to enter the skin at the midpoint of the transducer and at a 90-degree angle to the skin.

10. Pay attention to the depth of the joint capsule effusion during the procedure. Actively aspirate the syringe as the needle advances.

ANATOMICAL PITFALLS

Cartilage

While inserting the needle, a slow and steady movement helps avoid contact with bone and prevents damage to the articular cartilage. Because the cavity of the elbow joint can be small, a dry tap may indicate that the tip of the needle is outside the joint.

Ligaments and Tendons

Steroid injections make ligaments and tendons vulnerable to rupture. The ulnar and radial collateral ligaments, along with the annular ligament, form the joint capsule. A weakening of these ligaments ultimately leads to joint instability. The biceps brachii, triceps brachii, and common extensor tendons may also be affected.

Neurovascular Injury

Improper positioning of the patient and poor needle placement can lead to the injury of neurovascular structures surrounding the joint space. A medial approach to the elbow joint should be avoided because of the proximity of the ulnar nerve and superior ulnar collateral artery, which are at great risk of injury. An anterolateral or anteromedial approach can injure the radial and median nerves, respectively. To confirm that the needle is not within the lumen of a blood vessel, it is recommended to always aspirate with the syringe and ensure that there is no blood return before injecting medication.

Olecranon Bursa

The olecranon bursa is located posteriorly over the olecranon process. Olecranon bursitis may be confused with elbow joint effusion.

COMPLICATIONS

Elbow joint arthrocentesis is a relatively safe procedure. If correctly performed, complications are rare.

Procedural Pain

Severe pain during arthrocentesis usually results from the needle coming in contact with the highly innervated cartilaginous surfaces. If pain is encountered, the needle can be redirected or withdrawn. Either topical or local anesthesia or both should be used for the procedure.

Infection After Joint Injection

Although rare, an infection might develop if a needle is introduced into the joint through an area of cellulitis, severe dermatitis, or soft tissue infection, any of which are contraindications to arthrocentesis. Improper cleaning of the skin or lapses in sterile technique may also result in infection. When arthrocentesis for the diagnosis of a potentially septic joint is performed through infected skin, intravenous antibiotics should be administered immediately after the procedure, and the patient should be admitted to the hospital for the continuation of antibiotics.

Postinjection Flare

Some patients may experience an increase in joint pain after a steroid injection. Steroid crystals can induce an inflammatory crystal synovitis, beginning at approximately 6 to 12 hours after injection. Postinjection flare can persist for hours or days and presents with tenderness, warmth, and swelling of the joint. Antiinflammatory medications may reduce the occurrence of this reaction if taken immediately after the injection. If symptoms persist beyond 2 to 3 days, aspiration should be performed to rule out a septic joint.

Hemarthrosis

Bleeding is a rare complication except in patients with a bleeding diathesis. Most hemarthroses are small and self-limited and can be managed by observation alone. If a patient has a coagulopathy, it should be corrected.

CONCLUSION

Elbow joint aspiration is a safe clinical procedure that has both diagnostic and therapeutic utility. Its relative ease, minimal invasiveness, and few complications make it a very beneficial tool that can be used in the emergency department, operating room, or outpatient clinic.

Suggested Readings

Bernal-Lagunas R. Arthrocentesis. In: *Orthopedic Surgery in Patients with Hemophilia.* Italy: Springer Science+Business Media; 2008:63–68.

Boniface KS, Ajmera K, Cohen JS, Liu YJ, Shokoohi H. Ultrasound in emergency medicine: ultrasound-guided arthrocentesis of the elbow: a posterior approach. *J Emerg Med.* 2013;45:698–701.

Bork SC. *Elbow Arthrocentesis;* 2015. Available at http://emedicine.medscape.com/article/79975-overview#showall.

Cardone DA, Tallia AF. Diagnostic and therapeutic injection of the elbow region. *Am Fam Physician.* 2002;66:2097–2100.

Hansford BG, Stacy GS. Musculoskeletal aspiration procedures. *Semin Intervent Radiol.* 2012;29:270–285.

Mantuani D, Nagdev A. Ultrasound-guided elbow arthrocentesis. *ACEP Now.* 2013;32:9. Available at http://www.acepnow.com/article/ultrasound-guided-elbow-arthrocentesis.

Marhsall PD, Fairclough JA, Johnson SR, Evans EJ. Avoiding nerve damage during elbow arthroscopy. *J Bone Joint Surg.* 1993;75-B:129–131.

Thomsen TW. Arthrocentesis: Elbow (Emergency Medicine). Available at http://www.proceduresconsult.com/medical-procedures/arthrocentesis-elbow-EM-057-procedure.aspx#procedure.

Winegardner MF. Joint and bursal aspiration. In: Dehn RW, Asprey DP, eds. *Essential Clinical Procedures.* ed 3. Philadelphia: Elsevier; 2013:203–215.

REVIEW QUESTIONS

1. A 45-year-old man arrived at the emergency department with injuries to his left elbow after he fell in a bicycle race. Radiographic and MRI examinations show a fracture of the medial epicondyle and an injured ulnar nerve. Which of the following muscles is most likely to be paralyzed?

   A. Flexor digitorum superficialis
   B. Biceps brachii
   C. Brachioradialis
   D. Flexor carpi ulnaris
   E. Supinator

2. A mother tugs violently on her child's hand to pull him out of the way of an oncoming car, and the child screams in pain. Afterwards, the child cannot straighten his forearm at the elbow. When the child is seen in the emergency department, radiographic examination reveals a dislocation of the head of the radius. Which of the following ligaments is most likely directly associated with this injury?

   A. Annular
   B. Joint capsular
   C. Interosseous
   D. Radial collateral
   E. Ulnar collateral

3. A 58-year-old convenience store operator received a superficial bullet wound to the soft tissues on the medial side of the elbow in an attempted robbery. A major nerve was repaired at the site where it passed behind the medial epicondyle. Bleeding was stopped from an artery that accompanied the nerve in its path toward the epicondyle. Vascular repair was performed on this small artery because of its important role in supplying blood to the nerve. Which of the following arteries was most likely repaired?

   A. Profunda brachii
   B. Radial collateral
   C. Superior ulnar collateral
   D. Inferior ulnar collateral
   E. Anterior ulnar recurrent artery

4. A 43-year-old female tennis player visits an outpatient clinic for pain over the right lateral epicondyle of her elbow. Physical examination reveals that the patient has lateral epicondylitis. Which of the following tests should be performed during physical examination to confirm the diagnosis?

   A. Nerve conduction studies
   B. Evaluation of pain experienced during flexion and extension of the elbow joint
   C. Observing the presence of pain when the wrist is extended against resistance
   D. Observing the presence of numbness and tingling in the ring and little fingers when the wrist is flexed against resistance
   E. Evaluation of pain felt over the styloid process of the radius during brachioradialis contraction

5. A 29-year-old patient has a dislocated elbow in which the ulna and medial part of the distal humerus have become separated. Which class of joint is normally found between these two bones?

   A. Trochoid
   B. Ginglymus
   C. Enarthrodial
   D. Synarthrosis
   E. Sellar

Ingrown Toenail Removal

CHAPTER

31

INTRODUCTION

Onychocryptosis or ingrown toenail is a commonly encountered pathology of the foot. It arises when spicules from the nail plate irritate or penetrate the periungual skin as the nail plate grows distally. Penetration of the nail fold leads to an inflammatory response and hypertrophy of the tissue. In most patients, the lateral nail fold of the hallux, or great toe, is affected. These individuals present with pain, erythema, swelling of the nail fold, and possibly with infection. The pain may interfere with daily activities that require ambulation. Because of limited mobility and function, the quality of life can be compromised to varying degrees.

A number of underlying causes can give rise to ingrowing toenails. Among these are improper nail cutting, tight or ill-fitting footwear, trauma, poor foot hygiene, and anatomical abnormalities. Improperly trimmed nails can lead to spicule formation, whereas badly fitting shoes place pressure on the medial and lateral nail folds, deepening existing penetration. Trauma, either repetitive or inadvertent, can exacerbate the condition and increase the pain or discomfort felt by the patient. Fungal infection of the nail or bacterial infection of the nail fold can be precipitated by poor foot hygiene, leading to brittle nails, spicule formation, and purulent discharge. Lastly, anatomical factors such as thickening or thinning of the nail plate, pincer-shaped toenail, eversion of the hallux, and distal or lateral nail embedding may play a role in the pathogenesis of onychocryptosis.

Two major age groups with a high risk of developing ingrown toenails are adolescents and the elderly. Adolescents tend to have hyperhidrosis or increased perspiration, which leads to softening of the nail plate and nail folds. Splitting or breakage of the softened nails can result in spicule formation and penetration of the spicule into the softened nail folds. The elderly, on the other hand, experience thickening of the toenails due to natural aging processes. Reduced vision or mobility may impair their ability to properly trim thickened nails, which may promote ingrown toenails. In addition to these two groups, patients with conditions that predispose them to lower extremity edema (such as diabetes, peripheral vascular disease, renal disorders, and obesity) have a higher risk of developing onychocryptosis. The use of many different medications may also increase the risk for this condition.

CLINICALLY RELEVANT ANATOMY
Nail Unit

The nail unit consists of the nail plate, nail bed, nail matrix, and proximal, lateral, and medial nail folds (Fig. 31.1). The nail plate is the hard, keratinized portion that covers the nail bed. The root of the nail plate is embedded in the proximal nail fold, the middle is adherent to the nail bed, and the distal edge is free. With a growth rate of 0.2 mm per week, the nail plate takes 12 to 18 months for complete growth from the matrix to the distal edge. The nail matrix is the site of origin of the nail plate. The distal, white, semilunar portion of the matrix, known as the lanula, can be seen on the proximal border of the nail plate.

Blood Supply

Vascular supply of the digits of the foot arises from the dorsalis pedis and posterior tibial arteries. The posterior tibial artery bifurcates into the lateral and medial plantar branches. Digital branches of the lateral plantar artery supply the medial and lateral sides of the toes. The arcuate artery, a branch of the dorsalis pedis, supplies the adjacent sides of the second to fifth digits via the dorsal digital arteries. The first dorsal metatarsal artery, a branch of the dorsalis pedis, supplies the hallux.

Innervation

The sensory supply of the foot is from the tibial, sural, saphenous, superficial fibular, and deep fibular nerves. On the dorsal aspect of the foot, the sensory supply to the digits is provided by the dorsal digital nerves, which are branches of the superficial fibular nerve. It should be noted that a small portion of the skin between the first and second toes is supplied by the dorsal digital nerves arising from the deep fibular nerve. On the plantar aspect of the foot, the medial and lateral plantar nerves give rise to the common and the proper plantar digital nerves, which supply the toes.

INDICATIONS

Onychocryptosis treatment depends on the severity of the condition. Nail fold swelling, erythema, edema, and pain on palpation characterize mild onychocryptosis. Moderate onychocryptosis is marked by increased swelling, seropurulent drainage secondary to infection, and ulceration of the nail fold. Severe onychocryptosis can be distinguished by chronic inflammation, granulation tissue, and nail fold hypertrophy.

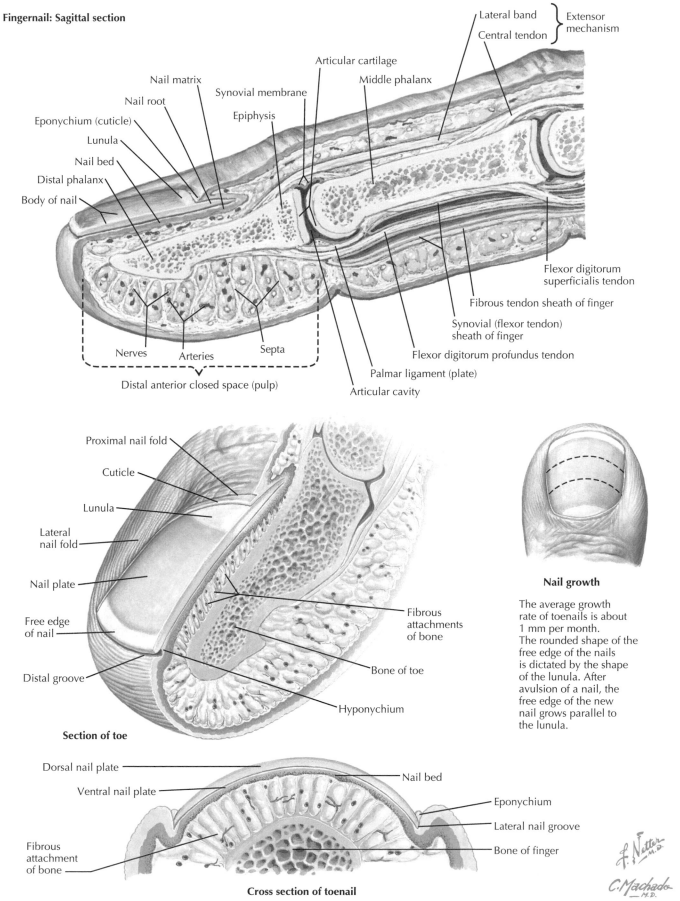

Fingernail: Sagittal section

Lateral band
Central tendon
} Extensor mechanism

Articular cartilage
Middle phalanx

Nail matrix
Synovial membrane
Nail root
Epiphysis
Eponychium (cuticle)
Lunula
Nail bed
Distal phalanx
Body of nail

Nerves
Arteries
Septa

Distal anterior closed space (pulp)

Flexor digitorum superficialis tendon
Fibrous tendon sheath of finger
Synovial (flexor tendon) sheath of finger
Flexor digitorum profundus tendon
Palmar ligament (plate)
Articular cavity

Proximal nail fold
Cuticle
Lunula
Lateral nail fold
Nail plate
Free edge of nail
Distal groove

Fibrous attachments of bone
Bone of toe
Hyponychium

Section of toe

Nail growth

The average growth rate of toenails is about 1 mm per month. The rounded shape of the free edge of the nails is dictated by the shape of the lunula. After avulsion of a nail, the free edge of the new nail grows parallel to the lunula.

Dorsal nail plate
Ventral nail plate
Nail bed
Eponychium
Lateral nail groove
Bone of finger
Fibrous attachment of bone

Cross section of toenail

FIGURE 31.1 Normal structure and function of the nail unit

Conservative therapy is indicated in patients with mild to moderate onychocryptosis. It consists of the following measures:

1. Trimming of the distal nail corner on the affected side
2. Antiseptic dressing
3. Astringent soaks
   a. Epsom salt solution
   b. 25% silver nitrate solution
   c. 10- to 20-minute soak of the affected foot in warm, soapy water several times daily
   d. Topical antibiotic ointment or mild- to high-potency topical steroid following the soak
4. Cotton wisp
   a. Placed under the ingrowing toenail using a nail elevator or small curette
5. Dental floss
   a. Inserted under the ingrown corner
6. Gutter splint
   a. Fashioned from a sterilized vinyl intravenous drip infusion tube slit from top to bottom
   b. Inserted at the ingrown nail edge and pushed down proximally to cover the spicule
   c. Secured with adhesive tape or acrylic resin
7. Acrylic nail
   a. Plastic nail platform placed under the nail
   b. Platform kept in place until the nail grows out (2 weeks to 3 months)

Surgical procedures are indicated for patients with severe ingrown toenails that do not respond to conservative treatment or that are recurrent. The nail plate and hypertrophied nail fold are excised. The most commonly used and successful procedure is a partial nail avulsion with phenol matricectomy. Other approaches include electrocautery and radiofrequency or carbon dioxide laser ablation of the nail matrix.

Additional indications for surgical treatment are onychomycosis (fungal infection of the nail); chronic, recurrent paronychia (inflammation of the nail fold); and onychogryposis (deformed, curved nail).

CONTRAINDICATIONS

Contraindications to partial or complete nail avulsion, with or without phenolization, are bleeding diatheses, allergy to local anesthetics, diabetes mellitus, and peripheral vascular disease. Pregnant patients are not good candidates for phenol ablation.

EQUIPMENT

Local anesthetic without epinephrine:
   Lidocaine 1% to 2% plain
   Bupivacaine 0.5% or ropivacaine 0.75% plain
5-mL syringe with 25- to 27-gauge needle
Sterile drape
Povidone-iodine solution
Alcohol wipes
Nonstick antiseptic gauze
Forceps
Beaver handle with #62 blade

English anvil nail splitter
Small curette
Sterile cotton-tipped applicator
Straight hemostat
Liquefied phenol BP (80% or 88%)
Isopropyl alcohol
Sterile saline
Digit tourniquet
Antiseptic dressing
Betadine ointment

PROCEDURE

See Fig. 31.2. Obtain patient consent and perform a time out.

1. Place the patient in the supine position with the knee flexed and foot flat on the table.
2. Clean the affected toe and immediate surroundings with povidone-iodine solution, and drape the foot so that the entire toe remains exposed.
3. Administer a digital ring block with local anesthetic.
4. Apply a tourniquet around the toe to exsanguinate the area.
5. Separate the affected side of the nail plate from the nail bed with a nail elevator.
6. Split the nail longitudinally, distally to proximally, with a nail splitter.
   a. Either split the nail with the splitter for the entire length of the nail or use the splitter for the first few millimeters and then use a scalpel to continue the cut toward the cuticle beneath the nail fold.
7. Remove the avulsed nail by gently twisting the nail plate upwards toward the midline and then pulling it distally.
   a. Make sure that no spicules or fragments are left behind in the nail bed.
   b. Gently curette the area to remove any remnants.
8. Dry the nail bed, and apply phenol solution to the bed with a cotton-tipped applicator in three 30-second applications.
   a. Apply 70% isopropyl alcohol to the nail bed immediately after the phenolization to neutralize the phenol.
9. Remove the tourniquet while applying pressure to stem residual bleeding.
10. Apply antibiotic ointment, and dress the treated area with sterile gauze and an antiseptic bandage.

Postoperative Care and Instructions

- Ask the patient to keep the foot elevated for 24 to 48 hours.
- Advise the patient to take over-the-counter analgesics for pain control.
- The patient can remove the dressing 24 hours after the procedure and repeat the following steps for 1 to 2 weeks:
  - Soak the foot in warm water twice daily.
  - Dry, apply antibiotic ointment, and dress the toe.
- The patient should wear loose-fitting shoes with low heels in order to prevent aggravation or recurrence of the condition.
- The patient should notify the physician of pain, swelling, or signs of infection. Toenails should be trimmed straight across in the future.

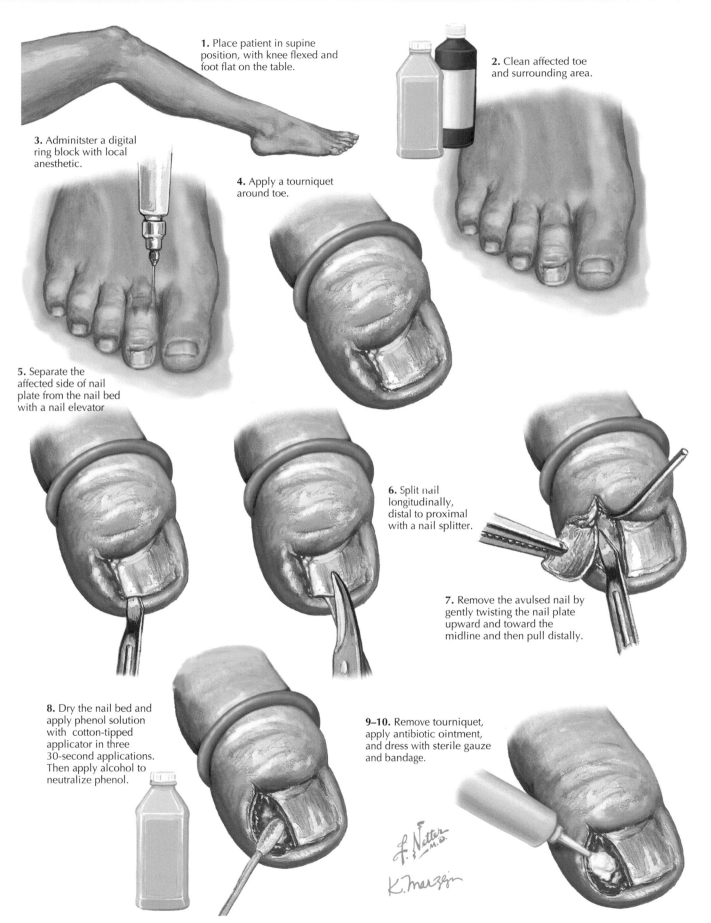

1. Place patient in supine position, with knee flexed and foot flat on the table.

2. Clean affected toe and surrounding area.

3. Adminitster a digital ring block with local anesthetic.

4. Apply a tourniquet around toe.

5. Separate the affected side of nail plate from the nail bed with a nail elevator

6. Split nail longitudinally, distal to proximal with a nail splitter.

7. Remove the avulsed nail by gently twisting the nail plate upward and toward the midline and then pull distally.

8. Dry the nail bed and apply phenol solution with cotton-tipped applicator in three 30-second applications. Then apply alcohol to neutralize phenol.

9–10. Remove tourniquet, apply antibiotic ointment, and dress with sterile gauze and bandage.

FIGURE 31.2 Ingrown toenail removal

ANATOMICAL PITFALLS

Structures at risk during the procedure are the blood vessels and nerves on the medial and lateral sides of the affected digit. Vasoconstrictive agents should not be used with anesthetics injected in the digits in order to avoid necrosis.

COMPLICATIONS

This simple, straightforward procedure has a low rate of failure and complications. The most likely complication arising from incomplete or ineffective matrix ablation or spicule removal is recurrence of the ingrown toenail. Paronychia, scarring, cellulitis, and osteomyelitis are also possible complications. Oozing due to phenol application can be controlled with potassium permanganate soaks or the application of 20% ferric chloride. Finally, an undesirable cosmetic appearance may result from the partial or total removal of the nail plate.

CONCLUSION

Onychocryptosis is a common condition that affects males and females of all ages. Arising from a variety of causes ranging from improperly trimmed toenails to footwear choice, the ingrown toenail generally causes pain and discomfort upon the application of pressure during daily activities. Conservative or surgical measures can be employed to treat the condition, depending on its severity. A number of studies have found that the lowest rate of recurrence is achieved with partial nail avulsion followed by phenol matricectomy. The procedure has a low complication rate and a high success rate, leading to good patient outcomes in the long term.

Suggested Readings

Bryant A, Knox A. Ingrown toenails: the role of the GP. *Am Fam Physician.* 2015;44(3):102–105.

Heidelbaugh J, Lee H. Management of the ingrown toenail. *Ame Fam Physician.* 2009;79(4):303–308.

Khunger N, Kandhari R. Ingrown toenails. *Ind J Dermatol Venereol Leprol.* 2012;78(3):279–289.

Nyberg S. Treating ingrown toenails. In: Dehn RW, Asprey DP, eds. *Essential Clinical Procedures.* ed 3. Philadelphia: Elsevier; 2013:323–327.

Thommasen H, Johnston C, Thommasen A. The occasional removal of an ingrowing toenail. *Can J Rural Med.* 2005;10(3):173–180.

REVIEW QUESTIONS

1. A 55-year-old woman is admitted to the emergency department. She complains of a chronically infected ingrown toenail of the great toe. Prior to removing the ingrown nail, an anesthetic is injected into the first web space. Which of the following nerves would be anesthetized at this location?

   A. Sural
   B. Superficial fibular
   C. Saphenous
   D. Tibial
   E. Deep fibular

2. A 25-year-old man presents to his local emergency department with complaints of pain in the toes and nail beds of his left foot. The physician wants to feel for arterial pulses in the foot. Which of the following arteries could be palpated?

   A. Dorsalis pedis
   B. Sural
   C. Fibular
   D. Deep plantar arch
   E. Anterior tibial

Knee Joint Aspiration

INTRODUCTION

Joint aspiration, also known as *arthrocentesis*, is a safe and minimally invasive clinical procedure in which a needle and syringe are used to collect synovial fluid from the joint capsule. This procedure can be used to establish a diagnosis, alleviate discomfort, drain infected fluid or blood, or inject medication into the joint space. As a diagnostic aid, arthrocentesis helps distinguish inflammatory arthropathies from osteoarthritis or crystal-induced arthritides. This chapter will focus on knee joint arthrocentesis.

If available, ultrasonography should be used as an adjunct. Recent studies suggest that ultrasound-guided arthrocentesis is superior to the classic anatomical landmark- and palpation-guided procedure. The use of ultrasonography greatly minimizes procedural pain, improves arthrocentesis success, yields more synovial fluid, allows for greater joint decompression, and improves clinical outcomes. Ultrasonography can be used to guide needle insertion under direct visualization. Alternatively, it can be used indirectly to visualize and mark the site targeted for needle insertion and estimate the depth and direction of needle placement.

If ultrasonography is not readily available, the procedure must be performed by palpation-guided arthrocentesis. When using anatomical landmarks, the risk of injury can be minimized by inserting the needle in the extensor surface of the joint while keeping the joint in minimal flexion. In either case, it is important to have a fundamental understanding of the clinically relevant anatomy to avoid injury to tendons, ligaments, muscles, and neurovascular structures when performing arthrocentesis of the knee.

CLINICALLY RELEVANT ANATOMY

The knee joint capsule, also known as an *articular capsule,* consists of an external fibrous layer and an internal synovial membrane. The fibrous layer is thin except for the thickened portions that make up the intrinsic ligaments of the knee.

Posteriorly, the fibrous layer surrounds the condyles and the intercondylar fossa. Distally, the fibrous layer attaches to the superior articular surface of the tibia. The synovial membrane lines all the surfaces of the articular cavity that are not covered by articular cartilage. It attaches to the peripheral margins of the articular cartilage, which covers the femoral and tibial condyles, posterior surface of the patella, and popliteal surface of the femur.

Bursae surround the knee, with anatomic variations in their arrangement (Fig. 32.1). The pes anserine and semimembranous bursae are of particular clinical significance. The pes anserine bursa is 4 to 5 cm distal to the anteromedial joint line and deep to the pes anserine, a common tendon comprising the tendons of the sartorius, gracilis, and semitendinosus muscles. The insertion of the tibial collateral ligament is deep to the anserine bursa. The semimembranosus bursa, located within the popliteal fossa, is a common cause of posterior knee joint swelling as a result of knee joint degeneration.

Several vital structures share a close anatomical relationship with the joint capsule, including menisci, ligaments, cutaneous nerves, muscles, and vessels, and are at risk of injury during knee joint aspiration. Hence, it is important to have a sound knowledge of the regional anatomy.

INDICATIONS

Before arthrocentesis is performed, periarticular entities, such as bursitis, cellulitis, contusion, and tendonitis, must be differentiated from articular processes. Typically, periarticular processes restrict the active range of motion more than the passive range and are localized to a specific area, whereas articular processes restrict both active and passive ranges of motion and often produce circumferential pain and swelling (Fig. 32.2).

Knee joint aspiration can be used for both diagnostic and therapeutic purposes.

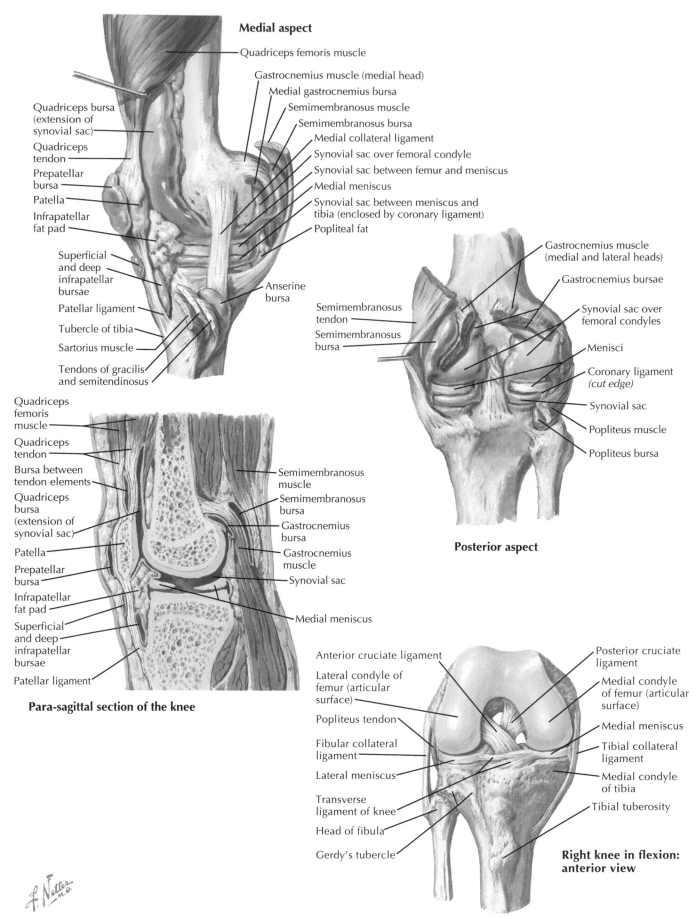

Medial aspect

Quadriceps femoris muscle
Gastrocnemius muscle (medial head)
Medial gastrocnemius bursa
Semimembranosus muscle
Semimembranosus bursa
Medial collateral ligament
Synovial sac over femoral condyle
Synovial sac between femur and meniscus
Medial meniscus
Synovial sac between meniscus and tibia (enclosed by coronary ligament)
Popliteal fat

Quadriceps bursa (extension of synovial sac)
Quadriceps tendon
Prepatellar bursa
Patella
Infrapatellar fat pad

Superficial and deep infrapatellar bursae
Patellar ligament
Tubercle of tibia
Sartorius muscle
Tendons of gracilis and semitendinosus

Anserine bursa

Gastrocnemius muscle (medial and lateral heads)
Gastrocnemius bursae
Synovial sac over femoral condyles
Menisci
Coronary ligament (cut edge)
Synovial sac
Popliteus muscle
Popliteus bursa

Semimembranosus tendon
Semimembranosus bursa

Posterior aspect

Quadriceps femoris muscle
Quadriceps tendon
Bursa between tendon elements
Quadriceps bursa (extension of synovial sac)
Patella
Prepatellar bursa
Infrapatellar fat pad
Superficial and deep infrapatellar bursae
Patellar ligament

Semimembranosus muscle
Semimembranosus bursa
Gastrocnemius bursa
Gastrocnemius muscle
Synovial sac
Medial meniscus

Para-sagittal section of the knee

Anterior cruciate ligament
Lateral condyle of femur (articular surface)
Popliteus tendon
Fibular collateral ligament
Lateral meniscus
Transverse ligament of knee
Head of fibula
Gerdy's tubercle

Posterior cruciate ligament
Medial condyle of femur (articular surface)
Medial meniscus
Tibial collateral ligament
Medial condyle of tibia
Tibial tuberosity

Right knee in flexion: anterior view

FIGURE 32.1 Anatomy of the knee

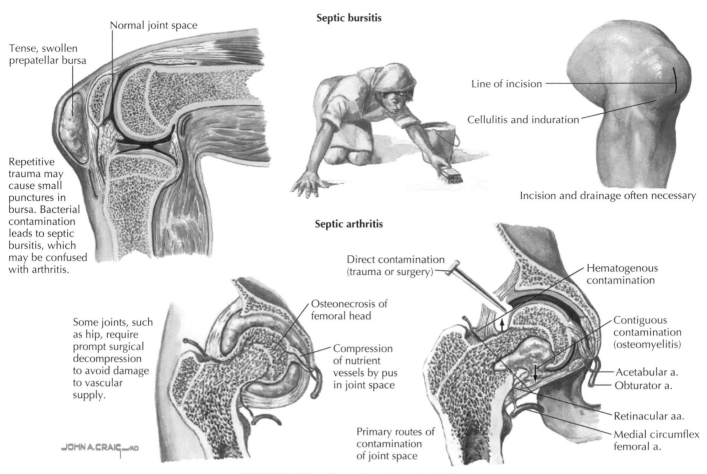

Normal joint space

Tense, swollen prepatellar bursa

Repetitive trauma may cause small punctures in bursa. Bacterial contamination leads to septic bursitis, which may be confused with arthritis.

Septic bursitis

Line of incision

Cellulitis and induration

Incision and drainage often necessary

Septic arthritis

Some joints, such as hip, require prompt surgical decompression to avoid damage to vascular supply.

Direct contamination (trauma or surgery)

Osteonecrosis of femoral head

Compression of nutrient vessels by pus in joint space

Primary routes of contamination of joint space

Hematogenous contamination

Contiguous contamination (osteomyelitis)

Acetabular a.

Obturator a.

Retinacular aa.

Medial circumflex femoral a.

JOHN A. CRAIG—MD

FIGURE 32.2 Septic bursitis and arthritis

Diagnostic Knee Joint Aspiration

Diagnostic knee joint aspiration is indicated when evaluating for chronic arthritis (rheumatoid arthritis, osteoarthritis), crystal-induced arthritis (gout, pseudogout), septic arthritis, articular inflammation of unknown origin, joint effusion, and hemarthrosis.

Aspirated synovial fluid is of high diagnostic value and can be analyzed for viscosity, glucose, total protein, uric acid, lactate, cell count, rheumatoid factor, mucin clots, and crystals. The fluid sample can undergo polymerase chain reaction studies, Gram stain, and culture for bacteria, mycobacteria, and fungi.

Therapeutic Knee Joint Aspiration

Therapeutically, knee joint aspiration is used to aspirate effusion or blood to relieve pain; improve mobilization of the joint; inject medications such as corticosteroids, antibiotics, or anesthetics; and drain septic effusions.

CONTRAINDICATIONS

There are few contraindications to knee joint aspiration. Relative contraindications include cellulitis, dermatitis, or skin infection overlying the site of needle entry; adjacent osteomyelitis; uncontrolled coagulopathy; and joint prosthesis. Suspected bacteremia is a relative contraindication, but arthrocentesis should still be performed if septic arthritis is suspected.

EQUIPMENT

Sterile gloves and drapes
Sterile gauze squares
Sterile hemostat
Sterile bandage
Tray table
Skin antiseptic solution: povidone-iodine or chlorhexidine
Syringes
    One small syringe (5 or 10 mL) for anesthetic
    Three large syringes (30 mL) for aspiration
Selection of needles: 18, 20, and 25 gauge
Local anesthetic (1% lidocaine)
Specimen tubes
Ultrasound, if available

PROCEDURE

Obtain patient consent and perform a time out. The knee joint may be entered through either a lateral or a medial approach. However, the lateral approach is more frequently used and is described here (Fig. 32.3, Video 32.1).

Lateral Approach

Explain the procedure and reassure the patient that it has very few risks. Inform the patient that there may be some pain during the injection of a local anesthetic and when the synovial cavity is entered.

1. Position the patient supine with the knee extended or held in slight flexion. If desired, place a rolled towel under the popliteal space to help support the knee.
2. Carefully examine, palpate, and identify the superolateral aspect of the patella. The needle should enter the skin 1 to 2 cm from the lateral edge of the superior third of the patella. This location provides the most direct route to the joint. If available, use ultrasonography to better visualize the knee joint.
3. Mark the skin with a pen at the site of injection.
4. Don the appropriate personal protective equipment. Wearing sterile gloves, sterilize the skin with antiseptic solution. Start at the site marked for the injection, and cleanse in concentric circles 2 to 3 inches (5 to 7.5 cm) in diameter around the site. Allow the application to dry and then reapply. If the patient is allergic to iodine, 70% alcohol can be used. Sterile drapes may be used but are not required.
5. Anesthetize the region with 1% lidocaine in a 5-mL or 10-mL syringe with a 25-gauge needle. Make a 2- to 3-cm wheal to anesthetize the skin and subcutaneous tissue at the insertion site. Insert the needle deeper, anesthetizing along the anticipated track of the arthrocentesis needle.
6. Place an 18- or 20-gauge needle on a 30-mL syringe, and use the nondominant hand to stretch the patient's skin. Insert the needle at a 45-degree angle to the sagittal plane, 1 cm posterior to the superolateral aspect of the patella. If needed, the patella can be grasped to aid entry of the needle. If available, the ultrasound transducer can be used to visualize the joint capsule and to help accurately direct the needle into the joint space.
7. Resistance will be felt at entry into the joint capsule. Once the needle has successfully entered the joint space, fluid aspiration can begin. If no fluid is seen entering the syringe, gently apply pressure over the patella to "milk" the joint. This allows the extraction of any excess fluid.
8. Once the syringe has filled, place a hemostat on the hub of the needle. With the needle stabilized, disconnect the syringe. If needed, a new syringe can be attached to drain more fluid or to deliver medication, such as a corticosteroid, into the joint space.
9. Slowly withdraw the needle and syringe from the joint space. Once the needle is withdrawn, place the safety cap over the needle and ensure proper disposal.
10. Apply pressure over the procedure site with gauze for a few minutes until the site is clear of fluid or blood. Dress with a sterile adhesive dressing.
11. The extracted fluid should be placed in properly labeled specimen tubes and sent promptly to the laboratory for analysis.

Medial Approach

The medial approach is identical to the lateral approach, except that the needle will enter the skin 1 to 2 cm from the medial edge of the superior third of the patella.

ANATOMICAL PITFALLS

Cartilage

While inserting the needle, a slow and steady movement helps in avoiding contact with bone and preventing damage to the articular cartilage.

Ligaments and Tendons

Steroid injections make ligaments and tendons more vulnerable to rupture. Repeated steroid injections into the joint can cause osteonecrosis and weaken capsular ligaments, ultimately leading to joint instability.

Neurovascular Injury

Improper positioning of the patient and poor needle placement can lead to the injury of neurovascular structures surrounding the joint space. The clinician must be aware of the proximity of nerves, arteries, and veins to the joint space because these structures are all at risk of injury when introducing a needle or injecting medication. To confirm that the needle is not within the lumen of a blood vessel, it is recommended to always aspirate and ensure that there is no blood return before injecting medication.

Prepatellar Bursa

The prepatellar bursa is located anterior to the patella. It is a superficial bursa with a thin synovial lining between the skin and patella. Prepatellar bursitis may be confused with knee joint effusion.

COMPLICATIONS

Knee joint arthrocentesis is a relatively safe procedure. If correctly performed, complications are rare.

Procedural Pain

Severe pain during arthrocentesis usually results from the needle coming in contact with the highly innervated cartilaginous surfaces. If pain is encountered, the needle can be redirected or withdrawn. Either topical or local anesthesia or both should be used for the procedure.

Infection After Joint Injection

Although rare, an infection might develop if a needle is introduced into the joint through an area of cellulitis, severe dermatitis, or soft tissue infection, any of which are contraindications to arthrocentesis. Improper cleaning of the skin or lapses in sterile technique may also result in infection. When arthrocentesis for

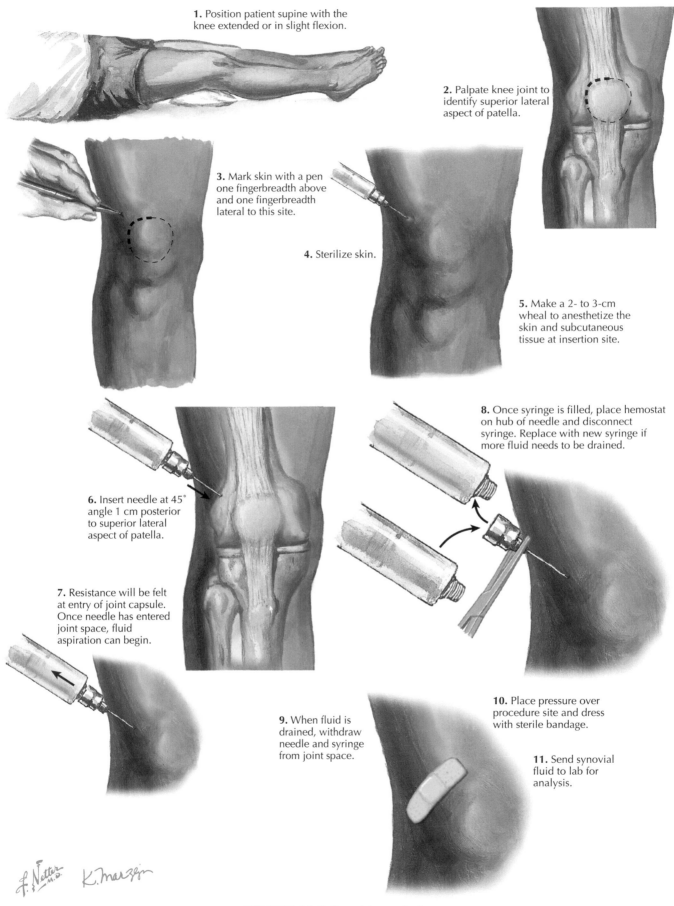

1. Position patient supine with the knee extended or in slight flexion.

2. Palpate knee joint to identify superior lateral aspect of patella.

3. Mark skin with a pen one fingerbreadth above and one fingerbreadth lateral to this site.

4. Sterilize skin.

5. Make a 2- to 3-cm wheal to anesthetize the skin and subcutaneous tissue at insertion site.

6. Insert needle at 45° angle 1 cm posterior to superior lateral aspect of patella.

7. Resistance will be felt at entry of joint capsule. Once needle has entered joint space, fluid aspiration can begin.

8. Once syringe is filled, place hemostat on hub of needle and disconnect syringe. Replace with new syringe if more fluid needs to be drained.

9. When fluid is drained, withdraw needle and syringe from joint space.

10. Place pressure over procedure site and dress with sterile bandage.

11. Send synovial fluid to lab for analysis.

FIGURE 32.3 Knee joint aspiration

the diagnosis of a potentially septic joint is performed through infected skin, intravenous antibiotics should be administered immediately after the procedure, and the patient should be admitted to the hospital for the continuation of antibiotics.

Postinjection Flare

Some patients may experience an increase in joint pain after a steroid injection. Steroid crystals can induce an inflammatory crystal synovitis, beginning at approximately 6 to 12 hours after injection. Postinjection flare can persist for hours or days and presents with tenderness, warmth, and swelling of the joint. Antiinflammatory medications may reduce the occurrence of this reaction if taken immediately after the injection. If symptoms persist beyond 2 to 3 days, aspiration should be performed to rule out a septic joint.

Hemarthrosis

Bleeding is a rare complication, except in patients with bleeding diathesis. Most hemarthroses are small and self-limited and can be managed with observation alone. If a patient has a coagulopathy, it should be corrected.

CONCLUSION

Knee joint aspiration is a safe clinical procedure used to collect synovial fluid from the joint capsule. Its relative ease, minimal invasiveness, and few complications make it a very beneficial tool that can be used in the emergency department, operating room, or outpatient clinic.

Suggested Readings

Ahmed I, Gertner E. Safety of arthrocentesis and joint injection in patients receiving anticoagulation at therapeutic levels. *Am J Med.* 2012;125:265–269.

Dunn AS, Turpie AG. Perioperative management of patients receiving oral anticoagulants: a systematic review. *Arch Intern Med.* 2003;163:901–908.

Partin W, Dorroh C. Emergency procedures. In: Stone C, Humphries RL, eds. *Current Diagnosis and Treatment: Emergency Medicine.* 7th ed; 2011.

Sanford SO. Arthrocentesis. In: Roberts JR, ed. *Roberts and Hedges' Clinical Procedures in Emergency Medicine.* 6th ed. Philadelphia: Elsevier; 2014:1075–1094.

Thomsen TW, Shen S, Shaffer RW, Setnik GS. Arthrocentesis of the knee. *N Engl J Med.* 2006;354:e19.

Winegardner MF. Joint and bursal aspiration. In: Dehn RW, Asprey DP, eds. *Essential Clinical Procedures*, 3rd ed. Philadelphia: Elsevier; 2013:203–215.

Zuber TJ. Knee joint aspiration and injection. *Am Fam Physician.* 2002;66:1497–1500.

REVIEW QUESTIONS

1. A 43-year-old man visits the outpatient clinic with a painful, swollen knee joint. The patient's history reveals chronic gonococcal arthritis. A knee aspiration is ordered for bacterial culture of the synovial fluid. A standard lateral suprapatellar approach is used and the needle passes proximal to and deep to the patella. Through which of the following muscles would the needle pass?

   A. Adductor magnus
   B. Short head of biceps femoris
   C. Rectus femoris
   D. Sartorius
   E. Vastus lateralis

2. A 58-year-old female employee of a housecleaning business visits the outpatient clinic with a complaint of constant, burning pain in her knees. Clinical examinations reveal "housemaid's knee." Which of the following structures is most likely affected?

   A. Prepatellar bursa
   B. Infrapatellar bursa
   C. Posterior cruciate ligament
   D. Patellar retinacula
   E. Lateral meniscus

Lumbar Puncture

INTRODUCTION

The first lumbar puncture (LP) was performed in 1891 to relieve increased intracranial pressure (ICP) in children with meningitis, although this is now contraindicated. Since then, LP has been performed to obtain relevant information for the diagnosis and treatment of a variety of infectious and noninfectious neurologic conditions. The cerebrospinal fluid (CSF) collected by LP has extraordinary value, especially in light of the many urgent, life-threatening conditions resulting from infections. However, LP may have adverse effects, so a careful preprocedural neurologic examination is necessary, since a focal deficit could be a sign of increased ICP. This increase in pressure can be caused by a mass lesion or an intracerebral bleed. Computed tomography (CT) of the head without contrast should be obtained in such circumstances prior to performing the LP. The results of an LP should be correlated with a proper history and physical examination and supportive laboratory tests. The LP procedure can be performed without imaging or with fluoroscopic or ultrasound guidance.

CLINICALLY RELEVANT ANATOMY

The anatomy relevant to LP involves the lumbar spine and spinal cord. The lumbar region of the spine consists of five vertebrae numbered in descending order from L1 to L5. These are the largest vertebral segments of the spine. The vertebral body size notably increases from L1 to L5 and is indicative of the increasing load placed on each vertebra. As a result, the L5 vertebra has the heaviest body, smallest spinous process, and thickest transverse process (Figs. 33.1 and 33.2). The primary functions of the vertebrae are to support the weight of the body on the pelvic region and to permit movement.

The spinal cord is a long neural structure that is an extension of the brainstem. The spinal cord usually extends down to the level of the intervertebral disc space between L1 and L2, where it becomes the conus medullaris and terminates in a fibrous extension known as the filum terminale (see Fig. 33.1).

The conus medullaris can be lower in children and infants, extending inferiorly to L3 and L4. As the child develops into an adult, the spinal column grows longer, so that the level of the conus medullaris rises with respect to the adjacent vertebrae. From the conus medullaris, the nerve branches that arise from the spinal cord are the cauda equina. Three layers of meningeal tissue, the dura, arachnoid, and pia mater, protect the spinal cord. From the surface, an LP needle must penetrate the skin, muscle, ligament, dura, and arachnoid to enter the subarachnoid space. The epidural space is filled with adipose tissue, whereas CSF is located in the subarachnoid space. The dura and arachnoid are extensions of the spinal meninges that continue past the conus medullaris and terminate at the second sacral vertebra. It is the subarachnoid space below the end of the spinal cord (ie, lumbar cistern) that is the target for an LP to collect CSF.

INDICATIONS

The indications for LP and CSF analysis include emergency and nonemergency situations. The most prevalent indication for LP is a suspicion of meningitis or other central nervous system (CNS) infections and conditions such as suspected subarachnoid hemorrhage in a patient with a CT scan negative for hemorrhage. Nonemergency indications for LP include evaluation for a variety of CNS conditions, such as syphilis, hydrocephalus, unexplained seizures, and demyelinating disorders. Additionally, LP may be used for therapeutic procedures such as spinal anesthesia, relief of idiopathic intracranial hypertension (previously called pseudotumor cerebri), intrathecal administration of medications, and contrast injection for myelography.

In the emergency department, LP is most often used to diagnose or exclude meningitis in patients with fever, headache, altered mental status, or meningeal signs. CSF analysis is highly sensitive and specific for bacterial and fungal meningitis. While the presence of fever alone is not an indication for LP, investigating a fever of unknown origin may require an LP to evaluate for CNS infections. Meningeal signs may

Vertebral Ligaments: Lumbar Region

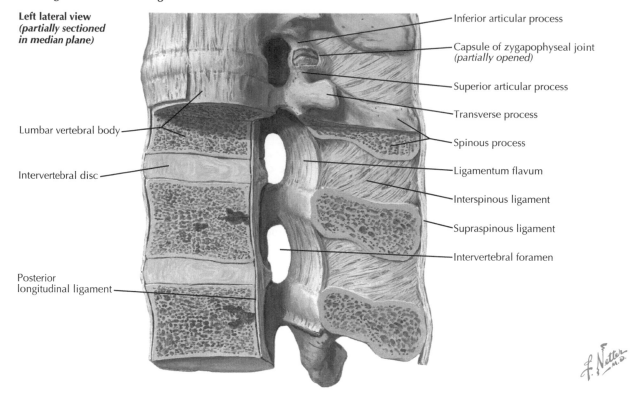

Left lateral view
(partially sectioned
in median plane)

Lumbar vertebral body

Intervertebral disc

Posterior
longitudinal ligament

Inferior articular process

Capsule of zygapophyseal joint
(partially opened)

Superior articular process

Transverse process

Spinous process

Ligamentum flavum

Interspinous ligament

Supraspinous ligament

Intervertebral foramen

Spinal Cord and Ventral Rami

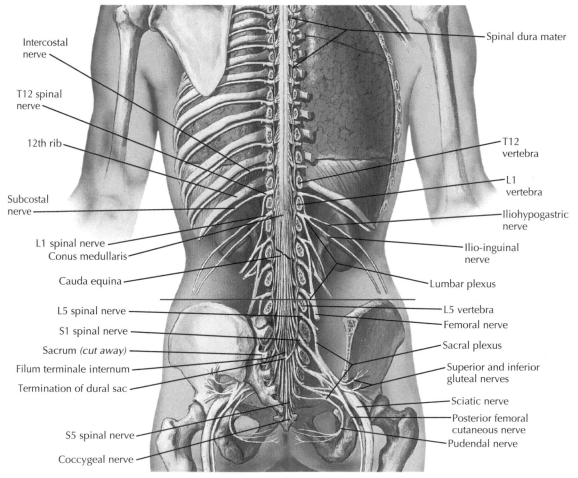

Intercostal
nerve

T12 spinal
nerve

12th rib

Subcostal
nerve

L1 spinal nerve
Conus medullaris

Cauda equina

L5 spinal nerve

S1 spinal nerve

Sacrum (cut away)

Filum terminale internum

Termination of dural sac

S5 spinal nerve

Coccygeal nerve

Spinal dura mater

T12
vertebra

L1
vertebra

Iliohypogastric
nerve

Ilio-inguinal
nerve

Lumbar plexus

L5 vertebra

Femoral nerve

Sacral plexus

Superior and inferior
gluteal nerves

Sciatic nerve

Posterior femoral
cutaneous nerve

Pudendal nerve

FIGURE 33.1 Anatomy of the vertebral column

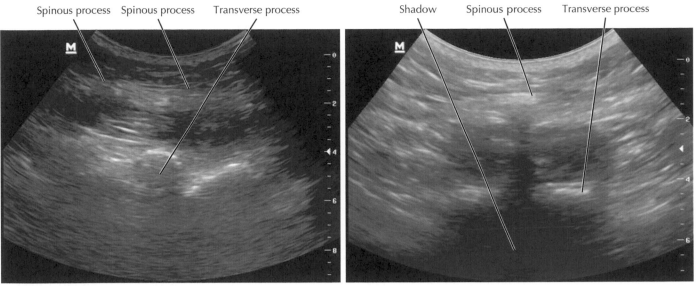

Midline spine: sagittal probe position   Midline spine: transverse probe position

FIGURE 33.2 Imaging of the spine

not be present in the early stages of the disease or in patients at the extremes of age, those who are immunocompromised or receiving antiinflammatory drugs, or those who have had partial antibiotic treatment. This is especially true in infants and young children, in whom fever, irritability, and vomiting are the most common symptoms. Other physical signs used in diagnosing meningitis include nuchal rigidity and the Kernig and Brudzinski signs.

Suspected subarachnoid hemorrhage is the second most common indication for LP in the emergency department. Although diagnosis may be made in the early stages of bleeding with noncontrast CT, blood in the CSF is highly sensitive for hemorrhage, especially since the sensitivity of CT decreases after 24 hours following the event. LP is useful for ruling out a suspected subarachnoid hemorrhage if the initial CT is negative.

CONTRAINDICATIONS

LP is absolutely contraindicated in patients with infection in the tissues near the puncture site. Relative contraindications are a suspected increase in ICP, thrombocytopenia, or coagulopathies.

Increased ICP is a contraindication because of the possibility of brain herniation, which LP may precipitate or aggravate with a decrease in pressure in the spinal compartment. This in turn may result in cardiorespiratory collapse, stupor, seizures, and death. Findings shown to be indicative of a poor outcome in patients with increased ICP who deteriorated after LP include focal findings on neurologic examination, papilledema, and suspected ICP on CT imaging. If possible, CT should be performed to prior to LP, but it should not delay appropriate treatment for suspected meningitis. In such cases, antibiotics, steroids, and other

treatment should not be withheld pending the LP. Routine CT should be completed in patients with one or more of the following risk factors: altered mental status, focal neurologic signs, papilledema, recent seizure, and immune compromise.

EQUIPMENT

The performance of LP requires minimal equipment. Local anesthetics may or may not be required, but it is advisable to use 1% to 2% lidocaine in conscious, awake patients. LP equipment comes in standardized kits, but it may be advisable to make extra equipment readily available at the bedside, including the following:

Ultrasound (if available)
Sterile gloves
Antiseptic or other sterile preparatory solution
Sterile drapes
Spinal needles
Specimen collection tubes
Anesthetic solution
Needles for anesthetic administration
Manometers (if pressure will be measured)
Syringes
Three-way stopcock
Sterile dressing

The choice of spinal needle depends on the operator, patient size, and the kit itself. Most kits supply a standard Quincke cutting needle. However, using smaller needles (22 gauge and higher) and those with atraumatic tips significantly lowers the incidence of post-LP headache compared with the use of standard spinal needles.

Procedure

See Fig. 32.3 and Video 32.1. Obtain patient consent and perform a time out. If ultrasound is available:

1. Place the patient in the lateral recumbent position with the hips, knees, and chin flexed toward the chest to allow maximal opening of the interlaminar spaces. If unable to lie in the lateral recumbent position, the patient may be allowed to sit up and lean forward to open the interlaminar spaces as widely as possible.

    a. Use a linear (procedural) high-frequency probe. For patients with a body mass index of over 30 kg/m², use a curvilinear (abdominal) low-frequency probe.

2. To determine the midline, find the L3-L4 or L4-L5 space (using an imaginary line connecting the highest points of the tops of the iliac crests) and place the probe sagitally along the axis of the spine. Sweep the probe medially and laterally to identify the spinous processes, which will appear as consecutive, hyperechoic, 1- to 3-cm long, rounded bony surfaces accompanied by a distal shadow. Mark the superior and inferior aspects of the probe, remove the probe, and draw a line to connect the dots. In older children and adults, LP may be performed in the L2-L3 interspace or as low as the L5-S1 interspace. In children younger than 12 months, LP should be performed below the L2-L3 interspace because of the potentially lower level of the conus medullaris.

    a. To determine the proper interspinous space, place the probe perpendicular to the marked midline. Slide it caudad and cephalad, and once again visualize the spinous processes. The shadow-free spaces above and below the spinous process are the desired interspinous spaces. Mark the center of this shadow-free space between L3 and L4 or L4 and L5 by drawing a line perpendicular to the midline.

    b. The meeting of two lines serves as the entry site for the needle. This completes the ultrasound-assisted portion of the procedure. Continue by prepping the patient using sterile technique.

    c. If ultrasound is not available, palpate the anatomical landmarks to determine where to insert the needle.

3. Use sterile gloves to prevent contamination and infection, and prepare all the equipment before proceeding. Thoroughly wash the hands and don a head covering, mask, gown, and sterile gloves before performing the procedure.

4. Prepare the puncture site using antiseptic solution to clean the skin in a circular manner, starting centrally and moving outward.

5. Place sterile drapes below and on the patient to obtain a sterile work field.

6. Anesthetize the area with lidocaine. Wait a few minutes to allow the anesthesia to take effect.

7. Stabilize the spinal needle on the index finger parallel to the bed, regardless of the patient's position.

8. Slowly penetrate the subcutaneous tissue with the needle using the thumbs, then angle the needle slightly toward the umbilicus.

9. Continue advancing the needle slowly and smoothly. Occasionally, a "pop" may be felt when the needle pierces the dura mater.

10. Remove the stylet to check for fluid return. If there is none, replace the stylet, advance or withdraw the needle a few millimeters, and recheck for fluid return. This process should be repeated until fluid is obtained. At that point, withdraw the stylet. A manometer may be used at this time to measure pressure.

11. Collect 8 to 15 mL of CSF. When fungal cultures are required, the amount may be increased to account for the slow growth of the organisms.

12. In general, collect the fluid in four tubes and label them in the order of collection.

13. When collection is complete, replace the stylet and remove the needle.

14. Apply a sterile dressing.

ANATOMICAL PITFALLS

A "dry tap" results from the LP needle being placed too shallowly so that it fails to enter the subarachnoid space. Conversely, if the needle is too deeply placed, the tip may traverse the subarachnoid space completely and enter a disc space anteriorly. Additionally, there is a risk of vessel damage with a needle placed too deeply, especially in young children and infants. Needles placed too laterally may miss the subarachnoid space completely.

COMPLICATIONS

Complications associated with LP include infection, bleeding from a traumatic tap, post-LP headache, and cerebral herniation. The most common complications are radicular backache near the LP site and headache. Headaches arise from CSF leakage and traction on the pain-sensitive meninges. These symptoms present as either frontal or occipital headaches, usually dissipate within 24 to 48 hours, and are exacerbated when the patient goes from a recumbent to a sitting position. Traumatic taps may occur with damage to venous structures in the subarachnoid space and may be prevented by proper training and technique. Bleeding may also result from anticoagulant therapy or coagulopathies. These complications rarely require treatment unless a spinal hematoma occurs, in which case magnetic resonance imaging evaluation and surgical treatment may be required. Iatrogenic epidermoid spinal tumors are a rare post-LP complication. These are prevented by keeping the stylet in the needle during skin penetration, thereby reducing the chance of introducing skin tissue into the spinal canal.

More severe complications of LP include infection and cerebral herniation; the latter is discussed under Contraindications. Meningitis is an uncommon complication. The most commonly isolated organisms in post-LP meningitis include *Streptococcus* species, *Staphylococcus*, and *Pseudomonas aeruginosa*. The infection may result from contaminated equipment, aerosolized particles from medical personnel, or

1. Place patient in lateral recumbent position with thighs and neck flexed.

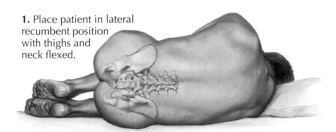

2. Palpate space between L3-L4 and mark on patient.

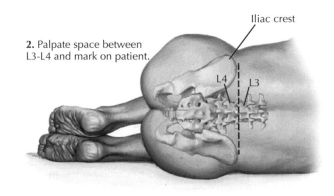

Iliac crest

L4　L3

3–6. Use sterile gloves for remainder of procedure. Prepare puncture site with antiseptic solution. Clean skin in a circular fashion, starting centrally. Drape patient to create sterile work field. Anesthetize the area.

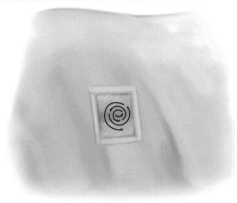

7. Stabilize the spinal needle on the index finger parallel to the bed.

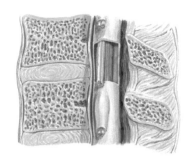

8. Slowly penetrate the subcutaneous tissue with the needle and then angle up slightly towards umbilicus.

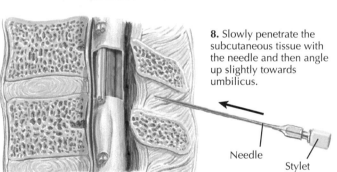

Needle

Stylet

9. Continue advancing needle until it pierces the dura. A "pop" may be felt.

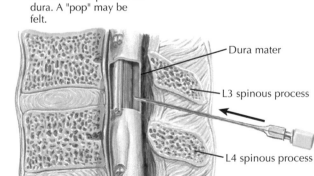

Dura mater

L3 spinous process

L4 spinous process

10–11. Once fluid is observed, the stylet may be withdrawn from the needle to allow for collection. The stylet may be removed incrementally to check for fluid return. If there is no fluid, replace stylet, move needle and recheck for fluid return. Repeat until fluid return occurs.

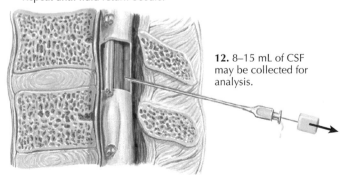

12. 8–15 mL of CSF may be collected for analysis.

13–14. Once samples are collected, replace stylet and remove needle. Apply sterile dressing.

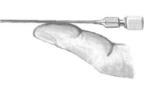

FIGURE 33.3 Lumbar puncture procedure

preexisting bacteremia in patients without preexisting meningitis. In addition, LP through a spinal epidural abscess may result in post-LP meningitis. Infections can be reduced with proper hand hygiene, sterile technique, and appropriate instrument sterilization.

CONCLUSION

LP is a relatively safe and extremely useful technique for the diagnosis of CNS infections, subarachnoid hemorrhages, and demyelinating disorders. LP should be performed after a proper history and neurologic examination and should not be performed before imaging of the brain in suspected cases of increased ICP. Although a relatively safe procedure, LP may have minor or major complications, most often postprocedural headache and back pain, but the most severe complications include infection and cerebral herniation.

Suggested Readings

American Academy of Neurology. Practice parameters: lumbar puncture (summary statement). Report of the Quality Standards Subcommittee. *Neurology.* 1993;43:625–627.

American College of Physicians. The diagnostic spinal tap. Health and Public Policy Committee. *Ann Intern Med.* 1986;104:880–886.

Baer ET. Post–dural puncture bacterial meningitis. *Anesthesiology.* 2006;105:381–393.

Baraff LJ, Byyny RL, Probst MA, et al. Prevalence of herniation and intracranial shift on cranial tomography in patients with subarachnoid hemorrhage and a normal neurologic examination. *Acad Emerg Med.* 2010;17:423–428.

Bonadio W. Pediatric lumbar puncture and cerebrospinal fluid analysis. *J Emerg Med.* 2014;46:141–150.

Ellenby MS, Tegtmeyer K, Lai S, Braner DA. Videos in clinical medicine: lumbar puncture. *N Engl J Med.* 2006;355:e12.

Eng RH, Seligman SJ. Lumbar puncture–induced meningitis. *JAMA.* 1981;245:1456–1459.

Gorelick PB, Biller J. Lumbar puncture: technique, indications, and complications. *Postgrad Med.* 1986;79:257–268.

Quincke HI. Lumbar puncture. In: Church A, ed. *Diseases of the nervous system.* New York: Appleton; 1909:223.

Sidman R, Connolly E, Lemke T. Subarachnoid hemorrhage diagnosis: lumbar puncture is still needed when the computed tomography scan is normal. *Acad Emerg Med.* 1996;3:827–831.

REVIEW QUESTIONS

1. A 3-year-old boy is brought to the emergency department with a severe headache, high fever, malaise, and confusion. Radiologic and physical examinations suggest a diagnosis of meningitis. An LP is ordered to confirm the diagnosis. Which vertebral level is the most appropriate location for the LP?

    A. T11 to T12
    B. L1 to L2
    C. L2 to L3
    D. L4 to L5
    E. T12 to L1

2. When an LP is performed to sample CSF, which of the following external landmarks is the most reliable for determining the position of the L4 vertebral spine?

    A. Inferior angles of the scapulae
    B. Highest points of the iliac crests
    C. Lowest pair of ribs bilaterally
    D. Sacral hiatus
    E. Posteroinferior iliac spines

3. A 15-year-old girl is suspected of having meningitis. To obtain a CSF sample by a spinal tap in the lumbar region, the tip of the needle must be placed in which of the following locations?

    A. In the epidural space
    B. Anterior to the anterior longitudinal ligament
    C. Superficial to the ligamentum flavum
    D. Between the arachnoid mater and dura mater
    E. In the subarachnoid space

4. A 24-year-old woman presents with a severe headache, photophobia, and back stiffness. Physical examination reveals positive signs for meningitis. The attending physician decides to perform an LP to determine if there is a pathogen in the CSF. What is the last structure the needle will penetrate before reaching the lumbar cistern?

    A. Arachnoid mater
    B. Dura mater
    C. Pia mater
    D. Ligamentum flavum
    E. Posterior longitudinal ligament

5. A 19-year-old patient presents to the emergency department with a high fever, severe headache, nausea, and stiff neck that have persisted for 3 days. The attending physician suspects meningitis and obtains a sample of CSF by LP. From which of the following spaces was the CSF collected?

    A. Epidural space
    B. Subdural space
    C. Subarachnoid space
    D. Pretracheal space
    E. Central canal of the spinal cord

6. A 3-day-old girl develops a fever. She is irritable and not feeding. As part of the workup for fever of unknown origin, LP is performed. This puncture must be performed below the spinal cord, which usually ends at which vertebral level in a patient this age?

    A. L1
    B. S1
    C. L3
    D. S3
    E. L5

Nasogastric Tube Placement

INTRODUCTION

Nasogastric intubation is a procedure that allows access to the stomach and gastrointestinal (GI) tract for the administration of medications, decompression of gastric contents, and assessment of GI injury or pathology. Nasogastric intubation involves the advancement of a soft, flexible, plastic tube via the nasal cavity to the nasopharynx and esophagus and into the stomach or small intestine. It is a common procedure performed in emergency departments, operating rooms, and medical clinics. What started out as a way to feed a paralyzed patient has evolved into a common method for treating bowel obstruction, diagnosing upper GI bleeding, providing nutrition, and giving medications.

Nasogastric intubation has a relatively low rate of complications, which usually involve misplacement of the tube, but it can be an uncomfortable procedure for the patient. When performed correctly, discomfort is minimized, as are complications. Therefore knowledge of the anatomy and procedural techniques is of utmost importance.

Tubing for enteral nutrition ranges from 3.5 Fr (1 Fr = 3.3 mm) to 16 Fr in diameter and 15 to 170 cm in length. Nasogastric decompression, administration of medications, and enteral nutrition require larger bores of 14 to 18 Fr and lengths from 60 to 122 cm. Nasogastric tube (NGT) size can be estimated by multiplying the endotracheal tube diameter (measured in millimeters) by 2.

CLINICALLY RELEVANT ANATOMY

The NGT is passed through the nasal cavity, nasopharynx, oropharynx, esophagus, and then into the stomach. The nasal cavity begins with the vestibule, a highly vascular region near the external nares. Deeper in the cavity is the respiratory region, with three nasal conchae to increase the surface area, thus improving the region's function of air conditioning. The nasal cavity consists of many small bones of the skull, including the ethmoid, sphenoid, frontal, vomer, nasal, maxillary, palatine, lacrimal bones, as well as the inferior nasal conchae (Fig. 34.1). The cribriform plate of the ethmoid bone creates the roof of the nasal cavity; damage to this bone can cause serious cerebral trauma and complications.

The mucosal lining of the nasal airway is quite delicate and easily damaged if proper care is not taken during NGT insertion. The vestibule and anterior portion of the nasal septum are highly vascular, making epistaxis (nosebleed)

a common complication of any procedures involving the nasal cavity. Three main arteries supply the nasal cavity via small branches: the ophthalmic artery gives off the anterior and posterior ethmoidal arteries, the maxillary artery provides the sphenopalatine and greater palatine arteries, and the facial artery gives off lateral nasal and septal branches. The sphenopalatine artery may cause serious epistaxis if ruptured. Injury to this vessel is a medical emergency, requiring cauterization or compression to control the bleeding.

The nasopharynx is located immediately beyond the nasal cavity and spans the region from the base of the skull to the inferior end of the soft palate. The pharyngeal opening of the pharyngotympanic (auditory or eustachian) tube is located in the nasopharynx. Although extremely rare, NGT entry into this structure has occurred. After the tube has passed through the nasopharynx, it reaches the oropharynx.

The oropharynx is inferior to the soft palate and posterior to the oral cavity. Slight discomfort may be associated with the gag reflex as the tube passes through the oropharynx (see Fig. 34.1). Once the NGT has passed the epiglottis, it enters the laryngopharynx, an area of procedural importance because the tube may travel along one of two pathways from this location. If the tube is advanced anteriorly, it is likely to be misplaced into the larynx. Excessive gagging, shortness of breath, and coughing generally accompany unintentional entrance into the larynx. If advanced posteriorly, the tube will properly enter the esophagus.

The esophagus is a long, muscular tube connecting the pharynx to the stomach. Two sphincters control the flow of food and fluid through it, one proximal near the pharynx and the other at the entrance to the stomach. Skeletal muscles allow for the voluntary control of swallowing at the upper esophageal sphincter. Unlike other portions of the GI tract, the esophagus lacks a thick serosal covering and is therefore more prone to puncture.

INDICATIONS

Nasogastric intubation is indicated for a number of therapies and diagnostic procedures. Gaining access to the stomach allows for the quick administration of medications, provision of enteral nutrition, acquisition of a sample of stomach contents, stomach lavage, and decompression to treat ileus or bowel obstruction. An NGT may be useful in the emergency settings to help reduce vomiting or aspiration by allowing gastric decompression.

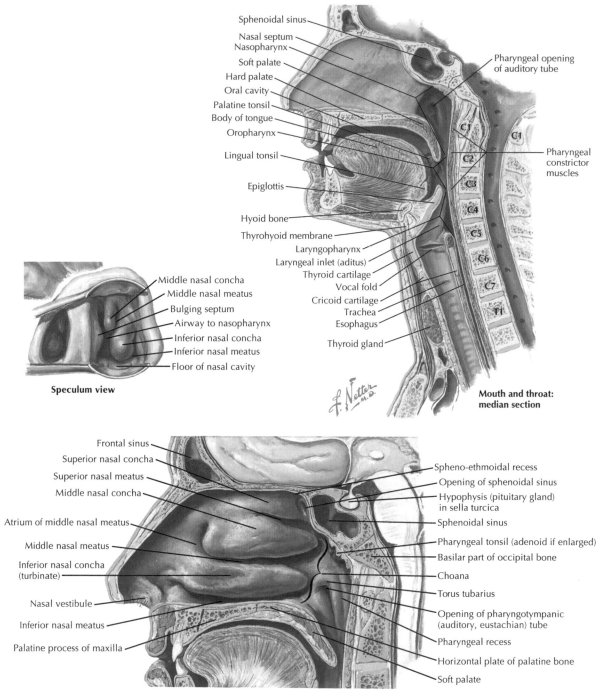

Speculum view

- Middle nasal concha
- Middle nasal meatus
- Bulging septum
- Airway to nasopharynx
- Inferior nasal concha
- Inferior nasal meatus
- Floor of nasal cavity

- Sphenoidal sinus
- Nasal septum
- Nasopharynx
- Soft palate
- Hard palate
- Oral cavity
- Palatine tonsil
- Body of tongue
- Oropharynx
- Lingual tonsil
- Epiglottis
- Hyoid bone
- Thyrohyoid membrane
- Laryngopharynx
- Laryngeal inlet (aditus)
- Thyroid cartilage
- Vocal fold
- Cricoid cartilage
- Trachea
- Esophagus
- Thyroid gland

- Pharyngeal opening of auditory tube
- Pharyngeal constrictor muscles

C1, C2, C3, C4, C5, C6, C7, T1

Mouth and throat: median section

- Frontal sinus
- Superior nasal concha
- Superior nasal meatus
- Middle nasal concha
- Atrium of middle nasal meatus
- Middle nasal meatus
- Inferior nasal concha (turbinate)
- Nasal vestibule
- Inferior nasal meatus
- Palatine process of maxilla

- Spheno-ethmoidal recess
- Opening of sphenoidal sinus
- Hypophysis (pituitary gland) in sella turcica
- Sphenoidal sinus
- Pharyngeal tonsil (adenoid if enlarged)
- Basilar part of occipital bone
- Choana
- Torus tubarius
- Opening of pharyngotympanic (auditory, eustachian) tube
- Pharyngeal recess
- Horizontal plate of palatine bone
- Soft palate

FIGURE 34.1 Lateral wall of nasal cavity and pharynx

Enteral Nutrition

NGTs are used to provide nutrition to patients who are unable to swallow or are at risk for aspiration. This is usually a temporary measure until a more definitive means of feeding the patient can be arranged or until the clinical situation reverses itself so that the NGT is no longer required. When using an NGT for feeding, make sure that the tube is properly aligned to avoid regurgitation and aspiration of the feeding. The use of an NGT for enteral nutrition is best minimized. Long-term enteral feeding tubes may require surgical placement using gastrostomy or jejunostomy to lessen the complications associated with NGTs.

Gastric Decompression

Patients with severe burns, small bowel obstruction, trauma, endotracheal intubation, sepsis, and a host of other medical issues are at an increased risk of developing paralytic ileus. In these cases, an NGT may be required for gastric decompression, and the tube is usually attached to a low-powered suction device. Removal of excess gastric fluid by

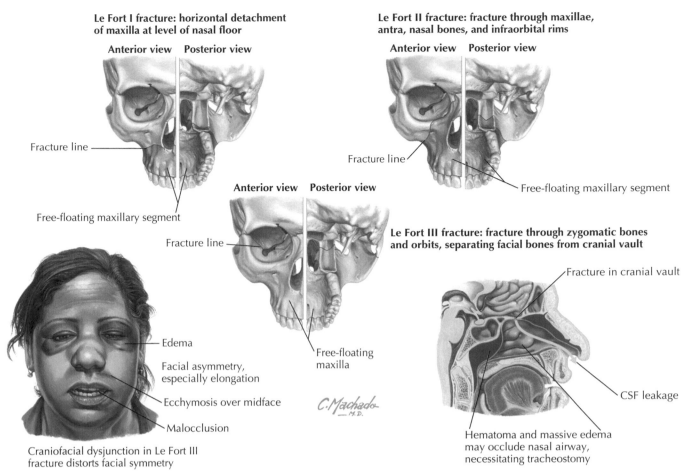

Le Fort I fracture: horizontal detachment of maxilla at level of nasal floor

Anterior view   Posterior view

Fracture line

Free-floating maxillary segment

Le Fort II fracture: fracture through maxillae, antra, nasal bones, and infraorbital rims

Anterior view   Posterior view

Fracture line

Free-floating maxillary segment

Anterior view   Posterior view

Fracture line

Free-floating maxilla

Edema

Facial asymmetry, especially elongation

Ecchymosis over midface

Malocclusion

Craniofacial dysjunction in Le Fort III fracture distorts facial symmetry

C. Machado
—M.D.

Le Fort III fracture: fracture through zygomatic bones and orbits, separating facial bones from cranial vault

Fracture in cranial vault

CSF leakage

Hematoma and massive edema may occlude nasal airway, necessitating tracheostomy

FIGURE 34.2 Contraindication: midface fractures

suction may help avoid vomiting and the aspiration of gastric contents.

Evaluation of Gastrointestinal Bleeding

NGTs have been used to assess the location and severity of GI bleeding, although endoscopy is now more commonly used. Aspiration of blood from an NGT traditionally indicates bleeding due to ulceration of the stomach or duodenum, gastritis, esophagitis, a Mallory-Weiss tear, or esophageal or gastric varices, all of which are examples of upper GI bleeding, which is defined as bleeding from a source proximal to the ligament of Treitz. Patients who present with melena or hematochezia and an NGT aspirate negative for blood are likely to have lower GI bleeding. Placement of an NGT in the presence of esophageal varices may cause significant bleeding and is thus generally not recommended in patients with known varices.

CONTRAINDICATIONS

Insertion of an NGT should be avoided in patients with significant facial or head trauma, recent midfacial or nasal surgery, and known GI conditions, including esophageal stricture or varices.

Basilar Skull Fracture and Midface Trauma

Severe facial and head trauma may include fractures of the base of the skull (Fig. 34.2). The cribriform plate lies in close proximity to the cranial vault. A tube can breach the intracranial compartment via four routes: a fractured cribriform plate, multiple fractures of the floor of the anterior cranial fossa, an abnormally thin cribriform plate (with or without trauma), or a thinned cribriform plate resulting from sinusitis. Midface trauma is therefore an absolute contraindication to the insertion of an NGT because passage of the tube through a fractured cribriform plate into the cranial cavity may cause greater and potentially fatal harm.

Bariatric Surgery

Because of the altered anatomy of the GI tract following bariatric surgery by either gastric bypass or a lap band, the insertion of an NGT should be avoided. The tube may cause perforation of the esophagus, stomach pouch, or jejunum. A bariatric surgeon should be consulted if the insertion of an NGT is required.

EQUIPMENT

NGT of the right size and type along with its connector.
There are two types of tubes: the Levin and Salem sump

tubes. The Levin tube is the simplest NGT with one lumen and multiple openings at the distal end for suction. The Salem sump tube is similar but has two lumens rather than one. The second lumen allows for ventilation during suctioning to avoid trapping the stomach wall with the suction. Salem sump tubes are the preferred choice for long-term gastric intubation with suctioning.

Lubricant

Syringe with a catheter tip

Suction tube and a suction device

0.5% phenylephrine nasal spray

Benzocaine-tetracaine spray

Benzoin tincture

Tape

PROCEDURE

Insertion of Nasogastric Tube

See Fig. 34.3 and Video 34.1. Obtain patient consent and perform a time out. The patient should be in a sitting position. Unconscious patients should be flat and supine or supine with the head slightly elevated.

1. Explain to the patient the steps of the procedure and the need for cooperation at some points.
2. Determine the length of tube necessary by estimating the nose-ear-xiphoid distance.
3. Lubricate the end of the tube.
4. Apply 0.5% phenylephrine nasal spray to both nostrils to prevent epistaxis. If intractable gagging occurs, spray benzocaine-tetracaine solution on the pharynx.
5. Insert the tube into the nostril along the floor of the nasal cavity and advance it posteriorly until it meets resistance.
6. Using slight pressure, aim the tube directly posterior until the tip reaches the nasopharynx and moves down into the oropharynx.
7. Have the patient take a sip of water with a straw; during the swallow, advance the tube into the esophagus. If done correctly, the patient may gag. However, if the patient coughs, it may indicate the tube is being advanced into the larynx or trachea. If this occurs, withdraw the tube and try again.
8. When the tube is in the esophagus, advance it into the stomach.
9. Once it is in the stomach, withdraw some gastric fluid with a syringe and inject air into the tube while listening over the left upper quadrant for the rush of air in the stomach.
10. Confirm the position of the tube with a chest radiograph.
11. Apply tincture of benzoin to the nose and secure the tube to the nose with tape. The tube should also be secured to the patient's gown to reduce tension. Securing the tube properly is a critical step, as improper tube alignment can put pressure on the nasal mucosa or alar cartilage, causing bleeding, dislodgment, or ischemia.

Alternative Methods and Tubes

Longer tubes are sometimes used, namely nasoduodenal and nasojejunal tubes. Alternatives include gastrostomy and jejunostomy tubes. If there is a contraindication to nasogastric intubation, an orogastric tube (ie, a tube inserted through the mouth) may serve the same purpose as nasogastric placement.

In anesthetized patients, tube insertion can be substantially more difficult. These patients are usually also endotracheally intubated, which makes NGT insertion more difficult because the patient is unable to assist by swallowing. Flexing the head and applying gentle pressure to lift the thyroid cartilage are techniques that may improve the success rate. In patients with cervical spine injury, flexing of the neck is contraindicated, but thyroid cartilage manipulation may be enough to allow successful NGT placement. After a failed first attempt, insertion should be tried again using a laryngoscope and Magill forceps to guide the tube.

ANATOMICAL PITFALLS

Misplacement of the tube can occur when it is placed too far anterior into the larynx, too distally into the duodenum, or too proximally in the distal esophagus.

COMPLICATIONS

Problems after NGT insertion are generally rare and can be avoided by careful insertion and continuous monitoring of the patient's status. Minor complications include mucosal tissue trauma and epistaxis or irritation of the nasal or esophageal lining. More serious complications include introduction of the tube into the respiratory tract or traumatic intracranial insertion with basilar skull fractures.

Aspiration

The presence of an NGT increases the likelihood of aspirating gastric contents. The tube alters the physiological action of the lower esophageal sphincter, thus allowing the reflux of gastric fluid, which may be aspirated into the lungs. Patients who suffer from aspiration are likely to develop pneumonitis or pneumonia as a result of gastric acid entering the lungs. Proper care to prevent aspiration-related complications includes keeping the patient in a semireclined position and vigilant suctioning. An NGT causes increased salivation and may impair the cough reflex, making aspiration more likely.

Tracheobronchial Complications

If the tube passes into a bronchus, resulting complications may include atelectasis, pulmonary abscess, pneumonitis, or pneumonia. Bronchial perforation and pneumothorax can also occur.

Nasogastric Tube Syndrome

Though uncommon, a serious and potentially fatal complication of NGT use is vocal cord paralysis with supraglottic edema, known colloquially as "nasogastric tube syndrome." The mechanical cause of this syndrome relates to erosion of the tube into or pressure on the larynx, worsened by movement of the larynx. Respiratory distress in the presence of

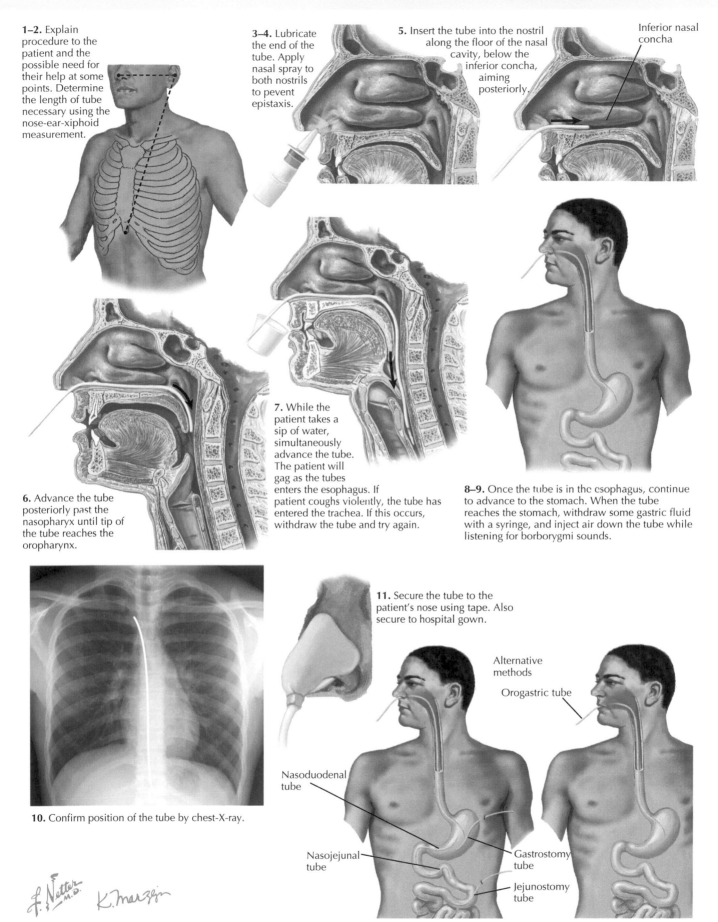

1–2. Explain procedure to the patient and the possible need for their help at some points. Determine the length of tube necessary using the nose-ear-xiphoid measurement.

3–4. Lubricate the end of the tube. Apply nasal spray to both nostrils to pevent epistaxis.

5. Insert the tube into the nostril along the floor of the nasal cavity, below the inferior concha, aiming posteriorly.

Inferior nasal concha

6. Advance the tube posteriorly past the nasopharynx until tip of the tube reaches the oropharynx.

7. While the patient takes a sip of water, simultaneously advance the tube. The patient will gag as the tubes enters the esophagus. If patient coughs violently, the tube has entered the trachea. If this occurs, withdraw the tube and try again.

8–9. Once the tube is in the esophagus, continue to advance to the stomach. When the tube reaches the stomach, withdraw some gastric fluid with a syringe, and inject air down the tube while listening for borborygmi sounds.

10. Confirm position of the tube by chest-X-ray.

11. Secure the tube to the patient's nose using tape. Also secure to hospital gown.

Alternative methods

Orogastric tube

Nasoduodenal tube

Nasojejunal tube

Gastrostomy tube

Jejunostomy tube

FIGURE 34.3 Nasogastric tube placement

an NGT should lead to the suspicion of NGT syndrome or placement in the trachea regardless of patient age.

Rhinitis and Maxillary Sinusitis

Seen most frequently in critically ill patients with long-term NGTs, nasogastric intubation can cause irritation and inflammation of the paranasal sinuses, most commonly the maxillary sinus. Though not well documented, there is literature noting the increased risk of rhinitis associated with NGT use.

CONCLUSIONS

There are several valid medical indications for NGT placement. Although considered safe, NGT insertion does have documented complications that should be understood prior to planned insertion.

Suggested Readings

Bontempo L. Maxillofacial disorders. In: Adams J, Barton E, Collings J, et al, eds. *Emergency Medicine*. Philadelphia: Elsevier; 2008:277–287.

Brousseau V, Kost K. A rare but seriuos entity: nasogastric tube syndrome. *Otolaryngol Head Neck*. 2006;(135):677–679.

Crystal C, Levsky M. Esophageal disorders. In: Adams J, Barton E, Collings J, et al, eds. *Emergency Medicine*. Philadelphia, PA: Elsevier; 2008: 301–311.

Dziewas R, Warnecke T, Hamacher C, et al. Do nasogastric tubes worsen dysphagia in patients with acute stroke? *BMC Neurol*. 2008;8:28.

Ferreras J, Junquera L, García-Consuegra L. Intracranial placement of a nasogastric tube after severe craniofacial trauma. *Oral Surg Oral Med Oral Pathol Oral Radiol Endod*. 2000:564–566.

Giantsou E, Gunning K. Blindly inserted nasogastric feeding tubes and thoracic complications in intensive care. *Health*. 2010;2(10):1135–1141.

Hansen J. *Netter's Clinical Anatomy*, 2nd ed. Philadelphia, PA: Elsevier; 2010.

Harmon J, Balakrishnan K, De Alarcon A, Hart C. The nasogastric tube syndrome in infants. *Int J Pediatr Otorhinolaryngol*. 2014;78:882–884.

Ilias A, Hui Y, Lin C, Chang C, Yu H. A comparison of nasogastric tube insertion techniques without using other instruments in anesthetized and intubated patients. *Ann Saudi Med*. 2013;33(5):476–481.

REVIEW QUESTIONS

1. A 73-year-old patient presents with neck pain, hoarseness, and weight loss over the previous 6 months. On laryngoscopy, a large tumor is identified on one of the true vocal folds. The ENT specialist is unable to pass the scope through the opening between the folds. What is the name of this opening?

   A. Piriform recess
   B. Vestibule
   C. Ventricle
   D. Vallecula
   E. Rima glottidis

2. Relative contraindications to NGT placement include the following except:

   A. Mid-face fractures
   B. History of laparoscopic gastric banding surgery
   C. Coma
   D. Cirrhotic patient vomiting blood

Paronychia Incision and Drainage

INTRODUCTION

Paronychia is defined as inflammation involving the lateral nail folds of the hands or feet. If the inflammation involves the proximal nail fold, it is termed *eponychia*. However, paronychia is often used for both conditions and is used as such here. There may or may not be an abscess on presentation. Depending on the severity of abscess and infection, incision and drainage may be necessary.

There is no specific test for paronychia (also spelled as perionychia), as the diagnosis is made clinically based on the appearance of a tender and swollen proximal or lateral nail fold. The condition can be either acute or chronic and can be caused by any factor that puts undue strain on the nail bed, such as excessive nail care, onychophagia (biting of nails), sucking the thumb, picking at or biting hangnails, or the frequent immersion of hands in water. Paronychias also occur more often in patients with diabetes mellitus or those who are immunocompromised.

CLINICALLY RELEVANT ANATOMY

The nail consists of the nail plate, matrix, and bed (Figs. 35.1 and 35.2). The nail plate, which is hard and keratinized, protects the nail matrix. The perionychium, consisting of proximal and lateral nail folds, surrounds the nail plate. The hyponychium is the area between the distal bed and nail plate. The nail matrix is protected by the nail plate and produces much of the nail volume. The nail matrix lies beneath the nail bed and contains blood vessels and nerves.

INDICATIONS

Acute paronychia is associated with the abrupt onset of edema, erythema, and tenderness in the nail folds. Acute paronychia with abscess formation requires incision and drainage. If the digit has been exposed to oral flora, as may be caused by nail biting or thumb sucking, paronychia may result from infection with flora of the skin or the oral cavity. The anaerobic bacteria involved may include *Peptostreptococcus, Fusobacterium, Prevotella,* and *Porphyromonas* species, and the aerobic bacteria may include *Streptococcus* or *Staphylococcus* species and *Eikenella corrodens.* If there is no exposure to oral flora, infection is likely caused by skin flora such as *Staphylococcus aureus* or *Streptococcus pyogenes.*

Chronic paronychia may have a similar appearance to acute paronychia, but in addition, there may be absence of the cuticle, nail dystrophy, or retraction of the nail fold. It is usually multifactorial in origin, is often associated with eczematous conditions, and can be exacerbated by episodes of acute paronychia. Although the specific inciting factor is not clearly defined, patients with chronic paronychia are often found to have *Candida albicans* or atypical mycobacteria in their proximal nail folds. Chronic paronychias may require management by a hand surgeon or dermatologist.

CONTRAINDICATIONS

There are no specific contraindications to the incision and drainage of a paronychia.

DIFFERENTIAL DIAGNOSIS

Conditions that must be distinguished from paronychia include felon, proximal onychomycosis, herpetic whitlow, acrodermatitis continua of Hallopeau, or infection of the nail with *Pseudomonas* species. A felon is an infection of the pulp of the distal phalanx and presents with the acute onset of swelling, redness, and extreme pain of the pulp of the fingertip. Unlike the other possible diagnoses, felon requires emergency incision and drainage to prevent permanent damage such as osteomyelitis and ischemic necrosis of the distal phalanx. Proximal onychomycosis generally results from a fungal infection and presents with an easily breakable nail plate, with minimal involvement of the nail folds. Herpetic whitlow is caused by herpes simplex virus infection and presents with vesicles, redness, extreme edema, and pain. A variant of pustular psoriasis, referred to as acrodermatitis continua of Hallopeau, an autoimmune disorder affecting the distal digits, has an unclear etiology. It presents with redness, scaling of the skin and nails, sterile pustules, and crusting. Pseudomonal infection of the nail results from prolonged exposure to water, may occur with chronic paronychia, and appears as a blue-green colored nail.

Treatment of paronychia depends on the severity of the infection. A mild to moderate case of acute paronychia without abscess can be managed with soaking or warm compresses to the affected digit for 20 minutes three times a daily, with or without topical antibiotic ointment after soaking. A more severe case may require oral antibiotic therapy. If an abscess has formed, incision and drainage are indicated. For chronic paronychia, the first treatment used should be topical corticosteroid application. If the paronychia remains unchanged, systemic antifungal treatment can be given. The patient should be advised to avoid water, allergens, and

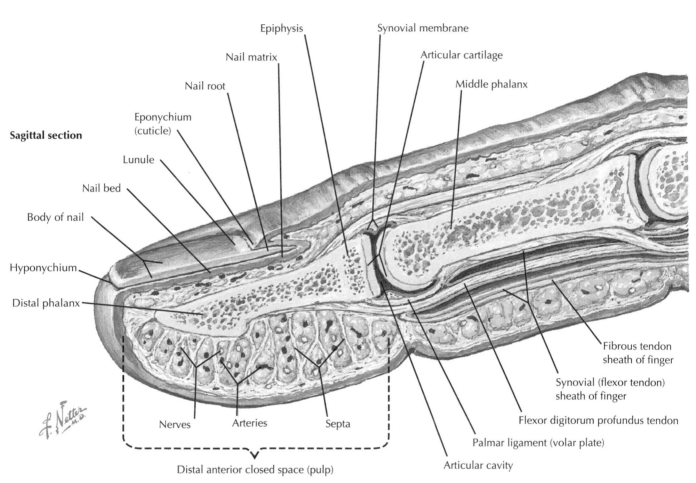

Sagittal section

Epiphysis

Synovial membrane

Nail matrix

Articular cartilage

Nail root

Middle phalanx

Eponychium
(cuticle)

Lunule

Nail bed

Body of nail

Hyponychium

Distal phalanx

Fibrous tendon
sheath of finger

Synovial (flexor tendon)
sheath of finger

Flexor digitorum profundus tendon

Palmar ligament (volar plate)

Articular cavity

Nerves   Arteries   Septa

Distal anterior closed space (pulp)

FIGURE 35.1 Anatomy of the fingers

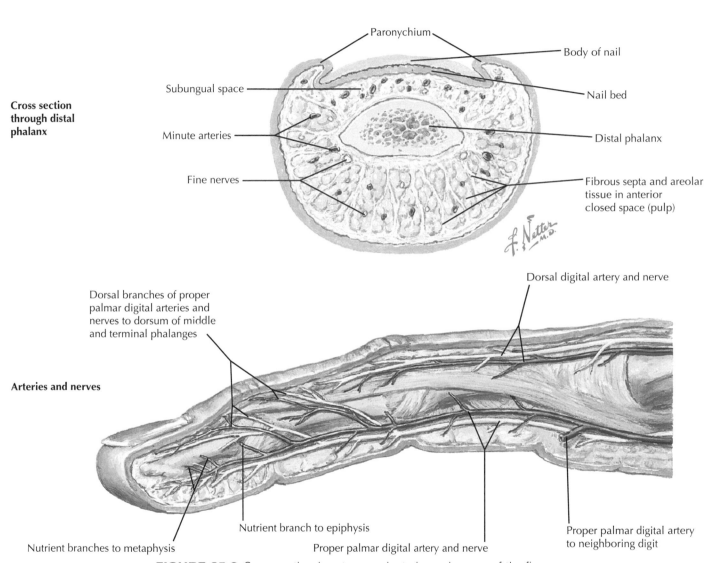

Cross section through distal phalanx

Paronychium

Body of nail

Subungual space

Nail bed

Minute arteries

Distal phalanx

Fine nerves

Fibrous septa and areolar tissue in anterior closed space (pulp)

Arteries and nerves

Dorsal digital artery and nerve

Dorsal branches of proper palmar digital arteries and nerves to dorsum of middle and terminal phalanges

Nutrient branches to metaphysis

Nutrient branch to epiphysis

Proper palmar digital artery and nerve

Proper palmar digital artery to neighboring digit

FIGURE 35.2 Cross-sectional anatomy and arteries and nerves of the finger

irritant exposure. If the inflammation is still unresponsive, a Gram stain and culture should be performed to check for a bacterial superinfection.

EQUIPMENT

Antiseptic solution, such as povidone-iodine or chlorhexidine
Local anesthetic solution (buffered if possible)
Anesthetic spray
Scalpel (or large-gauge needle)
Sterile gauze, gloves, and drape

PROCEDURE

See Fig. 35.3. Obtain patient consent, perform a time out, and wear the proper personal protective equipment.

1. Adequately cleanse the hand and affected finger with povidone-iodine solution, chlorhexidine, or alcohol, and place the hand on a sterile drape.
2. If the abscess is superficially located, local anesthetic may not be required. Drainage is performed by advancing a needle or the blunt end of the scalpel into the nail fold.
3. If there is too much pain or the abscess is deeper, anesthetic should be administered either by the application of ethyl chloride spray or by performing a digital block with the injection of local anesthetic.
4. A scalpel is inserted below the affected cuticle margin. Pus can be expressed from the incision site. For a unilateral abscess, the incision should be extended to the lateral nail fold on the affected side. The expressed material can be sent for culture.
5. Express as much purulence as possible from the abscess.
6. Once a satisfactory amount of purulence has been liberated, irrigate the sulcus of the paronychia. If the sulcus is large, pack it with fine gauze.
7. Leave the gauze in place for 24 to 48 hours to keep the incision open to allow for continued and complete drainage.
8. If the infected pocket extends below the nail, adequate drainage will require the removal of a portion of the infected nail, with gauze packing to prevent premature healing of the fold.
9. The stage and size of the paronychia will determine if antibiotics are required. This is done to ensure that if the portion of the nail that needs to be removed is part of the germinal matrix, it will grow back with the best cosmetic result.

Alternative Method

1. The nail fold can be elevated with the tip of a large-gauge needle and the abscess drained.
2. This method usually does not require antibiotics, and normal usage of the digit can be resumed in approximately 2 days.
3. The incised finger should be soaked frequently to maintain patency of the incision site and allow for complete drainage.
4. If the abscess is severe, treatment with antibiotics is recommended (5 days if incision and drainage is performed, 7 to 10 days if not).

ANATOMICAL PITFALLS

A thorough knowledge of digital anatomy is important for the successful drainage of a paronychia. Anatomical pitfalls include a variant innervation of the nail bed. There may also be inadvertent vascular injury. Injection of anesthetics should be avoid because it could seed the nearby vasculature of the digit with infectious organisms.

COMPLICATIONS

Complications of paronychia drainage include the need for repeat drainage due to inadequate healing, injury to the nail, and inadequate digital anesthesia.

CONCLUSION

Incision and drainage of the paronychia is a simple procedure that may be performed for a patient with an abscess that requires drainage.

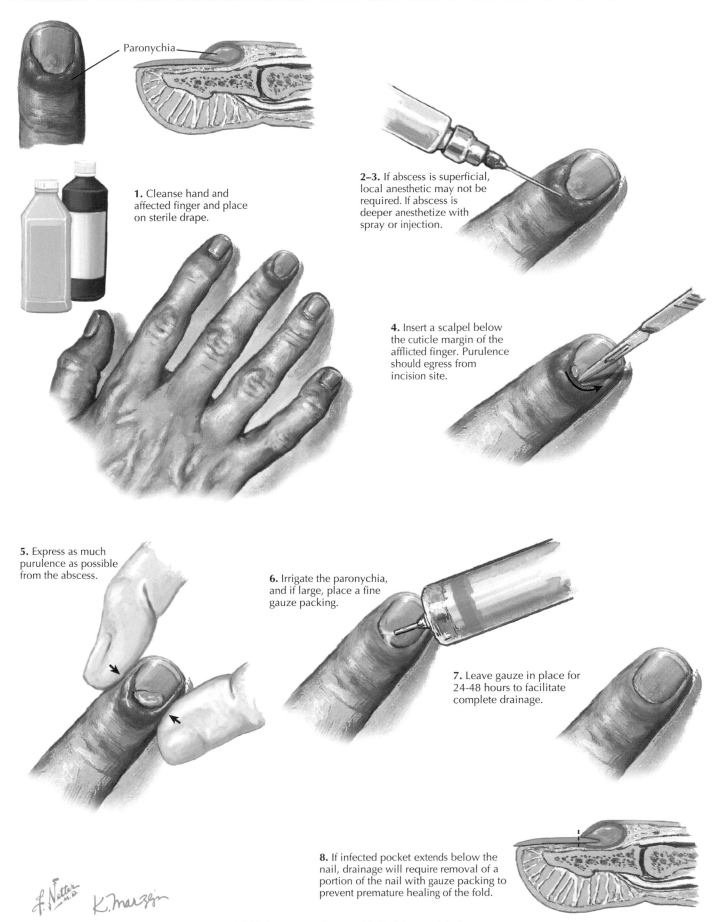

Paronychia

1. Cleanse hand and affected finger and place on sterile drape.

2–3. If abscess is superficial, local anesthetic may not be required. If abscess is deeper anesthetize with spray or injection.

4. Insert a scalpel below the cuticle margin of the afflicted finger. Purulence should egress from incision site.

5. Express as much purulence as possible from the abscess.

6. Irrigate the paronychia, and if large, place a fine gauze packing.

7. Leave gauze in place for 24-48 hours to facilitate complete drainage.

8. If infected pocket extends below the nail, drainage will require removal of a portion of the nail with gauze packing to prevent premature healing of the fold.

FIGURE 35.3 Paronychia incision and drainage

Suggested Readings

Colson AE, et al. Paronychia in association with indinavir treatment. *Clin Infect Dis.* 2001;32:140–143.

Rigopoulos D, et al. Acute and chronic paronychia. *Am Fam Physician.* 2008;77:339–346.

Rockwell PG. Acute and chronic paronychia. *Am Fam Physician.* 2001;15:1113–1116.

REVIEW QUESTIONS

1. A 65-year-old diabetic patient has a small but painful infection under the nail of his little finger. The emergency medicine physician diagnoses paronychia and proceeds to drain the abscess. Which of the following nerves is most likely mediating the pain sensation from the infection?

   A. Superficial radial
   B. Common palmar digital of the median
   C. Common palmar digital of the ulnar
   D. Deep radial
   E. Recurrent branch of the median

2. A 23-year-old man stuck himself with a sewing needle laterally near the fingernail of his thumb. Two days later, the nail is swollen and painful. The nerves that convey this pain lie in which of the following regions?

   A. Matrix of the nail
   B. Nail plate
   C. Lunule
   D. Hyponychium
   E. Nail bed

Skin Abscess Incision and Drainage

INTRODUCTION

A skin abscess is a localized accumulation of exudative material in the dermis or subcutaneous tissue (Fig. 36.1). It often presents with the typical signs of inflammation: redness, tenderness, and warmth. The most common pathogen is *Staphylococcus aureus*. Methicillin-resistant *Staphylococcus aureus* (MRSA) has emerged from being a hospital-acquired pathogen to being ubiquitous in the outpatient setting. The causative agents for any particular infection may depend on the location where the infection is found on the body. Aerobic bacteria, particularly *Staphylococcus* and *Streptococcus* species, are more commonly isolated from abscesses on the trunk, neck, hand, and legs. Anaerobic gram-positive cocci, such as *Fusobacterium* and *Bacteroides* species, are most commonly isolated from the head, fingers and nail bed, and perineum.

CLINICALLY RELEVANT ANATOMY

An abscess that is difficult to incise safely because of its close proximity to important or delicate structures should be evaluated carefully before treatment or should be referred to a surgeon. Examples include abscesses on the lateral and posterior neck that may have arisen from congenital cysts or abscesses located in the nasolabial region of the face. Treatment of facial abscesses in general may depend on the patient's preference. Some may prefer repeated aspirations with incision and drainage to manage abscesses located in cosmetically important areas. Surgical consultation is advisable in such cases. Incision is particularly avoided in the nasolabial area to minimize the risk of septic phlebitis and subsequent intracranial infection through the cavernous sinus. It is safer to treat nasolabial abscesses with warm compresses and broad-spectrum antibiotics. Emergency consultation or urgent follow-up with an otolaryngologist is advised for these infections. Abscesses in close anatomic proximity to important nerves or blood supply, such as on the hand (with the exception of paronychias and felons), perirectal area, or breast, are also at a greater risk for complications and should be referred to a surgeon, if available, for initial evaluation.

INDICATIONS
Incision and Drainage

The primary treatment for skin abscesses is incision and drainage. Needle aspiration alone does not provide adequate drainage for the complete resolution of an abscess. A randomized clinical study of 101 cases of skin abscesses compared these two methods. Among those treated with incision and drainage, 80% resolved within 1 week, compared with only 26% of cases treated with needle aspiration. However, there are circumstances in which fine-needle aspiration may be more appropriate because scarring could be an issue. In these cases, a surgeon should be consulted for care and follow-up.

Empiric Antibiotic Treatment

Although antibiotics are necessary under certain conditions as stated below, there is no evidence supporting their routine use after incision and drainage to augment recovery or improve outcome.

MRSA infections, although resistant to penicillin, are often cured by incision and drainage alone. However, there are several clinical situations when antibiotics would be administered in the setting of an abscess.

CONTRAINDICATIONS

A case of subcutaneous swelling with and without extensive surrounding erythema is often obviously an abscess, and treatment can therefore proceed without uncertainty. However, abscesses sometimes have overlapping clinical presentations with other soft tissue infections, particularly cellulitis. In such cases, it is a challenge to determine whether there is an occult abscess. If there is marked cellulitis with no distinct area of fluctuance, incision and drainage should not be attempted. Bedside ultrasound, if available, is helpful in distinguishing such entities.

Abscesses that are very large, have multiple interconnections, or are recurrent should be evaluated by a surgeon, as they may involve an unusual underlying etiology or be associated with fistulas. Mycotic abscesses should not be incised and drained. A patient with an abscess accompanied by sepsis should be evaluated emergently by a surgeon.

BEDSIDE ULTRASONOGRAPHY

Imaging is not routinely used in diagnosing subcutaneous abscesses except where a foreign body may be present. While the accurate diagnosis and management of abscesses can often be done based on clinical examination alone, several recent studies demonstrate that performing an ultrasound

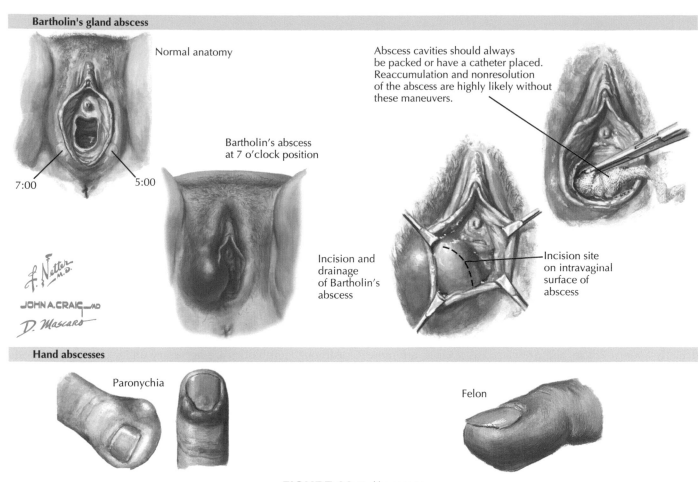

Bartholin's gland abscess

Normal anatomy

7:00   5:00

Bartholin's abscess at 7 o'clock position

Incision and drainage of Bartholin's abscess

Abscess cavities should always be packed or have a catheter placed. Reaccumulation and nonresolution of the abscess are highly likely without these maneuvers.

Incision site on intravaginal surface of abscess

Hand abscesses

Paronychia

Felon

FIGURE 36.1 Abscesses

before attempting incision and drainage increases accuracy and, in some instances, avoids harm to the patient. Therefore emergency bedside ultrasound should be used whenever available for all abscesses. The use of a high-frequency linear probe to visualize superficial structures is very helpful in diagnosing soft tissue infections and can identify abscesses in cases that may superficially appear to be cellulitis alone (Fig. 36.2). A study of emergency department patients with cellulitis found that management plans were altered in about 50% of cases after using bedside sonography. This imaging technique may therefore provide valuable guidance in managing abscesses.

Ultrasound is helpful even in clear-cut cases by revealing important structures located close to the abscess. It may also help to distinguish between an abscess and a discrete area of fluctuance actually caused by other types of subcutaneous fluid. Muscles, tendons, vessels, and nerves can all be distinctly identified by ultrasonography.

EQUIPMENT

Equipment stand, adequate lighting
Goggles or other eye protection
Povidone-iodine antiseptic solution
Local anesthesia (1% lidocaine), 3- to 10-mL syringe, and 25- to 30-gauge needles
Sterile drapes, gloves, and gauze
Scalpel with No. 11 blade
Irrigating syringe (30 to 60 mL) and large-bore plastic catheter
Sterile saline solution
Packing tape (plain or with iodoform)
Small forceps
Small curved hemostat
Scissors
Culture swabs
Wound dressing

PROCEDURE

Obtain patient consent, don appropriate personal protective equipment, and perform a time out. Incision and drainage of soft tissue abscesses should be performed either in the emergency department or in the operating room. The choice of site for the procedure may depend on the size and location of the abscess

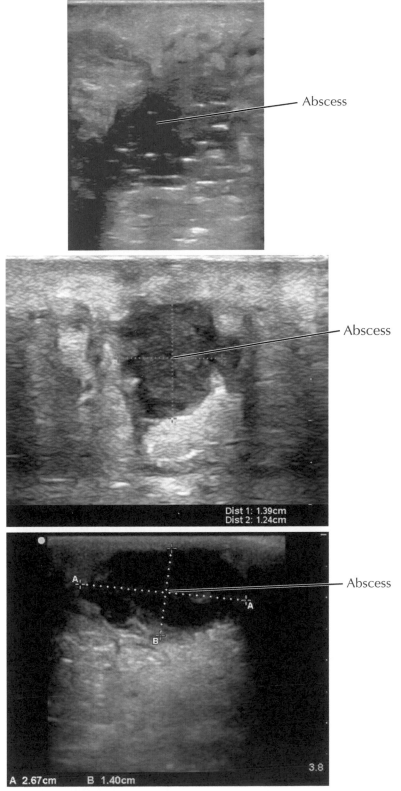

FIGURE 36.2 Ultrasound imaging of abscesses

as well the ability to administer adequate anesthesia. Abscesses that are very deep in the soft tissue or those in close proximity to important structures are better managed in an operating room. The affected area is usually very sensitive, and local anesthetics alone may not be well tolerated by some individuals. These agents are often ineffective in the low pH of infected tissue. Certain patients may therefore require conscious sedation in the emergency department or general or regional anesthesia, which would necessitate management in the operating room.

See Fig. 36.3.

1. Position the patient so that the affected area is fully exposed. Using povidone-iodine, gently clean the area, starting from the tip of the abscess and moving outward on the surrounding skin in a circular motion.
2. Apply anesthesia by positioning a 25- or 30-gauge needle parallel to the skin and injecting lidocaine just under the skin. Start at the top of the wound and repeat the process until the entire area that is to be incised has been anesthetized.
3. Incise the dome of the abscess with a No. 11 scalpel blade. (Note that the scalpel should be used for incision only and not for probing the wound.) Make a linear incision over the crest and along the total length of the abscess, extending it into the cavity. This facilitates thorough drainage of the abscess and allows for the complete removal of loculations. The incision should be made along the natural contours and creases of the skin to minimize scarring.
4. As the abscess begins to drain spontaneously, use a culture swab to gently swab the area. Label the specimen and send it for culture and sensitivity. The sensitivity results are important if antibiotics are indicated after the procedure for any of the following conditions:
   - Severe local infection
   - Immunocompromise
   - History of recurrent or multiple abscesses
   - Systemic signs of infection
   - Failure of initial antibiotic treatment
   - Extremes of age
5. After allowing the abscess to drain spontaneously, use a hemostat wrapped in gauze to probe carefully, sweeping all sides of the cavity to evaluate its depth and break up any loculations. If necessary, administer additional anesthesia into deeper tissues and through the edges of the cut skin to achieve better pain management.
   NOTE: The removal of purulent material can also be achieved using a suction tool with a blunted end or, in smaller abscesses, a simple cotton swab. Customarily, this process is done with the operator's finger, but while this may allow for easier assessment of the cavity, it may also be unsafe and should only be attempted when there is absolute certainty that the abscess does not contain a sharp foreign body. This is especially important in the management of cutaneous abscesses in intravenous drug users.
6. Generously irrigate the cavity with a sterile saline solution to ensure the optimum removal of necrotic material.
7. Depending on the location and size of the abscess, use forceps or a hemostat to loosely pack the wound with packing strip gauze. If iodoform rather than plain gauze is used, warn the patient that there will be a brief stinging sensation after packing.
   NOTE: The purpose of this step is to keep the wound open to encourage the continued drainage of the exudate. It is also done to promote healing from the base to the surface. If the skin were to heal first and enclose an empty space, the abscess might recur. The packing should be done loosely because a tightly packed wound may cause pain and further necrosis of the cavity wall.
8. Lightly apply an absorbent dressing to the wound. If the area affected is an extremity, the patient should be told to keep it elevated. If necessary, prescribe analgesics at the end of the operation. Discuss with the patient and his or her family regarding the best pain management strategy after discharge.
9. If the patient is being managed as an outpatient, set a follow-up appointment and provide information on how to care for the wound at home.

Follow-up Care

In most cases, the patient should have a follow-up appointment. If packing was used, the patient should be seen in 48 hours if healing well. If the abscess was on the face, the patient should return in 24 hours. The patient can be instructed to remove the packing just prior to the appointment. This is aided by soaking the part, which helps reduce the pain of removing the packing. Depending on the location of the procedure, this may require a sitz bath. Reliable patients should be able to monitor the wound at home. If it is a shallow cavity, the base can be gently cleaned daily with peroxide-soaked cotton swabs. The area is then irrigated with normal saline and a dry dressing applied. The schedule for changing the dressing and follow-up visits should be guided by the clinical scenario. Generally, follow-up may be discontinued after all signs of inflammation have disappeared and granulation tissue is developing normally.

ANATOMICAL PITFALLS

Knowledge of surrounding anatomical structures during the incision and drainage of abscesses can prevent complications. For example, the underlying cutaneous neurovascular supply should be appreciated. Additionally, deeper structures that could be injured by the injection of anesthetics or the skin incision must be considered.

COMPLICATIONS

Injury to underlying anatomical structures is a complication of incising and debriding abscesses. Both the underlying cutaneous neurovascular supply as well as deeper tissue structures must be considered during such procedures. In addition, the spreading of infected material to deeper tissue planes or open vessels must be avoided so that systemic infection does not occur.

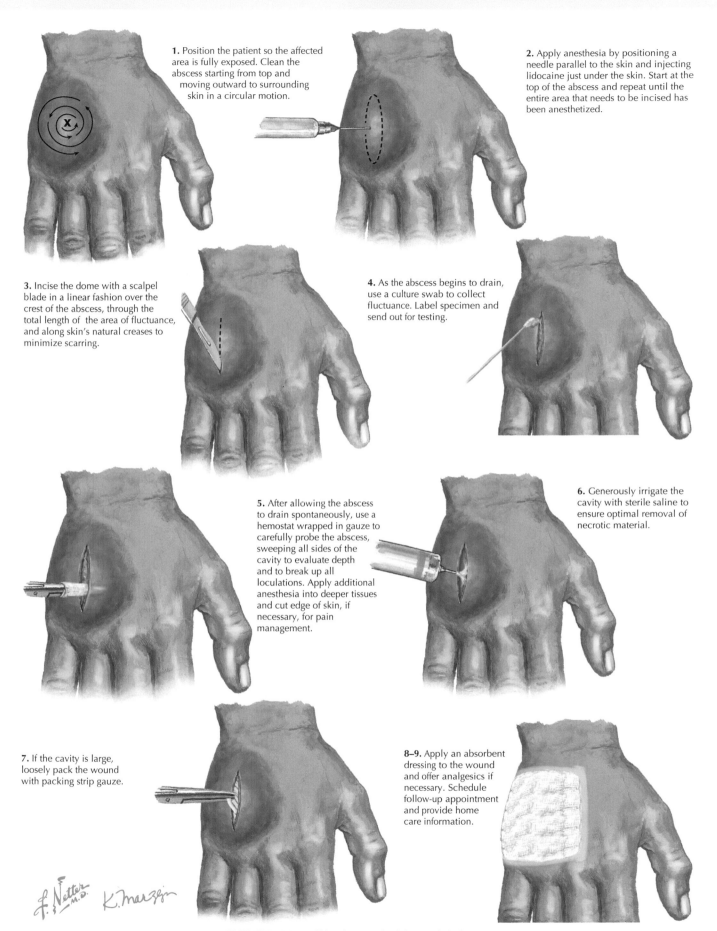

1. Position the patient so the affected area is fully exposed. Clean the abscess starting from top and moving outward to surrounding skin in a circular motion.

2. Apply anesthesia by positioning a needle parallel to the skin and injecting lidocaine just under the skin. Start at the top of the abscess and repeat until the entire area that needs to be incised has been anesthetized.

3. Incise the dome with a scalpel blade in a linear fashion over the crest of the abscess, through the total length of the area of fluctuance, and along skin's natural creases to minimize scarring.

4. As the abscess begins to drain, use a culture swab to collect fluctuance. Label specimen and send out for testing.

5. After allowing the abscess to drain spontaneously, use a hemostat wrapped in gauze to carefully probe the abscess, sweeping all sides of the cavity to evaluate depth and to break up all loculations. Apply additional anesthesia into deeper tissues and cut edge of skin, if necessary, for pain management.

6. Generously irrigate the cavity with sterile saline to ensure optimal removal of necrotic material.

7. If the cavity is large, loosely pack the wound with packing strip gauze.

8–9. Apply an absorbent dressing to the wound and offer analgesics if necessary. Schedule follow-up appointment and provide home care information.

FIGURE 36.3 Skin abscess incision and drainage

CONCLUSION

Abscess incision and drainage is a simple procedure that can be safely performed on a patient with a soft tissue abscess.

Suggested Readings

Abrahamian FM, Shroff SD. Use of routine wound cultures to evaluate cutaneous abscesses for community-associated methicillin-resistant *Staphylococcus aureus. Ann Emerg Med.* 2007;50(1):66.

Blaivas M, Adhikari S. Unexpected findings on point-of-care superficial ultrasound imaging before incision and drainage. *J Ultrasound Med.* 2011;30:1425–1430.

Butler KH. Incision and drainage. In: Robert JR, Hedges JR, eds. *Clinical Procedures in Emergency Medicine*, 5th ed. Philadelphia: Saunders; 2010:657–691.

Fitch MT, Manthey DE, McGinnis HD, et al. Videos in clinical medicine. Abscess incision and drainage. *N Engl J Med.* 2007;357(19):e20.

Gaspari RJ, Resop D, Mendoza M, et al. A randomized controlled trial of incision and drainage versus ultrasonographically guided needle aspiration for skin abscesses and the effect of methicillin-resistant *Staphylococcus aureus. Ann Emerg Med.* 2011;57(5):483–491.

Rajendran PM, Young D, Maurer T, et al. Randomized, double-blind, placebo-controlled trial of cephalexin for treatment of uncomplicated skin abscesses in a population at risk for community-acquired methicillin-resistant *staphylococcus aureus* infection. *Antimicrob Agents Chemother.* 2007;51(11):4044–4048.

Wright TN, Gilligan L, Zhurbich O, Davenport DL, Draus Jr JM. Minimally invasive drainage of subcutaneous abscesses reduces hospital cost and length of stay. *South Med J.* 2013;106(12):689–692.

REVIEW QUESTIONS

1. A male infant was brought to the emergency department with a 3-day history of a rash on his legs. There was no history of fever, sore throat, or rash on any other part of the body. Physical examination revealed a temperature of 37°C and painless, fluid-filled blisters on the legs. The skin around the blisters was red and itchy. A few broken blisters were covered by yellow-colored crusts. The diagnosis of bullous impetigo was made. Which of the following is the etiologic agent most likely causing this condition?

    A. *Streptococcus pyogenes*
    B. *Streptococcus pneumoniae*
    C. *Staphylococcus aureus*
    D. *Staphylococcus epidermidis*
    E. *Streptococcus agalactiae*

2. For the patient in Question 1, which of the following medications will most likely be the first choice?

    A. Macrolides
    B. Erythromycin
    C. Cephalosporins
    D. Aminoglycoside
    E. Tetracyclines

3. Before performing incision and drainage for an abscess, a surgeon should be consulted in which of the following scenarios?

    A. 4-cm fluctuant mass on the anterior right neck
    B. 4-cm fluctuant mass overlying the left knee
    C. 4-cm fluctuant mass on the left buttock
    D. 4-cm fluctuant mass on the right forearm
    E. 4-cm fluctuant mass in the left axilla

Shoulder Joint Aspiration

INTRODUCTION

The technical aspects of aspiration of the shoulder joint are not as well represented in the literature as those for aspiration of the large joints of the lower limb. This is likely related to the higher incidence of pathology in those joints, with the shoulder joint being less commonly afflicted with infections and crystal arthropathies.

Advances in ultrasound have added a noninvasive adjunct to support invasive procedures with increased safety and decreased morbidity. Compared with other imaging modalities, ultrasound, with its lack of radiation exposure, provides a noninvasive, easily learned, cost-effective, accessible tool to facilitate invasive procedures. It permits the rapid assessment of internal structures and has therefore become commonplace in the emergency department. Its use decreases the failure rate of procedures compared with those performed without ultrasound.

In musculoskeletal pathology, ultrasound plays a pivotal role in the diagnosis and management of several entities. Excellent resolution of musculoskeletal structures can be achieved, with clear differentiation of soft tissue, bony structures, and pathology. Ultrasound guidance can be used both before and during a procedure. In contrast, other testing modalities visualize the anatomical structures before the procedure; therefore the location can be marked, but the procedure is then performed without direct visualization.

This chapter discusses ultrasound-guided shoulder aspiration. It is a procedure that has both diagnostic and therapeutic value and is relatively safe and simple to execute.

CLINICALLY RELEVANT ANATOMY

The unique anatomy of the shoulder is responsible for it being the most mobile joint in the body. The shoulder enables upper limb adduction, abduction, flexion, extension, external and internal rotation, and 360-degree circumduction. It is a ball-and-socket joint encased in a fibrous capsule lined with synovium. To counteract the instability associated with its wide range of motion, the joint is held in place by many muscles, tendons, and ligaments and is stabilized by the glenoid labrum (Figs. 37.1 and 37.2).

The shoulder is responsible for connecting the upper extremity to the axial skeleton. The shoulder girdle (composed of the clavicle and the scapula) articulates with the head of the humerus. Several articulations are formed between these bones, comprising the entire shoulder joint

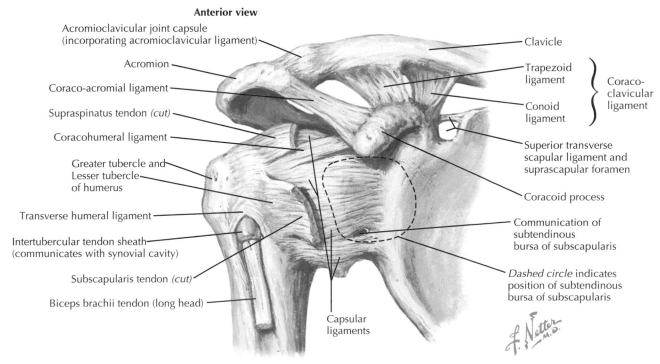

Anterior view

Acromioclavicular joint capsule (incorporating acromioclavicular ligament)

Acromion

Coraco-acromial ligament

Supraspinatus tendon *(cut)*

Coracohumeral ligament

Greater tubercle and Lesser tubercle of humerus

Transverse humeral ligament

Intertubercular tendon sheath (communicates with synovial cavity)

Subscapularis tendon *(cut)*

Biceps brachii tendon (long head)

Clavicle

Trapezoid ligament

Conoid ligament

} Coracoclavicular ligament

Superior transverse scapular ligament and suprascapular foramen

Coracoid process

Communication of subtendinous bursa of subscapularis

Dashed circle indicates position of subtendinous bursa of subscapularis

Capsular ligaments

FIGURE 37.1 Shoulder (glenohumeral joint)

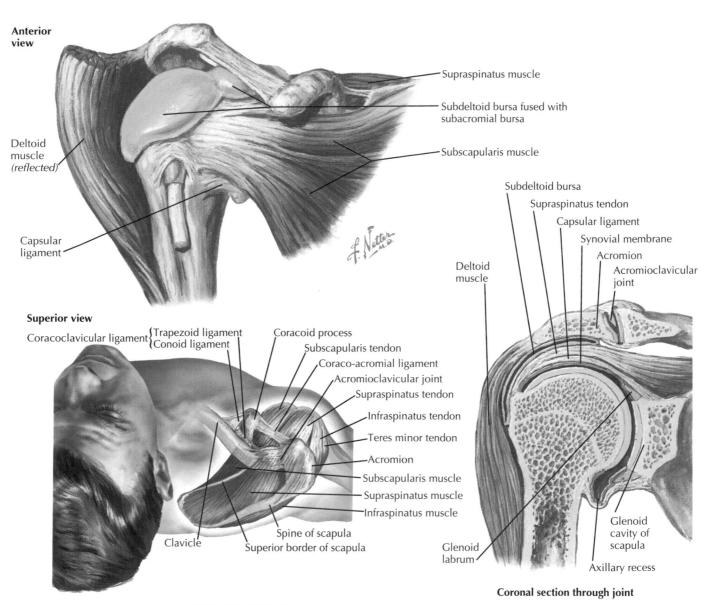

Anterior view

Deltoid muscle (reflected)

Capsular ligament

Supraspinatus muscle

Subdeltoid bursa fused with subacromial bursa

Subscapularis muscle

Superior view

Coracoclavicular ligament {Trapezoid ligament / Conoid ligament}

Coracoid process

Subscapularis tendon

Coraco-acromial ligament

Acromioclavicular joint

Supraspinatus tendon

Infraspinatus tendon

Teres minor tendon

Acromion

Subscapularis muscle

Supraspinatus muscle

Infraspinatus muscle

Spine of scapula

Superior border of scapula

Clavicle

Subdeltoid bursa

Supraspinatus tendon

Capsular ligament

Synovial membrane

Acromion

Acromioclavicular joint

Deltoid muscle

Glenoid labrum

Glenoid cavity of scapula

Axillary recess

Coronal section through joint

FIGURE 37.2 Shoulder: anterior, superior, and coronal views

complex. These are the acromioclavicular, glenohumeral, and sternoclavicular joints. The glenohumeral joint is the main ball-and-socket joint of the shoulder. The glenoid labrum is a lip of fibrocartilaginous tissue that forms a ring around the edge of the glenoid cavity, effectively deepening it to house the humeral head.

The structures responsible for shoulder stability include muscles, tendons, and ligaments. The glenohumeral joint is stabilized by four rotator cuff muscles, all originating on the scapula, and their tendinous attachments. The supraspinatus, infraspinatus, and teres minor insert into the greater tubercle of the humerus. The subscapularis inserts into the lesser tubercle of the humerus.

The superior, middle, and inferior glenohumeral ligaments provide additional reinforcement to the shoulder joint, resisting dislocating forces.

The glenohumeral joint is the most common site for sonographic-guided intervention. The axillary recess represents the most inferior portion of the glenoid capsule and lies between the teres minor and subscapularis muscles. The anterior portion of the joint capsule, extending between the coracoid process and the subscapularis muscle and tendon, forms the subscapular recess. The rotator interval is a triangular space between the supraspinatus and subscapularis muscles. The superior glenohumeral ligament and the glenohumeral capsular tissue are contained in this interval. This extension of the capsule within the rotator interval forms a synovial-lined sheath that houses the tendon of the long head of the biceps.

INDICATIONS

Acute Joint With Effusion

Numerous pathologic entities can lead to acute joint effusions, including infectious, traumatic, crystal-induced, hematologic, degenerative, rheumatologic, neoplastic, or idiopathic conditions. More commonly seen conditions are infectious or crystalline disease and trauma.

Patients with septic joints may present with signs of localized inflammation in the joint, such as warmth, tenderness, swelling, and decreased and painful range of motion. Systemic symptoms such as fever, chills, and rigor may also be present. Septic joints can potentially lead to rapid joint destruction as well as bacteremia and hence must be identified as early as possible. In other causes of monoarticular arthropathies, such as crystal-induced disease, localized symptoms are also common.

Synovial fluid is used to differentiate septic joints from other causes of arthralgia. Synovial fluid findings supporting the diagnosis of septic arthritis are positive cultures and a markedly elevated white blood cell count with neutrophil predominance. Culture and sensitivity studies allow antibiotic treatment to be tailored to the specific cause of the infection. Early drainage and targeted intravenous antibiotic therapy decrease the chance of permanent joint damage as well as the need for invasive procedures. Crystal-induced arthropathies can be diagnosed by the specific characteristics of crystals seen on microscopy. Since expansion of the joint capsule is restricted by the tissues stabilizing it, collections of inflammatory and infectious material within the capsule may place pressure on the nearby tissues. Shoulder aspiration is effective in quickly relieving this type of pain.

Calcific Tendinitis

Calcific tendinitis is caused by the deposition of carbonate-apatite crystals in the rotator cuff tendons. This may cause acute or chronic pain and is responsible for 7% of cases of shoulder pain. Though it may cause days missed from work, it is usually self-limited, even after a period of severe pain. It may be treated with nonsteroidal antiinflammatory drugs, ultrasound, and subacromial steroid injections early in the course of the disease. These conservative options provide symptomatic and often permanent or long-term relief. Other treatment alternatives include surgery, acetic acid iontophoresis, shockwave lithotripsy, and percutaneous aspiration of the calcifications. Percutaneous needle aspiration and lavage of calcifications has been shown to be effective in the short and long term, with results similar to and better than those published for other techniques.

CONTRAINDICATIONS

Due to the relatively simple nature of shoulder joint aspiration, not many contraindications exist. The presence of cellulitis over the area of needle insertion is an absolute contraindication because it might introduce infection into a previously sterile joint.

A bleeding diathesis is a relative contraindication, as aspiration might result in iatrogenic hemarthrosis. Though the overall risk may not be high, the amount of hemorrhage in patients with bleeding disorders can be unpredictable. Anticoagulant therapy is considered a relative contraindication by some. There are studies, however, that report arthrocentesis to be safe in patients receiving chronic warfarin therapy at therapeutic levels.

Confirmed bacteremia is a relative contraindication. Shoulder aspiration in a patient with confirmed bacteremia theoretically poses a risk of seeding bacteria into the joint space. The bacteria cultured from the blood would also be presumed to be the same as those causing the joint space infection.

EQUIPMENT

Ultrasound machine and probe. A high-frequency (greater than 7 MHz) linear-array probe is preferred for joint aspiration. It provides sufficient depth of view and excellent resolution of structures. The quadrilateral-shaped image allows many nearby structures to be observed simultaneously, along with the location of the needle, as it is advanced. Sterile covers for the ultrasound probe are usually not required.

Sterile gloves, surgical gauze, and drapes

Skin cleaning fluid: alcohol or iodine solution

3.5-inch, 18-gauge spinal needle; larger needles (up to 14 gauge) can be used to aspirate thick fluids

Syringes: 10 to 50 mL, depending on the anticipated volume of the fluid to be aspirated

1% lidocaine solution

Collection containers for lab specimens

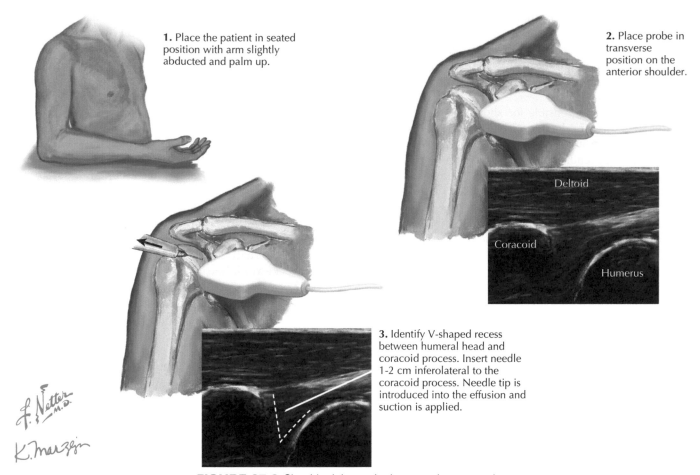

1. Place the patient in seated position with arm slightly abducted and palm up.

2. Place probe in transverse position on the anterior shoulder.

Deltoid

Coracoid

Humerus

3. Identify V-shaped recess between humeral head and coracoid process. Insert needle 1-2 cm inferolateral to the coracoid process. Needle tip is introduced into the effusion and suction is applied.

FIGURE 37.3 Shoulder joint aspiration: anterior approach

PROCEDURE

Explain the procedure, obtain consent, and perform a time out. Adhere to proper sterile technique. Sterile gear should be worn, and the area should be appropriately cleaned and draped. Care should be taken to avoid contact between the sonography gel and the needle.

Approaches to Joint Effusion Aspiration

Anterior Approach

See Fig. 37.3.

1. With the patient seated, extend and slightly abduct the arm with the palm facing up. Alternatively, the patient may lie supine with the arm held in partial external rotation. This position allows the long head of the biceps brachii to be relocated lateral to the site of aspiration. More of the joint is also exposed.

2. Place the ultrasound probe transversely over the anterior shoulder at the level of the coracoid process. Just below the skin and subcutaneous tissue, a "starry sky" pattern is seen. This represents the deltoid muscle. Deep to the deltoid, the hyperechoic, curved periosteum of the humeral head can be seen. The anterior surface of the medial aspect of the coracoid process is also visualized. Joint effusions will be seen in this area as anechoic collections of fluid.

3. Identify the V-shaped recess between the humeral head and the coracoid process. With the transducer in the transverse orientation, insert the needle 1 to 2 cm inferolateral to the coracoid process. The needle tip is introduced into the effusion and suction is applied under sonographic guidance.

Posterior Approach

See Fig. 37.4.

1. With the patient seated, the elbow is flexed and the forearm placed on the thigh in the neutral position.

2. Place the probe on the posterior aspect of the shoulder, just below the acromion. Again, the deltoid muscle is visualized just below the skin and subcutaneous tissue. Deep to the deltoid are the triangular, hypoechoic infraspinatus muscle and the hyperechoic tendon as they travel laterally over the humeral head. The humeral head and glenoid rim, which is a more medially and superficially located hyperechoic structure, can be observed deep to the probe. The hyperechoic scapula may also be seen medial and deep to the humeral head. Anechoic-appearing effusions will appear in the groove between the humeral head and the dorsal glenoid rim.

3. Hold the transducer in the transverse orientation; it may be rotated or tilted slightly to obtain the best image of the

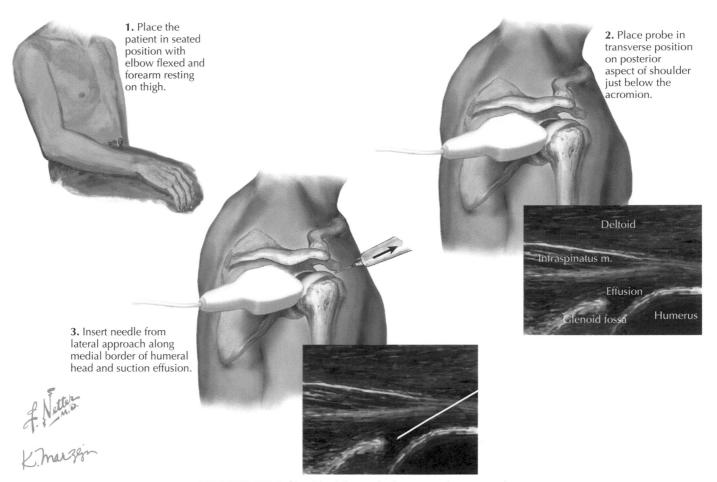

1. Place the patient in seated position with elbow flexed and forearm resting on thigh.

2. Place probe in transverse position on posterior aspect of shoulder just below the acromion.

3. Insert needle from lateral approach along medial border of humeral head and suction effusion.

Deltoid

Infraspinatus m.

Effusion

Glenoid fossa

Humerus

FIGURE 37.4 Shoulder joint aspiration: posterior approach

joint space. Locate the effusion within the aforementioned groove. Insert the needle using a lateral approach. This permits a long-axis view of the needle as it enters the joint. Ensure that the needle is seen entering the groove along the medial border of the humeral head to avoid the circumflex scapular vessels and suprascapular nerves traveling near the medial aspect of the glenoid rim.

Aspiration for Calcific Tendinitis

For calcifications in the supraspinatus and infraspinatus tendons, the patient is seated and the arm is rotated externally with the hand placed behind the back. For calcifications in the subscapularis tendon, the arm is externally rotated with the hand supine and resting on the thigh.

The skin is cleaned and sterilized. A 20-gauge needle is introduced via an anterior caudocranial approach. This is done under ultrasound guidance using a freehand technique, with the needle being inserted following the plane of the sound waves. The angle of the needle insertion places the syringe below the calcification. The needle is then connected to a syringe filled with 1% lidocaine.

After injecting a local anesthetic into the route toward the calcification, the tip of the needle is introduced into the calcification. Direct aspiration is avoided because of the possibility of occlusion of the needle. Instead, a small amount of saline

is injected into the calcification, followed by the release of the plunger. This allows the backflow of calcium-containing fluid into the syringe. This is repeated until the fluid in the syringe becomes cloudy, at which point it is replaced by a new syringe. The procedure is continued until the fluid no longer becomes cloudy. If multiple calcifications exist in the same shoulder, the process may be carried out for each one.

Triamcinolone, 40 mg, is injected into the subacromial-subdeltoid bursa to prevent bursitis. Aspiration by this method takes about 15 minutes.

ANATOMICAL PITFALLS

During ultrasound of the posterior aspect of the shoulder, hypoechoic fluid may be noted beneath the deltoid muscle but superior to the supraspinatus tendon. This represents subacromial bursitis and should not be confused with an effusion. Bursitis will not be seen on the anterior view of the shoulder.

In the posterior approach to shoulder aspiration, one must be aware of the neurovascular anatomy of the region. The route of the suprascapular nerve takes it close to the joint capsule of the shoulder, toward which it also gives off branches. The circumflex scapular vessels as well as the posterior circumflex humeral vessels course near to the glenohumeral joint. For safe arthrocentesis, the needle must be advanced along the medial border of the humeral head.

COMPLICATIONS

Ultrasound-guided aspiration of the shoulder joint is a relatively safe procedure that is well tolerated by the vast majority of patients. Complications are uncommon and are usually not severe when they do occur. In order to minimize the complications of this procedure, one must carefully identify surrounding vessels, nerves, tendons, and muscles and adhere to aseptic technique.

Introduction of an infection into a previously sterile joint is the greatest concern in this procedure. Careful cleaning and draping of the area and the use of sterile gear minimize this risk. Because of the seriousness of potential infection, strict aseptic practices should be followed in all aspirations. As with all other procedures, conscious sedation may be needed for certain patients.

Recurrence is a possibility for both effusions and calcific tendinitis. In calcific tendinitis, recurrence can last for weeks after the procedure but is usually followed by a gradual disappearance of the calcifications. This may be due to the change within the tissue after removal of the calcifications.

CONCLUSION

Before ultrasound technology became popular, joint injections and aspirations were mainly performed using only anatomical landmarks. Sonography has decreased the failure rates of these procedures. It also allows for the postponement or replacement of more invasive procedures.

The shoulder joint is not the most commonly aspirated joint, but emergency physicians must have knowledge of the procedure for when the need arises. A relatively safe procedure, it has major diagnostic and therapeutic value. Thus, this procedure should be part of the skills training of every emergency physician.

Suggested Readings

Barr L, Hatch N, Roque PJ, Wu TS. Basic ultrasound-guided procedures. *Crit Care Clin*. 2014;30:275–304.

Bettencourt RB, Linder MM. Arthrocentesis and therapeutic joint injection: an overview for the primary care physician. *Prim Care*. 2010;37:691–702.

Bouffard JA, Lee SM, Dhanju J. Ultrasonography of the shoulder. *Semin Ultrasound CT MR*. 2000;21:164–191.

Daley EL, Bajaj S, Bisson LJ, Cole BJ. Improving injection accuracy of the elbow, knee, and shoulder does injection site and imaging make a difference? A systematic review. *Am J Sports Med*. 2011;39:656–662.

del Cura JL, Torre I, Zabala R, Legórburu A. Sonographically guided percutaneous needle lavage in calcific tendinitis of the shoulder: short-and long-term results. *Am J Roentgenol*. 2007;189:W128–W134.

del Cura JL. Ultrasound-guided therapeutic procedures in the musculoskeletal system. *Curr Probl Diagn Radiol*. 2008;37:203–218.

Glenohumeral capsule and ligaments. In: Bain G, Itoi E, Di Giacomo G, Sugaya H, eds. *Normal and Pathological Anatomy of the Shoulder*. New York: Springer Heidelberg; 2015.

Gonçalves B, Ambrosio C, Serra S, Alves F, Gil-Agostinho A, Caseiro-Alves F. US-guided interventional joint procedures in patients with rheumatic diseases—when and how we do it? *Eur J Radiol*. 2011;79:407–414.

Hansford BG, Stacy GS. Musculoskeletal aspiration procedures. *Semin Intervent Radiol*. 2012;29:270–285.

Kishner S, Munshi S, Black J, Gest T. *Shoulder Joint Anatomy*; 2015. Available from http://emedicine.medscape.com/article/1899211-overview.

Lin JT, Adler RS, Bracilovic A, Cooper G, Sofka C, Lutz GE. Clinical outcomes of ultrasound-guided aspiration and lavage in calcific tendinosis of the shoulder. *HSS J*. 2007;3:99–105.

Thumboo J, O'Duffy JD. A prospective study of the safety of joint and soft tissue aspirations and injections in patients taking warfarin sodium. *Arthritis Rheum*. 1998;41:736–739.

REVIEW QUESTIONS

1. Ultrasound examination of the shoulder of a 62-year-old woman clearly demonstrated erosion of the tendon within the glenohumeral joint. Which of the following tendons was eroded?

   A. Glenohumeral
   B. Long head of triceps brachii
   C. Long head of biceps brachii
   D. Infraspinatus
   E. Coracobrachialis

2. The right shoulder of a 78-year-old woman had become increasingly painful over the past year. Abduction of the right arm caused her to wince from the discomfort. Palpation of the deltoid muscle by the physician produced exquisite pain. Imaging studies reveal intermuscular inflammation extending over the head of the humerus. Which of the following structures was most likely inflamed?

   A. Subscapular bursa
   B. Infraspinatus muscle
   C. Glenohumeral joint cavity
   D. Subacromial bursa
   E. Teres minor muscle

3. A 43-year-old man visits the outpatient clinic with a painful shoulder. Physical examination reveals a painful arc syndrome due to supraspinatus tendinopathy. Which of the following conditions will most likely be present during physical examination?

   A. Painful abduction from 0 to 15 degrees
   B. Painful abduction from 0 to 140 degrees
   C. Painful abduction from 70 to 140 degrees
   D. Painful abduction from 15 to 140 degrees
   E. Painful abduction from 40 to 140 degrees

Transurethral (Foley Catheter) and Suprapubic Urinary Bladder Catheterization

INTRODUCTION

Urinary bladder catheters are used for the drainage and collection of urine into a drainage bag. Transurethral catheterization involves the placement of a catheter through the urethra, whereas suprapubic catheterization is the insertion of a catheter through the anterior abdominal wall into the urinary bladder.

The Foley catheter, inserted through the urethra, was invented by the surgeon Frederic Foley in the 1930s. Short (21 cm) and long (40 to 45 cm) catheters are available. Larger-diameter catheters (20 to 24 Fr) are used for the drainage of clots and hematuria. Once the catheter is inserted into the bladder, a balloon is inflated to maintain its position. Two sizes of balloon are available, 5 mL and 20 to 30 mL. The larger balloons are recommended after surgery or for women with weak pelvic floor musculature.

Catheters are made from latex, silicone, plastic, or Teflon. Latex is cost effective and is used more often. However, if used long term, it is associated with urethral inflammation and strictures, as well as being contraindicated for individuals with latex allergy. Therefore, when prolonged use is required, silicone catheters are recommended.

CLINICALLY RELEVANT ANATOMY

Transurethral Placement

The male urethra is a narrow fibromuscular tube that carries urine and semen from the bladder and ejaculatory ducts, respectively, to the exterior of the body. It is up to 20 cm long and extends from the neck of the bladder to the meatus on the glans penis. It is divided into three parts, the prostatic, membranous, and spongy segments (Figs. 38.1 and 38.2).

The prostatic urethra is about 3 cm long and traverses the prostate gland from the base to the apex. It is the most dilatable and widest part of the urethra. The membranous urethra is about 1.25 cm long, lies within the urogenital diaphragm, and is surrounded by the sphincter urethrae muscle. This is the least dilatable portion. The spongy or penile urethra is about 15.75 cm long and is enclosed in the bulb and corpus spongiosum of the penis. The external meatus is the narrowest portion of the urethra. The portion that lies within the glans penis is dilated to form the fossa terminalis (navicular fossa). The bulbourethral glands open into the penile urethra below the urogenital diaphragm.

The penis is composed of two corpora cavernosa and the corpus spongiosum, which surrounds the urethra. In the penis, the erectile bodies are surrounded by Buck's fascia, dartos fascia, and skin.

The female urethra, which is about 3.8 cm long, is a tubular structure that extends from the neck of the bladder and terminates at the vaginal vestibule, about 2.5 cm below the clitoris. It traverses the sphincter urethrae and lies anterior to the vagina. At the sides of the external urethral meatus are the small openings of the paraurethral gland ducts.

Suprapubic Placement

The urinary bladder is located in the anterior pelvis, enveloped by extraperitoneal fat and connective tissue. It is separated from the pubic symphysis by an anterior prevesical space known as the retropubic space (of Retzius). The dome of the bladder is covered by peritoneum, and the bladder neck is fixed to neighboring structures by reflections of the pelvic fascia and by the true ligaments of the pelvis. Palpation or percussion can confirm a distended bladder; however, bedside ultrasound imaging should always be performed if available to confirm the bladder position.

INDICATIONS

Bladder catheterization should only be done when it is necessary to relieve urinary retention or to monitor fluid status. If a sterile urine sample is all that is needed, straight catheterization should be performed. This uses a catheter without a balloon and is immediately removed after the sample is taken. For men who require the monitoring of fluid output, a condom catheter, a condom attached to tubing and a collection bag, can be used. This avoids the complications of an indwelling catheter. Catheters must be placed using aseptic technique and removed as soon as clinically indicated to avoid infections and possible subsequent sepsis.

Diagnostic

Diagnostic catheterization is a nonemergency procedure used for the collection of sterile urine or the measurement and monitoring of urine output. This is often necessary for critically ill patients or during surgery to assess fluid status. Placement of a catheter may also be required after certain operations for the genitourinary tract or nearby structures.

Therapeutic

Therapeutic catheterization may be performed for emergencies or for less urgent reasons. It is used for the management of acute urinary retention or bladder outlet

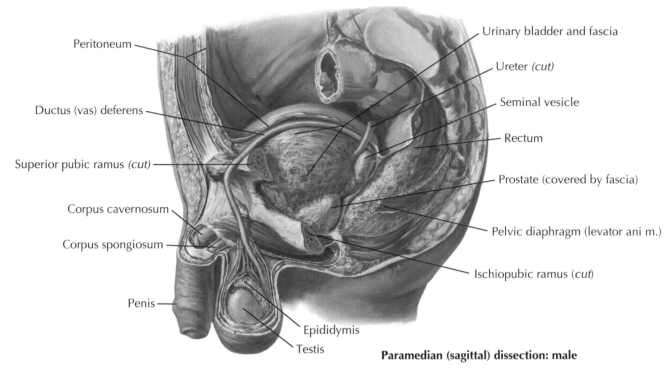

Peritoneum

Ductus (vas) deferens

Superior pubic ramus *(cut)*

Corpus cavernosum

Corpus spongiosum

Penis

Epididymis

Testis

Urinary bladder and fascia

Ureter *(cut)*

Seminal vesicle

Rectum

Prostate (covered by fascia)

Pelvic diaphragm (levator ani m.)

Ischiopubic ramus *(cut)*

Paramedian (sagittal) dissection: male

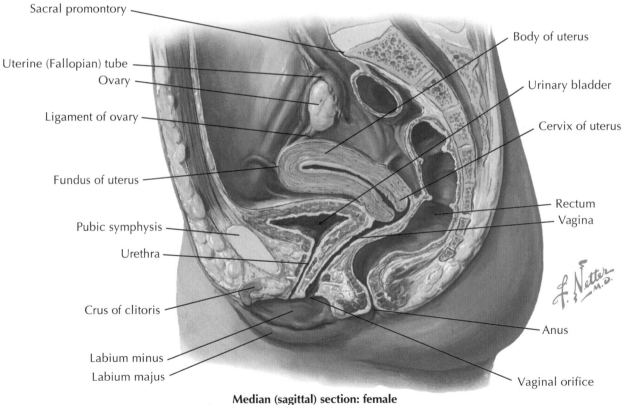

Sacral promontory

Uterine (Fallopian) tube

Ovary

Ligament of ovary

Fundus of uterus

Pubic symphysis

Urethra

Crus of clitoris

Labium minus

Labium majus

Body of uterus

Urinary bladder

Cervix of uterus

Rectum

Vagina

Anus

Vaginal orifice

Median (sagittal) section: female

FIGURE 38.1 The bladder and urethra

Female: frontal section

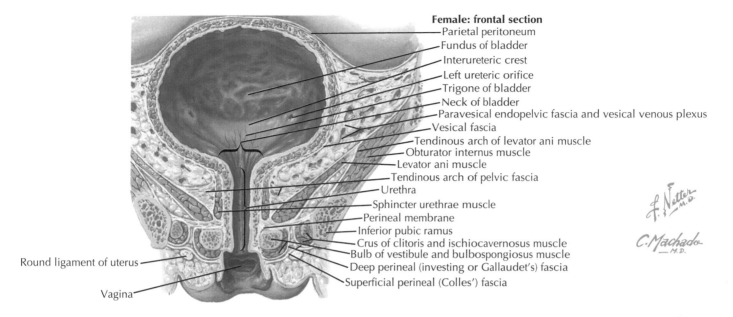

Parietal peritoneum
Fundus of bladder
Interureteric crest
Left ureteric orifice
Trigone of bladder
Neck of bladder
Paravesical endopelvic fascia and vesical venous plexus
Vesical fascia
Tendinous arch of levator ani muscle
Obturator internus muscle
Levator ani muscle
Tendinous arch of pelvic fascia
Urethra
Sphincter urethrae muscle
Perineal membrane
Inferior pubic ramus
Crus of clitoris and ischiocavernosus muscle
Bulb of vestibule and bulbospongiosus muscle
Deep perineal (investing or Gallaudet's) fascia
Superficial perineal (Colles') fascia

Round ligament of uterus

Vagina

Male: frontal section

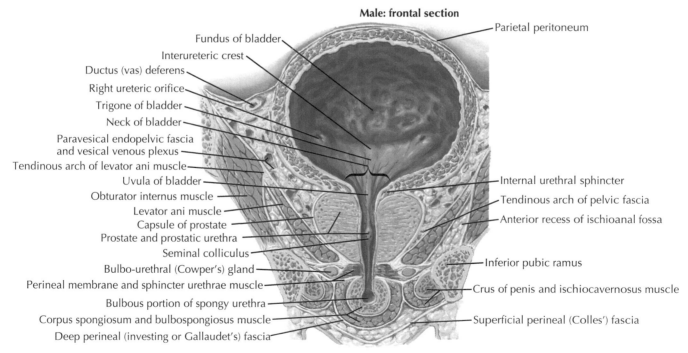

Fundus of bladder
Interureteric crest
Ductus (vas) deferens
Right ureteric orifice
Trigone of bladder
Neck of bladder
Paravesical endopelvic fascia and vesical venous plexus
Tendinous arch of levator ani muscle
Uvula of bladder
Obturator internus muscle
Levator ani muscle
Capsule of prostate
Prostate and prostatic urethra
Seminal colliculus
Bulbo-urethral (Cowper's) gland
Perineal membrane and sphincter urethrae muscle
Bulbous portion of spongy urethra
Corpus spongiosum and bulbospongiosus muscle
Deep perineal (investing or Gallaudet's) fascia

Parietal peritoneum
Internal urethral sphincter
Tendinous arch of pelvic fascia
Anterior recess of ischioanal fossa
Inferior pubic ramus
Crus of penis and ischiocavernosus muscle
Superficial perineal (Colles') fascia

FIGURE 38.2 Urinary bladder: female and male

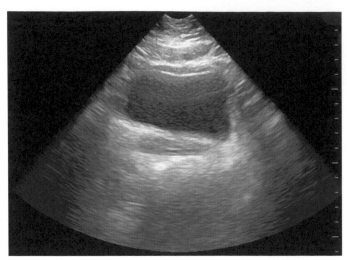

FIGURE 38.3 Transverse bladder ultrasound image

obstruction to avoid hydronephrosis. It is also used for hematuria with clots, hygiene care for immobilized patients, or the decompression of a neurogenic bladder. It may be necessary for urinary incontinence following the failure of conservative behavioral, pharmacologic, and surgical therapy or in the presence of open wounds in the sacral and perineal regions. It may also be used for continuous bladder irrigation.

Suprapubic catheterization is indicated for patients in whom transurethral catheterization is contraindicated. This approach may be used, for example, in cases of urethral rupture or stricture or trauma, a mass at the neck of the bladder, benign prostatic hypertrophy, or prostatic cancer. It may also be necessary for patients with urinary incontinence from muscle weakness or a congenital defect that prevents them from feeling the need to urinate.

CONTRAINDICATIONS
Transurethral Placement

The absolute contraindication to transurethral catheterization is urethral injury, usually occurring after pelvic trauma or a straddle-type injury. If there is blood at the urethral meatus or gross hematuria due to trauma, the urethra should be evaluated with a retrograde urethrogram to rule out the presence of a tear. Relative contraindications include urethral strictures, recent urinary tract surgery, and the presence of an artificial sphincter.

Suprapubic Placement

Suprapubic catheterization is absolutely contraindicated when the bladder cannot be accurately located by palpation or ultrasonography (Fig. 38.3). Relative contraindications include unexplained hematuria or an uncorrected coagulopathy. Prior pelvic or lower abdominal surgery (for conditions such as pelvic or bladder cancer) is also a contraindication because of the possibility of bowel adhesions.

EQUIPMENT
Transurethral

Foley catheter of the appropriate size, material, and contour
Urinary drainage bag and connecting tube
Sterile lubricant
Antiseptic solution and sterile cotton balls to sterilize the male urethral meatus and the female perineum
Sterile syringe, 5 to 10 mL, filled with enough sterile water to inflate the catheter balloon, usually 5 mL
Sterile gloves and drapes

Suprapubic

Antiseptic for skin sterilization
Sterile cap, mask, gloves, and gown
1% lidocaine with a 10-mL syringe and 25-gauge, 1-cm and 22-gauge, 4-cm needles
Sterile towels or sterile drapes
No. 11 scalpel blade, mounted
Catheter-clad needle (such as an angiocath), 14 gauge, 30 cm, or other percutaneous suprapubic catheter sets. A central venous catheter kit can also be used if no other equipment is available.
50-mL syringe
Closed urinary drainage system
Silk suture (3-0) on a curved cutting needle
Needle holder
Suture scissors
Antibacterial ointment
Sterile gauze sponges, 5 × 5 cm², and tape
Rolled bath towel for placement under the patient's hips

PROCEDURE

Obtain patient consent and perform a time out.

Transurethral Procedure
Male

See Fig. 38.4 and Video 38.1. The patient should be lying supine. Appropriate personal protective equipment should be donned.

1. Assemble all necessary equipment.
   a. Open the catheter tray and catheter and position them on a sterile field so that all required materials are readily accessible.
   b. Apply some lubricant on the sterile field.
   c. Put on sterile gloves and drape the perineal area.
   d. Ensure the catheter container is open and the lubricating jelly is accessible.
   e. Moisten the cotton swabs with antiseptic.
   f. Be sure that the syringe is filled with enough sterile water to inflate the balloon.
2. Using the left hand (standing on the patient's right side), grasp the penis so that the shaft is in the palm and the glans of the penis is free but secure. The penis should be held at a right angle to the abdomen. The left hand should remain in this position for the remainder of the

1. Assemble and prepare all necessary equipment:
   a. Open catheter tray and selected catheter and place on sterile field
   b. Place lubricant on the sterile field
   c. Put on sterile gloves
   d. Ensure that catheter is open
   e. Moisten cotton swabs with antiseptic
   f. Fill syringe with sterile water to inflate balloon

The male patient should be in supine position.

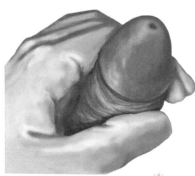

2. Stand at patient's right side. With left hand, grasp penis so that shaft is in the palm and the glans is free but secure, and perpendicular to the abdomen. The left hand remains in this position until step 8.

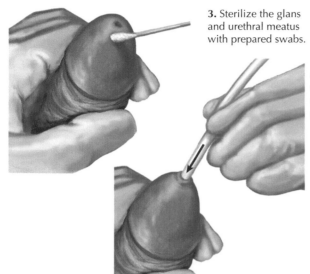

3. Sterilize the glans and urethral meatus with prepared swabs.

4–5. Grasp the Foley catheter in the right hand and coat tip with lubricant. Insert the catheter into the urethral meatus and advance through urethra to base of penis with successive, steady movements.

6–7. Advance the catheter through the membranous and prostatic urethrae into the bladder. Continue to advance to the hilt to ensure that the balloon is not inflated in the urethra. Release the penis and prepare to inflate balloon.

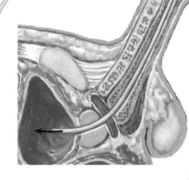

8. Inflate the balloon with sterile water and withdraw the catheter until balloon is pulled snuggly against the trigone.

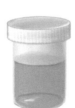

9. Obtain a specimen for appropriate tests and connect drainage bag to the catheter. Secure catheter to upper thigh with tape, leaving adequate slack.

FIGURE 38.4 Transurethral (Foley catheter) urinary bladder catheterization: male

procedure because it is no longer sterile. For uncircumcised patients, retract the foreskin over the glans.

3. Sterilize the glans and urethral meatus with swabs dipped in antiseptic solution.
4. Grasp the Foley catheter in the right hand and coat the tip with lubricating jelly.
5. Insert the catheter into the urethral meatus and advance it down the urethra to the base of the penis with successive, steady movements.
6. Advance the catheter through the membranous and prostatic urethrae into the bladder.
7. Advance the catheter to the hilt (even if urine is obtained earlier) to ensure that the balloon is not inflated in the urethra. As soon as the catheter has been advanced to this point, release the penis to free both hands for inflation of the balloon.

8. Inflate the balloon with about 5 mL of sterile water and withdraw the catheter until the balloon is pulled snugly against the trigone of the bladder.
9. Obtain a specimen for appropriate tests, including routine urinalysis. Connect the urinary drainage system bag to the catheter, and tape the catheter to the upper thigh, leaving some slack. Remember to retract the foreskin back over the glans if the patient is uncircumcised.

Female

See Fig. 38.5 and Video 38.2. The patient should be in the lithotomy position to maximize exposure of the periurethral region. If she is comatose or under anesthesia, flex her knees and hips, and allow the thighs to abduct.

Steps 1a to 1f are the same as those described above for males.

1. Assemble and prepare all necessary equipment:
   a. Open catheter tray and selected catheter and place on sterile field
   b. Place lubricant on the sterile field
   c. Put on sterile gloves
   d. Ensure that catheter is open
   e. Moisten cotton swabs with antiseptic
   f. Fill syringe with sterile water to inflate balloon

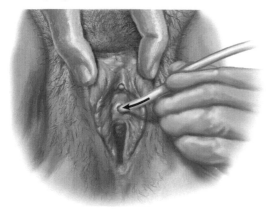

The female patient should be in the lithotomy position.

2–3. Stand at patient's right side. Using the left hand, spread the labia minora and identify the clitoris. Cleanse the entire area, labia and urethral meatus, with prepared swabs. The left hand continues to hold the labia apart for the rest of the procedure.

Clitoris
Urethral meatus

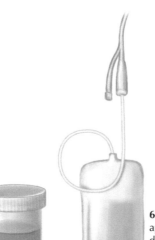

Advance until urine returns. Continue to advance another 4-5 cm to make sure the balloon is well within the bladder.

4. Grasp the catheter in the right hand and coat the tip and proximal portion with lubricant. Insert the catheter into the urethral meatus, just below the clitoris.

5. Inflate the balloon with sterile water and withdraw the catheter gently until the balloon is pulled snuggly against the trigone.

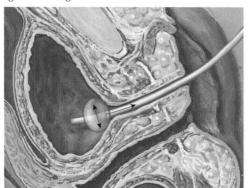

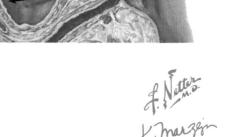

6–7. Obtain a specimen for appropriate tests and connect drainage bag to the catheter. Secure catheter to upper thigh with tape, leaving adequate slack.

FIGURE 38.5 Transurethral (Foley catheter) urinary bladder catheterization: female

1. Using the left hand (standing on the patient's right side), spread the labia minora and identify the clitoris. Thoroughly cleanse the entire area with swabs soaked in antiseptic solution. Clean the labia with anterior to posterior strokes using two successive swabs, and then cleanse the urethral meatus using another two successive swabs.
2. The left hand continues to hold the labia apart for the rest of the procedure.
3. Grasp the catheter with the right hand, coat the tip and proximal portion with lubricating jelly, and insert the catheter into the urethral meatus, just below the clitoris. Advance the catheter until urine returns, then advance it 4 to 5 cm farther to make sure that the balloon is well within the bladder.

4. Inflate the balloon with about 5 mL of sterile water and withdraw the catheter gently until the balloon is pulled snugly against the trigone.
5. Collect a small amount of urine in a sterile container for appropriate studies, including routine urinalysis. Connect the catheter to the urinary drainage bag.
6. Tape the Foley catheter and the urinary drainage tube to the upper thigh, leaving enough slack.

Suprapubic Procedure

The patient should be supine with a rolled-up towel placed under the hips.

1. Assemble all necessary equipment.
2. Locate the distended bladder by ultrasound. If ultrasound is not available, palpation and percussion should be performed to locate the bladder.

3. Prepare the area just above the pubic symphysis by clipping the pubic hair and sterilizing the skin. Extend the sterile field with drapes.

4. The point of needle insertion is 1.2 cm from the superior edge of the pubic symphysis in the midline.

5. Using 1% lidocaine in a 10-mL syringe with a 25-gauge needle, anesthetize the skin at the point of insertion. Switch to a 22-gauge needle to anesthetize the subcutaneous tissue and anterior wall of the bladder.

6. Make a 0.5-cm transverse incision over the anesthetized skin with the No. 11 scalpel blade.

7. The technique for placing the catheter depends on the type of catheter used:

   a. *Catheter-clad needle*:
      1. Attach a 50-mL syringe to a 14-gauge, 30-cm catheter-clad needle.
      2. Insert the catheter unit through the skin incision and advance caudally with a smooth, deliberate motion at a 50- to 60-degree angle to the abdominal surface.
      3. Maintaining gentle suction with the syringe will cause the aspiration of urine as soon as the bladder cavity has been entered.
      4. Once the bladder has been entered, slip the catheter tip off the needle by holding the hub of the needle in the left hand and advancing the catheter with the right hand.
      5. Advance the catheter about 6 to 8 cm.
      6. Attach the catheter to the sterile intravenous tubing connected to the empty intravenous bag or bottle that is to receive the urine.
      7. Suture the catheter in place at the insertion site with 3-0 silk suture. Wind the ends of the suture around the catheter at least three times to secure it to the abdominal wall.
      8. Apply antibacterial ointment to the insertion site, cover it with sterile 5 × 5 cm² gauze sponges, and tape in place.
      9. Tape all connections.

   b. *Central venous catheter kit*: Use the Seldinger technique, a guidewire procedure, to insert the catheter.

   c. *Percutaneous suprapubic catheter*: Follow the manufacturer's instructions for use.

ANATOMICAL PITFALLS

Benign Prostatic Hyperplasia

In some cases, catheterization can be difficult, especially in men with benign prostatic hyperplasia or with a false urethral passage. A certain degree of persistence in attempting to place the catheter is acceptable, but if too many attempts are made, there is a chance of rupturing the urethra or creating a false passage. If attempts do fail, a suprapubic catheter should be placed instead.

One way to reduce complications is by using a larger catheter, which tends to be stiffer and provides more forceful dilation of the prostatic urethra. The larger, blunt tip will follow the true lumen of the urethra rather than entering smaller false passages.

Another method involves lubricating the urethra using a 30- to 50-mL sterile catheter-tipped syringe to inject lubricating jelly down the urethra with gentle pressure. Then try inserting the catheter again.

One can also consider lubricating the urethra with the catheter as it is being passed. Fill a syringe with 30 to 50 mL of lubricating jelly, insert the tip of the syringe into the catheter, and fill the catheter with jelly. As the catheter is being passed, use the syringe to inject lubricant, which will lubricate the entire length of the catheter and aid in dilating the urethra just ahead of the catheter tip.

To facilitate insertion, a coudé catheter can be used. This has a curved tip that can navigate through a urethra narrowed by processes such as benign prostatic hyperplasia. The tip should be directed anteriorly to facilitate its passage through the prostatic urethra.

Trauma

Foley catheters are inserted during resuscitation in patients with major trauma. Prior to insertion, a rectal examination should be considered in any male with major blunt trauma to ensure that the prostate gland is firmly attached to the surrounding tissues. A free-floating prostate gland or gross blood escaping from the urethra is indicative of a urethral rupture until proven otherwise. In these cases, a suprapubic rather than a Foley catheter should be placed.

COMPLICATIONS

Mechanical problems such as leakage, catheter blockage, and inability to pass a catheter are common. With suprapubic catheter placement, there is a risk of bladder bleeding or of bowel injury when the bladder is not fully distended or after routine catheter change. Long-term complications include skin erosion and chronic leakage.

The most common complications are urinary tract infections and bacteriuria. Recurrent urinary tract infections from chronic catheter use can lead to acute or chronic pyelonephritis and sepsis. Urea-splitting bacteria, such as *Proteus mirabilis*, are commonly associated with the formation of bladder stones.

Spontaneous rupture of the urinary catheter balloon can occur, leaving retained balloon fragments in the bladder. A cystoscopy should be performed to remove the fragments because they can cause urethral obstruction.

A more frequently encountered complication of indwelling catheters is the formation of a fistula between the bladder, small intestine, colon, rectum, or vagina. Risk factors include prolonged catheterization, malignancy, inflammation, radiotherapy, and trauma.

Although rare, bladder perforation may occur.

CONCLUSION

Bladder catheterization is used in both emergency and routine clinical situations. Useful for diagnostic and therapeutic procedures, transurethral and suprapubic catheterization require the knowledge of male and female anatomy. An understanding of catheter technology and routine catheter care can help reduce mechanical problems and the incidence of infection. Routine maintenance of urinary catheters to reduce the risk of complications includes proper hygiene of the pericatheter region, maintenance of unobstructed urine flow, frequent and proper emptying of the closed catheter drainage system, and proper specimen collection.

Suggested Readings

Daneshgari F, Krugman M, Bahn A, Lee RS. Evidence-based multidisciplinary practice: improving the safety and standards of male bladder catheterization. *Medsurg Nurs.* 2002;11(5):236–241. 246.

Hadfield-Law L. Male catheterization. *Accid Emerg Nurs.* 2001;9(4):257–263.

Hart S. Urinary catheterization. *Nurs Stand.* 2008;22(27):44–48.

Hollingsworth JM, Rogers MA, Krein SL, et al. Determining the noninfectious complications of indwelling urethral catheters: a systematic review and meta-analysis. *Ann Intern Med.* 2013;159:401–410.

Igawa Y, Wyndaele JJ, Nishizawa O. Catheterization: possible complications and their prevention and treatment. *Int J Urol.* 2008;15:481–485.

Newman DK. The indwelling urinary catheter: principles for best practice. *J Wound Ostomy Continence Nurs.* 2007;34(6):655–661.

Ortega R, Ng L, Sekhar P, Song M. Videos in clinical medicine. Female urethral catheterization. *N Engl J Med.* 2008;358(14):e15.

Selius BA, Subedi R. Urinary retention in adults: diagnosis and initial management. *Am Fam Physician.* 2008;77(5):643–650.

REVIEW QUESTIONS

1. While performing a voiding cystourethrogram on a 45-year-old man, the urologist inserted the catheter too forcefully and accidentally damaged the wall of the membranous portion of the urethra in the deep perineal compartment (urogenital diaphragm). Which of the following structures would most likely be traumatized at this location?

   A. Bulbospongiosus muscle
   B. Sphincter urethrae (compressor urethrae)
   C. Corpus cavernosus penis (crus)
   D. Ischiocavernosus muscle
   E. Opening of the bulbourethral duct

2. A 62-year-old man is admitted to the emergency department due to increasing difficulty urinating over a period of several months. Physical examination reveals prostatic hypertrophy. After several unsuccessful attempts to catheterize the penile urethra, the urologist orders drainage of the urinary bladder by the least invasive procedure, avoiding entry into the peritoneal cavity or the injury of any major vessels or organs. Which of the following spaces must be traversed by the needle to reach the bladder?

   A. Ischioanal fossa
   B. Perineal body
   C. Retropubic space (of Retzius)
   D. Superficial perineal cleft
   E. Deep perineal pouch

3. A 45-year-old man is admitted to the emergency department after a violent car crash. Physical examination reveals that the patient suffered a "straddle" injury to the perineum. An MRI examination reveals extravasation of urine and blood from a torn bulbar urethra into the superficial perineal cleft. Which of the following fasciae provide boundaries for this space?

   A. Camper's fascia and Scarpa's fascia
   B. Perineal membrane and external perineal fascia of Gallaudet
   C. Colles' fascia and external perineal fascia of Gallaudet
   D. Perineal membrane and superior fascia of urogenital diaphragm
   E. Urogenital diaphragm and apex of prostate gland

4. A 15-year-old is admitted to the emergency department 2 days after crashing his bicycle. MRI examination reveals severe edema of the scrotum and abdominal wall and extravasated urine. Which of the following structures is most likely ruptured?

   A. Spongy urethra
   B. Preprostatic urethra
   C. Prostatic urethra
   D. Urinary bladder
   E. Ureter

CHAPTER 1. Endotracheal Intubation

1. **E.** The rima glottidis is the opening between the vocal folds and the arytenoid cartilages. The piriform recess is the recess lateral to the laryngeal opening of the laryngopharynx. The vestibule is the region between the epiglottis and rima glottidis. The ventricle is the area between the true and false vocal cords. The vallecula is a bilateral recess anterior to the epiglottis at the base of tongue.

2. **C.** The trachea lines up anatomically with the right main stem bronchus.

3. **A.** Auscultation should be performed over five points to ensure that the endotracheal tube is properly placed. If advanced too far, it may be in the right main stem bronchus, causing decreased or absent breath sounds on the left. Absent breath sounds could also indicate a pneumothorax due to traumatic intubation or barotrauma caused by mechanical ventilation.

CHAPTER 2. Intercostal Nerve Block

1. **C.** To avoid damaging the lungs, a chest tube should be placed below the level of the lungs in the costodiaphragmatic recess, entering through the eighth or ninth intercostal space. At the midclavicular line, the costodiaphragmatic recess is between the sixth and eighth intercostal spaces, at the midaxillary line between the eighth and tenth intercostal spaces, and at the paravertebral line between the tenth and twelfth ribs.

2. **C.** The parietal pleura is innervated by the intercostal nerves, which are somatic nerves and thus very sensitive to pain. Therefore the parietal pleura is the deepest layer that must be anesthetized to reduce pain during thoracentesis or chest tube placement.

3. **A.** One is least likely to damage important structures by making an incision or pushing a chest tube into the thorax over the upper border of the rib. The intercostal vein, artery, and nerve, in that order (VAN structures), lie at the inferior border of each rib. Entering through the middle of the intercostal space does not eliminate the risk of piercing important structures. Passing between the internal and external intercostal muscles or between the intercostal muscles and the posterior intercostal membrane does not allow entry into the pleural cavity.

4. **E.** In thoracocentesis, a needle is inserted into the pleural space to evacuate air or fluid that has become trapped. The pleural reflection lines extend posteriorly as far as T12 and indicate where the fluid accumulates. To drain all of the fluid efficiently, the needle must be placed into the costodiaphragmatic recess, the lowest point of the pleura. Inserting the needle into the eleventh intercostal space ensures that the lung is not damaged, because it does not normally extend this far inferiorly. Inserting the needle at all the other levels risks damaging the lung and will not remove all fluid from the space as effectively.

5. **A.** Pleuritic pain is caused by inflammation of the parietal pleura, which is mainly supplied by the intercostal nerves. The phrenic nerve only supplies the central part of the parietal pleura. The vagus nerve supplies visceral efferents and afferents to the lungs and visceral pleura but not to the parietal pleura. Likewise, the cardiopulmonary nerves do not carry somatic afferent fibers. The recurrent laryngeal nerve is a branch of the vagus nerve and does not innervate the lungs.

6. **D.** Flail chest is characterized by paradoxical breathing movements that are caused by multiple rib fractures. The sensory innervation to the intercostal spaces and the underlying parietal pleura is supplied by the corresponding intercostal nerves. The phrenic nerve provides motor innervation to the diaphragm and sensory innervation to the diaphragmatic and mediastinal parietal pleura and pericardium. The vagus nerves provide parasympathetic innervation to the thoracic viscera and to the gastrointestinal tract up to the left colic flexure distally. The cardiopulmonary nerves carry sympathetic innervation from the T1 to T4 levels to the thoracic organs and afferent pain fibers from these organs. Thoracic splanchnic nerves carry sympathetic innervation to the abdomen.

CHAPTER 3. Mask Ventilation

1. **E.** An infection of the submandibular space is usually the result of a dental infection in the mandibular molar area in the floor of the mouth (Ludwig angina). If the patient is not treated promptly with antibiotics, the pharyngeal and submandibular swelling can lead to asphyxiation. Quinsy, also known as peritonsillar abscess, is a pus-filled inflammation of the tonsils that can occur due to tonsillitis. Ankyloglossia, also known as tongue-tied, is a congenital defect that results in a shortened lingual frenulum, which can affect speech. Torus palatinus is a benign bony growth on the hard palate; a torus mandibularis is a similar growth on the inside of the mandible. Such growths are usually benign and do not typically cause pain. A ranula is a mucocele found on the floor of the mouth, often resulting from dehydration in older individuals, which leads to the inspissation of salivary secretions. It can be caused by local trauma, but a ranula is usually asymptomatic.

2. **B.** The posterior cricoarytenoid muscle is the only abductor of the larynx that opens the rima glottidis and rotates the arytenoid cartilages laterally. All of the other listed muscles are adductors and thus do not open the airway.

CHAPTER 4. Thoracostomy

1. **C.** To avoid damaging the lungs, a chest tube should be placed below the level of the lungs in the costodiaphragmatic recess, entering through the eighth or ninth intercostal space. At the midclavicular line, the costodiaphragmatic recess is between the sixth and eighth intercostal spaces, at the midaxillary line between the eighth and tenth intercostal spaces, and at the paravertebral line between the tenth and twelfth ribs.

2. **C.** The parietal pleura is innervated by the intercostal nerves, which are somatic nerves and thus very sensitive to pain. Therefore the parietal pleura is the deepest layer that must be anesthetized to reduce pain during thoracentesis or chest tube placement.

3. **D.** The order traversed is skin, external intercostal muscles, internal intercostal muscles, innermost intercostal muscle, and parietal pleura. The tube should not traverse the visceral pleura.

CHAPTER 5. Thoracentesis

1. **E.** A tension pneumothorax is caused by injury to the lung that results in air accumulation within the pleural cavity. The site of the wound acts as a one-way valve, allowing air to enter the pleural cavity but not to leave it. The lack of negative pressure in the pleural cavity causes the lung to collapse. Flail chest, emphysema, and hemothorax will not necessarily lead to air in the pleural cavity. The tension pneumothorax occurred during a violent fall. Therefore this is not likely to be a spontaneous pneumothorax, which is a result of nontraumatic rupture of the pleura.

2. **A.** One is least likely to damage important structures by making an incision or pushing a chest tube into the thorax over the upper border of the rib. The intercostal vein, artery, and nerve, in that order (VAN structures), lie at the inferior border of each rib. Entering through the middle of the intercostal space does not eliminate the risk of piercing important structures. Passing between the internal and external intercostal muscles or between the intercostal muscles and the posterior intercostal membrane does not allow entry into the pleural cavity.

CHAPTER 6. Tracheostomy, Tracheotomy, Cricothyroidotomy

1. **C.** The most likely structures one would encounter while performing a midline incision below the isthmus of the thyroid gland are the inferior thyroid vein and the thyroidea ima artery. The inferior thyroid vein drains into the left brachiocephalic vein, which crosses superficially just inferior to the isthmus. The thyroidea ima artery is an anatomical variant that may arise from the aortic arch, vertebral artery, or other regional arteries. The middle thyroid veins drain the thyroid gland to the internal jugular vein and lie superior to the incision site. The inferior thyroid arteries branch from either subclavian artery and meet the thyroid gland at an oblique angle. They would not be ligated with a midline incision. The brachiocephalic veins are inferior to the incision site.

2. **C.** An incision at the level of the third and fourth tracheal cartilages usually has the fewest complications during a tracheotomy. The isthmus of the thyroid gland (a richly vascular structure) is usually at the level of the second tracheal cartilage, and this incision is just inferior to that. However, other vascular structures such as a thyroidea ima artery or tributaries of the external jugular veins are at risk during a tracheotomy, requiring care in performing the procedure.

3. **C.** The cricothyroid artery is a small branch of the superior thyroid artery. It anastomoses with the cricothyroid artery of the opposite side at the upper end of the median cricothyroid ligament, a common site for establishing an emergency airway. The cricothyroid artery can be pushed into the airway during a cricothyroidotomy and may cause hemorrhaging. If it bleeds directly into the trachea, it may be unnoticed by medical personnel, putting the patient at risk for the fatal aspiration of blood.

4. **B.** Cricothyroidotomy is an emergency procedure used to provide an airway in cases of laryngeal obstruction. It is performed by making an incision in the cricothyroid membrane, which is located between the thyroid and cricoid cartilages.

CHAPTER 7. Cardiac Pacing

1. **B.** The sinu-atrial (SA) node functions as the primary intrinsic pacemaker of the heart, setting the cardiac rhythm. An artificial pacemaker assists in producing a regular rhythm when the SA node is not functioning normally. The atrioventricular (AV) node receives depolarization signals from the SA node. The signal is delayed within the AV node, providing time for the atria to contract, and is then propagated through the bundle of His and Purkinje fibers.

2. **C.** Artificial pacemakers are commonly used to treat patients with weak or failing cardiac conduction systems. The electrode at the tip of the pacemaker is threaded through the subclavian vein to the superior vena cava into the right atrium and then to the right ventricle, where it stimulates Purkinje fibers to cause ventricular contraction. The right and left atria do not contain Purkinje fibers and would therefore not be useful in artificially pacing the heart. The left ventricle is more difficult to access. The superior vena cava is not related to cardiac pacing.

3. **B.** As the electrode approaches the ventricles, the QRS complex gains in amplitude. At the level of the tricuspid valve, the P wave is positive. As the sensing electrode passes into the right ventricle, the P wave begins to diminish in size and the QRS complex increases.

CHAPTER 8. Cardioversion and Defibrillation

1. **A.** The indications for emergency synchronized electrical cardioversion include hemodynamic instability owing to supraventricular tachycardia, atrial flutter, atrial fibrillation, or monomorphic ventricular tachycardia. When the rhythm is too rapid, QRS complexes may not be detected by the defibrillator and a shock will not be delivered. These rhythms require high-energy unsynchronized shocks. Cardioversion and defibrillation are contraindicated in dysrhythmias that are already in a homogenous depolarization state because of enhanced automaticity, as in digitalis toxicity or catecholamine-induced arrhythmia. In these situations, providing external energy will be ineffective and can potentially lead to ventricular tachycardia or fibrillation.

2. **D.** The indications for emergency synchronized electrical cardioversion include hemodynamic instability owing to supraventricular tachycardia, atrial flutter, atrial fibrillation, or monomorphic ventricular tachycardia with a pulse.

3. **B.** The indications for emergency synchronized electrical cardioversion include hemodynamic instability owing to supraventricular tachycardia, atrial flutter, atrial fibrillation, or monomorphic ventricular tachycardia with a pulse. Synchronized cardioversion requires conscious sedation.

4. **A.** Atrial flutter can be stable or unstable. It usually presents with atrial rates between 240 and 350 beats/min. These rapid atrial rates, similar to atrial fibrillation, are caused by electrical activity that moves in a self-perpetuating loop within the atrium. The impact of atrial flutter depends upon the ventricular rate and hence the patient's cardiac output. Since not all atrial impulses will be conducted to the ventricles, the faster the atrial rate, the less effective the conduction and the more negative the effect on cardiac output, causing unstable atrial flutter. The patient may present with palpitations, chest pain or discomfort, shortness of breath, lightheadedness or dizziness, nausea, vomiting, hypotension, a feeling of impending doom, or symptoms of heart failure. Unstable atrial flutter should be treated with synchronized cardioversion rather than medication since it may degenerate into atrial fibrillation or a terminal rhythm. It can be associated with

thrombus formation, heart failure, and further cardiovascular instability and collapse. Decompensation can be prevented by early cardioversion. Stable atrial flutter is more sensitive to direct-current cardioversion than atrial fibrillation and usually requires a lower-energy shock. Usually, 20 to 50 J is enough to convert atrial flutter to sinus rhythm. Unstable atrial flutter requires a higher initial shock of 50 to 100 J.

CHAPTER 9. Diagnostic Peritoneal Lavage

1. **E.** The linea alba is formed by the intersection of the aponeuroses of the abdominal muscles between the right and left rectus abdominis muscles. It is located at the midline of the body. The midaxillary line is oriented vertically, running in a straight line down from the axilla. The arcuate line (of Douglas) is a curved horizontal line that represents the lower edge of the posterior tendinous portion of the rectus abdominis sheath. An incision at this line will not separate the rectus abdominis sheaths. The semilunar line is an imaginary vertical line below the nipples that usually parallels the lateral edge of the rectus sheath. The tendinous intersections of the rectus abdominis muscles divide the muscle into sections and are usually not well defined. An incision along these intersections would not divide the two rectus sheaths.

2. **D.** The extraperitoneal fascia is the deepest layer, adjacent to the parietal peritoneum of the anterior abdominal wall. The transversalis fascia is located deep to the abdominal musculature and associated aponeuroses. The anterior wall of the rectus sheath is the layer just deep to Scarpa's fascia and superficial to the rectus abdominis muscle anteriorly.

3. **A.** The patient is unstable and should have an E-FAST, if available. E-FAST exams can be performed at bedside while initial resuscitation is simultaneously being conducted. It can also be repeated at a moment's notice. The clinical scenario coupled with finding fluid in the peritoneum can lead to life-saving treatment. E-FAST exams can aid in the diagnosis of intraperitoneal bleeding from blunt trauma or an ectopic pregnancy, as well as pericardial effusion or tamponade and pneumothorax. They are not sensitive for solid-organ injury or a retroperitoneal bleed. Diagnostic peritoneal lavage is invasive, has a high risk of complications, takes longer to perform, and cannot be repeated. Unstable patients should not be moved to the CT suite. Even when a patient requires emergency surgery, E-FAST can demonstrate the need to place a chest tube or perform pericardiocentesis prior to moving the patient, in addition to giving the surgeon guidance as to possible intraabdominal bleeding.

4. **B.** An international normalized ratio of 4 indicates coagulopathy, which is a contraindication to performing diagnostic peritoneal lavage as it could cause more bleeding and further cardiovascular instability.

CHAPTER 10. Extended Focused Assessment With Sonography for Trauma

1. **A.** Examination of the pericardium and heart is performed with a subcostal or subxiphoid view. In the suprasternal approach, the transducer is placed in the suprasternal notch with the long axis of the transducer oriented parallel to the trachea; this allows visualization of the ascending aorta and its branches. With the parasternal approach, the transducer is placed near the sternum in the left third or fourth intercostal space, showing the right ventricular outflow tract and interventricular septum.

2. **B.** In a supine patient, fluid often accumulates in the pouch of Morison, the most dependent space in the abdomen. The hepatorenal space is located behind the liver and in front of the parietal peritoneum covering the right kidney. The vesicouterine and rectouterine spaces are also potential areas of fluid accumulation; however, this occurs when the patient is erect rather than supine.

3. **D.** The spleen is a large lymphatic organ that rests against the diaphragm and the ninth to eleventh ribs in the left hypochondriac area. Splenic laceration is often associated with severe blood loss and shock. Nearly all of the liver is located in the right hypochondrium and epigastrium, although some protrudes into the left hypochondrium below the diaphragm. The left kidney lies retroperitoneally at approximately the level of the T11 to L3 vertebrae. The ilium is the upper portion of the hip bone and contributes to the bony pelvis. The ileum is the distal portion of the small intestine.

4. **A.** The spleen lies under the left lobe of the liver superior to the kidneys and adjacent to the ninth to eleventh ribs. The pain that the patient experienced with respiratory motion was likely due to the rib fracture. The lungs are located completely within the thoracic cavity, above the level of the twelfth rib. The kidney lies at the twelfth rib. The liver is located on the right, around the level of the fifth to tenth ribs. The pancreas is predominantly located in the middle of the body, medial to the kidneys at the level of the eleventh to twelfth ribs.

5. **A.** Absence of pleural sliding implies the presence of a pneumothorax. The lung pulse is a vertical movement of the pleural line synchronous with the cardiac rhythm. A lines are horizontal echogenic lines located between the rib shadows. B lines arise at the border between aerated and compressed lung. E lines are vertical lines extending from the areas of subcutaneous emphysema deep into the chest.

CHAPTER 11. Fasciotomy

1. **B.** The common fibular (peroneal) nerve winds around the neck of the fibula before dividing into superficial and deep branches that innervate the lateral and anterior compartments of the leg, respectively. These compartments are responsible for dorsiflexion and eversion of the foot, and injury to these nerves results in deficits in these movements. The tibial nerve lies superficially in the popliteal fossa. This nerve innervates the posterior compartment of the leg, so compression in this area results in the loss of plantar flexion and weakness of inversion. The lateral compartment of the leg is innervated by the superficial fibular (peroneal) nerve and is mainly involved in eversion of the foot. The cutaneous branches of the superficial fibular (peroneal) nerve emerge through the deep fascia in the anterolateral aspect of the leg and supply the dorsum of the foot. The anterior compartment of the leg is innervated by the deep fibular (peroneal) nerve and is mainly involved in dorsiflexion of the foot. The medial malleolus is an inferiorly directed projection from the medial side of the distal end of the tibia. The tibial nerve runs near the groove behind the medial malleolus, and compression at this location results in the loss of flexion, adduction, abduction of the second to fifth toes, and abduction of the great toe.

2. **C.** Compartment syndrome is characterized by increased pressure within a confined fascial compartment, which impairs the blood supply, resulting in pallor. Venous thrombosis does not characteristically cause pain but may cause fatal pulmonary embolism. Thoracic outlet syndrome affects nerves in the brachial plexus, the

subclavian artery, and blood vessels between the neck and axilla, far above the cast. Raynaud disease affects blood flow to the digits when they are exposed to temperature changes or stress. The fracture at the radial groove probably resulted in a radial nerve injury, but it would not be responsible for these symptoms.

CHAPTER 12. Nosebleed Management

1. **D.** Kiesselbach's (also called Little's) plexus is an anastomosis of four arteries, the anterior ethmoidal, sphenopalatine, superior labial, and greater palatine arteries, at the anterior nasal septum. The two largest contributors, however, are the septal branches of the sphenopalatine (from the maxillary artery) and superior labial arteries (branches of the facial artery, which in turn is a branch of the external carotid artery).

2. **A.** The most common cause of epistaxis is digital manipulation. This is compounded in the winter months by hot, dry home environments. Hypertension is not a cause of epistaxis. Although hemophilia and immune thrombocytopenic purpura may worsen bleeding, it is still likely that digital manipulation initiates the epistaxis. Bleeding most often arises from Kiesselbach's plexus, or Little's area, an anastomotic network of vessels located at the anterior cartilaginous septum. It receives its blood supply from both the internal and external carotid arteries. Many of the arteries supplying the septum have anastomotic connections at this site.

CHAPTER 13. Pericardiocentesis

1. **A.** With the subxiphoid approach, the needle passes up through the diaphragm to the fibrous pericardium. Most of the diaphragmatic surface of the heart comprises the right ventricle, the chamber that would therefore be entered if a needle is inserted too far. The other chambers of the heart would not lie in the direct path of the needle unless there was severe pathology such as cardiomegaly.

2. **E.** Cardiac tamponade is a condition in which fluid accumulates in the pericardial cavity. It can result from pericardial effusion or from the leakage of blood from the heart or proximal portions of the great vessels. The increased pressure within the pericardial sac leads to decreased cardiac filling during diastole and therefore reduced systolic blood pressure. Because of the reduced pumping capacity of the heart, there is increased pressure in the venous system, leading to distention of the jugular veins. Pericardiocentesis is the correct answer, as none of the other options listed resolve the cause of the cardiac compromise.

3. **B.** During pericardiocentesis, the needle is inserted below the xiphoid process or in the left fifth intercostal space, in the midclavicular line. The most effective way of draining the pericardium is by penetrating the thoracic wall at its lowest point anatomically; thus the third intercostal space would be too superior in position. The sixth and seventh intercostal spaces are locations that are not used clinically because of the increased likelihood of injury to the pleura or lungs and other complications.

4. **A.** The most common complication of pericardiocentesis is a dry tap, which may occur if the needle is blocked by clotted blood or a skin plug. With a parasternal approach, probing of the anterior costal cartilage can block the needle. Dry taps are resolved by repositioning or irrigating the needle. In some cases, the pericardial effusion may be located posterolaterally, and it would be difficult to tap the fluid through a subxiphoid or parasternal approach. An apical approach could help avoid a dry tap when the fluid is located posteriorly or laterally.

5. **C.** The patient is suffering from cardiac tamponade, which involves filling of the pericardial cavity with fluid that restricts cardiac function. The classic signs of tamponade, referred to as "Beck's triad," include (1) a small, quiet heart, because of compression from the fluid-filled pericardial sac and muffling of the heart sounds; (2) decreased pulse pressure resulting from a reduced difference between systolic and diastolic pressure, because the tamponade restricts the ability of the heart to fill in diastole; and (3) increased central venous pressure, because venous blood cannot enter the compressed heart. None of the other answers provided fit the definition.

CHAPTER 14. Central Venous Catheterization

1. **D.** The subclavian vein traverses between the clavicle and first rib and is the most superficial structure to be damaged after a fracture of the clavicle. The subclavian artery runs posterior to the subclavian vein, and although in the appropriate location, it would probably not be damaged because of its deep anatomical position. The cephalic vein is a tributary of the axillary vein after ascending on the lateral side of the arm, superficial and lateral to the site of injury. The lateral thoracic artery is a branch of the axillary artery and runs lateral to the pectoralis minor. It travels inferiorly and medially from its point of origin and is not near the clavicle during its descent. The internal thoracic artery arises from the first part of the subclavian artery before descending deep to the costal cartilages. Its point of origin from the subclavian artery is lateral to the clavicular injury, whereas its course behind the costal cartilages is medial to the clavicular fracture.

2. **A.** With the supraclavicular approach, contralateral rotation of the head and neck away from the site provides open access to allow the introducer needle to be placed along the lateral border of the clavicular head of the sternocleidomastoid muscle. The needle should be inserted superiorly and behind the clavicle, just lateral to the clavicular head of the sternocleidomastoid muscle.

3. **A.** The femoral vein may be accessed by introducing the needle at a 45-degree angle in a cephalic direction toward the umbilicus, approximately 1 cm medial to the femoral artery pulse. Ideally, the femoral artery pulse should be palpated 2 cm beneath the inguinal ligament. Pressure from palpation may compress the femoral vein and impede cannulation, so the pressure should be released but the fingers left on the skin to serve as a visual reference to the underlying anatomy.

CHAPTER 15. Peripheral Arterial Line Placement

1. **B.** The radial pulse is best located on the forearm, just proximal to the wrist joint. At this point, the radial artery travels on the distal radius, between the flexor carpi radialis and brachioradialis tendons. The palmaris longus tendon travels more medially to the radial artery and above the flexor retinaculum. The flexor pollicis longus tendon is a deeper structure in the forearm and is also located medial to the radial artery.

2. **B.** The radial artery enters the palm through the anatomic snuffbox. The artery then pierces the two heads of the first dorsal interosseous muscle and enters the deep aspect of the palm. The flexor pollicis longus tendon runs on the palmar aspect of the hand and the radial artery on the dorsal aspect before entering the deep aspect of the palm, and therefore the radial artery does not run below this tendon. The radial artery does not run between the first and second interosseous muscles, which therefore cannot be used as landmarks for identifying the artery. Finally, the

artery does not run between the first dorsal interosseous and the adductor pollicis longus muscles.

3. **D.** The radial pulse is palpated lateral to the tendon of the flexor carpi radialis, where the artery can be compressed against the distal radius. The radial pulse can also be felt in the anatomic snuffbox, between the tendons of the extensor pollicis brevis and extensor pollicis longus muscles, where it can be compressed against the scaphoid.

CHAPTER 16. Peripheral Intravenous Cannulation

1. **A.** The three chief structures in the cubital fossa, from lateral to medial, are the biceps brachii tendon, brachial artery, and median nerve. The common and anterior interosseous arteries arise distal to the cubital fossa. The ulnar and radial arteries derive from the bifurcation of the brachial artery distal to the cubital fossa.

2. **A.** The basilic vein can be used for dialysis, especially when the cephalic vein is judged too small, as in this case. The basilic vein can be elevated from its position as it passes through the fascia on the medial side of the arm. The cephalic vein passes more laterally up the arm. The lateral cubital vein is a tributary of the cephalic vein, and the medial cubital vein joins the basilic vein, both of which are rather superficial in position. The medial antebrachial vein courses up the midline of the forearm ventrally.

3. **A.** The femoral vein lies medial to the femoral artery in the femoral sheath, which has lateral, intermediate, and medial compartments. The lateral compartment contains the femoral nerve. The medial compartment encloses the femoral canal and consists of lymphatic tissue and a lymph node, plus areolar tissue. The intermediate compartment contains the femoral vein.

CHAPTER 17. Venous Cutdown

1. **D.** The great saphenous vein is commonly used in venous cutdown procedures. Because branches of the saphenous nerve cross the vein in the distal part of the leg, the nerve can easily be injured, causing postoperative discomfort. The saphenous nerve is responsible for cutaneous innervation on the medial surface of the leg and the medial side of the foot. Injury to this nerve will result in a loss of sensation and can create chronic dysesthesias in the area. The common fibular (peroneal) nerve bifurcates at the neck of the fibula into the superficial and deep fibular (peroneal) nerves, which innervate the lateral and anterior compartments of the leg, respectively. These nerves are lateral and therefore not associated with the great saphenous vein. The lateral sural nerve is a cutaneous nerve arising from the junction of branches from the common fibular (peroneal) and tibial nerves. It innervates the skin on the posterior aspect of the leg and lateral side of the foot.

2. **A.** The basilic vein can be used for dialysis or venous cutdown, especially when the cephalic vein is judged to be too small, as in this case. The basilic vein can be elevated from its position as it passes through the fascia on the medial side of the arm. The cephalic vein passes more laterally up the arm. The lateral cubital vein is a tributary of the cephalic vein, and the medial cubital vein joins the basilic vein, both of which are rather superficial in position. The medial antebrachial vein courses up the midline of the forearm ventrally.

3. **C.** The median cubital vein is a superficial vein that lies on the biceps brachii aponeurosis. The biceps brachii aponeurosis is a flat sheet of connective tissue that fans from the medial side of the biceps brachii tendon to blend with the deep fascia of the biceps brachii muscle. It reinforces the cubital fossa and protects the brachial artery, which runs beneath it.

CHAPTER 18. Dislocated Hip Reduction

1. **C.** The iliofemoral ligament is the most important ligament reinforcing the joint anteriorly, resisting both hyperextension and lateral rotation at the hip joint. The pubofemoral ligament reinforces the joint inferiorly and limits extension and abduction. The ischiofemoral ligament reinforces the joint posteriorly and limits extension and medial rotation. Negative pressure in the acetabular fossa has nothing to do with resisting hyperextension of the hip joint but does help resist dislocation of the head of the femur. The gluteus maximus muscle extends and laterally rotates the thigh; it does not particularly resist hyperextension.

2. **C.** An intracapsular femoral neck fracture causes avascular necrosis of the femoral head because the fracture damages the radicular branches of the medial and lateral circumflex arteries that pass beneath the ischiofemoral ligament and pierce the femoral neck. Until an individual reaches about 6 to 10 years of age, the blood supply to the head of the femur is provided by a branch of the obturator artery that runs with the ligament of the head of the femur. Thereafter, the artery of the ligament of the femoral head is insignificant. Intertrochanteric fracture of the femur would not damage the blood supply to the head of the femur but would cause complications because the greater trochanter is an attachment site for several gluteal muscles. Thrombosis of the obturator artery could result in muscular symptoms, although there are several collateral sources of blood supply in the thigh. Comminuted fracture of the extracapsular femoral neck would not ordinarily imperil the vascular supply.

3. **D.** The ligament of the femoral head conveys a small blood vessel to supply the head of the femur primarily in childhood. The ligament is stretched during abduction and lateral rotation of the hip joint and has an important role in stabilizing an infant's hip joint before walking. It has the potential to increase stability of the joint in hip reconstruction performed in children to address developmental hip dysplasia. The strength of this ligament is comparable to the anterior cruciate ligament of the knee. The iliofemoral ligament (the Y ligament of Bigelow) on the anterior aspect of the hip bone resists hyperextension of the hip joint. The pubofemoral ligament arises from the pubic bone and is located on the inferior side of the hip joint; it resists abduction of the joint. The ischiofemoral ligament is a triangular band of strong fibers that arises from the ischium and winds upward and laterally over the femoral neck, strengthening the capsule posteriorly. The transverse acetabular ligament attaches to the margins of the acetabular notch, and the ligament of the head of the femur arises from it. Although the transverse acetabular ligament is fibrous rather than cartilaginous, it is regarded as part of the acetabular labrum.

4. **B.** A femoral neck fracture is a contraindication to closed reduction. Manipulating the extremity can cause further injury to the bones, blood vessels, and nerves. This injury requires open reduction and internal fixation.

CHAPTER 19. Dislocated Finger Reduction

1. **E.** The extensor tendons of the fingers insert distally on the distal phalanx of each digit. If the tendon is avulsed or the proximal part of the distal phalanx is detached, the distal interphalangeal joint is pulled into total flexion by the unopposed flexor digitorum profundus. This result gives the digit the appearance of a mallet. In a boutonnière deformity, the central portion of the extensor tendon expansion is torn over the proximal interphalangeal (PIP) joint, allowing the tendon to move toward the palm, causing the tendon to act as a flexor of the PIP joint. This causes the distal interphalangeal

(DIP) joint to be hyperextended. Swan-neck deformity involves the slight flexion of metacarpophalangeal (MCP) joints, hyperextension of PIP joints, and slight flexion of DIP joints. This condition most often results from shortening of the tendons of the intrinsic muscles, as in rheumatoid arthritis. Dupuytren contracture results from a connective tissue disorder in the palm, usually causing irreversible flexion of digits 4 and 5. Claw hand occurs with lesions to the median and ulnar nerves at the wrist. All intrinsic muscles are paralyzed, including the extensors of the interphalangeal joints. The MCP joint extensors, supplied by the radial nerve, and the long flexors of the fingers, supplied more proximally in the forearm by the median and ulnar nerves, are intact and are unopposed, pulling the fingers into the "claw" appearance.

2. **A.** This proximal injury to the median nerve would paralyze all of the long flexors of the digits, except for the distal interphalangeal flexors of digits 4 and 5, thereby swinging the "balance of power" to the muscles that extend the digits, all of which are innervated by the radial nerve. The intrinsic hand muscles can aid in flexion of the metacarpophalangeal joints, and they are innervated by the ulnar nerve. However, they are too small to compensate for the extensor forces exerted on the fingers.

CHAPTER 20. Dislocated Knee Reduction

1. **B.** This type of injury can result in the "unhappy triad" (of O'Donoghue), with damage to the medial collateral ligament (MCL), anterior cruciate ligament (ACL), and medial meniscus. A blow to the lateral side of the knee stretches and tears the MCL, which is attached to the medial meniscus. The ACL is tensed during knee extension and can therefore tear after the MCL is ruptured. The remaining choices describe structures on the lateral surface of the knee, which are not usually injured by this type of trauma.

2. **C.** When the popliteus contracts, it rotates the distal portion of the femur in a lateral direction. It also draws the lateral meniscus posteriorly, thereby protecting this cartilage as the femoral condyle glides and rolls backward during flexing of the knee. This action of the popliteus allows the knee to flex and therefore unlock. The biceps femoris is a strong flexor of the leg and laterally rotates the knee when it is in a position of flexion. The gastrocnemius is a powerful plantar flexor of the foot. The semimembranous, similar to the biceps femoris, is a component of the hamstring muscles and is involved in extending the thigh and flexing the leg at the knee joint. The rectus femoris is the strongest quadriceps femoris muscle involved in extending the leg at the knee.

3. **A.** The "unhappy triad" (of O'Donoghue) refers to injury of the medial collateral ligament, medial meniscus, and anterior cruciate ligament. Sudden, forceful thrusts against the lateral side of the knee put tension on the medial collateral ligament, which can then rupture. The medial meniscus is attached to the medial collateral ligament such that it then tears. The anterior cruciate ligament resists hyperextension of the knee and is thus the third structure that breaks in the unhappy triad.

4. **D.** A bucket-handle tear is often associated with rupture of the anterior cruciate ligament. Both the medial and lateral menisci are subject to rotational injuries and may be torn. The medial meniscus is much more liable to injury because it is attached to the fused deep layer of the medial collateral ligament and joint capsule. The lateral meniscus is separated from the fibular collateral ligament and is external to the capsule of the knee joint. Commonly seen in football players' knees, meniscal tears are usually diagnosed by magnetic resonance imaging or arthrosco-

py. The presenting symptoms of tearing may be pain and swelling or locking of the knee, suggesting a bucket-handle tear in which a partly detached cartilage wedges between the tibia and femur, inhibiting further movement. Sometimes a momentary click can be heard during flexion and extension movements of the knee. Although meniscectomy can successfully resolve the symptoms of a torn meniscus, there is currently greater emphasis on repairing small tears. Meniscal cysts can form secondary to meniscal tears, some of which can also be treated arthroscopically.

5. **A.** A lateral blow to the knee often produces an injury referred to as the "unhappy triad," involving damage to the anterior cruciate ligament, medial meniscus, and medial collateral ligament. The medial meniscus and medial collateral ligament are often damaged together as they are tightly attached to each other. The lateral collateral ligament and lateral meniscus would not be damaged because a blow to the lateral knee would not put strain on these structures. Damage to the posterior cruciate ligament would produce a positive posterior "drawer sign," and it is typically damaged during a blow to the medial side of the knee. The posterior cruciate ligament is stronger than the anterior one and is only typically damaged when a person falls on the tibial tuberosity of a flexed knee. The semitendinosus tendon is located on the medial side of the knee but is not attached closely to the other structures, and it is not taut in this type of injury.

CHAPTER 21. Dislocated Shoulder Joint Reduction

1. **D.** The supraspinatus is one of the rotator cuff muscles. Its tendon is relatively avascular and is often injured when the shoulder is dislocated. This muscle initiates abduction of the arm, and damage to it impairs this movement. The coracobrachialis muscle, which runs from the coracoid process to the humerus, functions in adduction and flexion of the arm. The main function of the triceps brachii is to extend the elbow, and damage to its long head would not affect abduction. The pectoralis minor functions as an accessory respiratory muscle and serves to stabilize the scapula. It is not involved in abduction. The teres major adducts and medially rotates the arm.

2. **E.** The coracoacromial ligament contributes to the coracoacromial arch, preventing superior displacement of the head of the humerus. Because this ligament is very strong, it is rarely damaged. Instead, it can cause inflammation or erosion of the tendon of the supraspinatus muscle as the tendon passes back and forth under the ligament. The acromioclavicular ligament, connecting the acromion with the lateral end of the clavicle, is not in contact with the supraspinatus tendon. The coracohumeral ligament is located too far anteriorly to impinge upon the supraspinatus tendon. The glenohumeral ligament is located deep to the rotator cuff muscles and would not contribute to injury of the supraspinatus muscle. The transverse scapular ligament crosses the scapular notch and is not in contact with the supraspinatus tendon.

3. **B.** In shoulder separation, the acromioclavicular or coracoclavicular ligaments or both can be partially or completely torn through. If the acromioclavicular joint is interrupted, the distal end of the clavicle may deviate upward in a complete separation while the arm droops away inferiorly, causing a palpable "step off" that can sometimes be seen. Displacement of the head of the humerus is shoulder dislocation, not separation. The coracoacromial ligament is not torn in shoulder separation, although it is sometimes used in the repair of the torn coracoclavicular ligament. Disruption of the glenoid labrum often accompanies shoulder dislocation.

4. **D.** The acromioclavicular ligament connects the clavicle to the coracoid process of the scapula. Separation of the shoulder, that is, dislocation of the acromioclavicular joint, is associated with damage to the acromioclavicular ligament (the capsule of the joint) and, in more severe injuries, disruption of the coracoclavicular ligaments (conoid and trapezoid portions). The glenohumeral ligament may be injured by an anterior dislocation of the humerus but is not likely to be injured with a separated shoulder. The coracoacromial ligament, transverse scapular ligament, and tendon of the long head of the triceps brachii are not likely to be injured with separation of the shoulder.

5. **A.** The axillary nerve is a direct branch of the posterior cord of the brachial plexus and wraps around the surgical neck of the humerus to innervate the teres minor and deltoid muscles. With this anatomical arrangement, the axillary nerve is tightly tethered to the proximal humerus. When the head of the humerus is dislocated, it often puts traction on the axillary nerve.

CHAPTER 22. Occipital Nerve Block

1. **C.** The trapezius is innervated by the accessory nerve (cranial nerve XI). The obliquus capitis muscle is innervated by the suboccipital nerve, which also supplies the rectus capitis posterior major and minor. The greater occipital nerve supplies the semispinalis capitis.

2. **A.** The third occipital nerve is the medial branch of the dorsal ramus of C3. It pierces the trapezius muscle medially in the neck below the external occipital protuberance and supplies the skin of the nuchal region. The greater and lesser occipital nerves lie lateral to the midline and are less likely to be affected in this patient. The suboccipital nerve lies within and supplies the muscles of the suboccipital triangle. The accessory nerve supplies the trapezius and sternocleidomastoid muscles and has no cutaneous supply.

CHAPTER 23. Digital Nerve Block

1. **C.** The common palmar digital branch comes off the superficial branch of the ulnar nerve and supplies the skin of the little finger and medial side of the ring finger. The superficial branch of the radial nerve provides cutaneous innervation to the radial (lateral) dorsum of the hand and thumb, index finger, and lateral middle finger over the proximal phalanx. The common palmar digital branch of the median nerve innervates most of the lateral aspect of the palmar hand and the dorsal aspect of the second and third fingers as well as the lateral part of the fourth digit. The deep radial nerve supplies the extensor carpi radialis brevis and supinator muscles and continues as the posterior interosseous nerve. The recurrent branch of the median nerve supplies the abductor pollicis brevis, flexor pollicis brevis, and opponens pollicis muscles.

2. **C.** The recurrent branch of the median nerve innervates the thenar muscles (opponens pollicis, abductor pollicis brevis, and flexor pollicis brevis) and is not responsible for any cutaneous innervation. Damage to the palmar cutaneous branches of the median nerve or the ulnar nerve would not cause weakness of opposition of the thumb because they are principally sensory in function. The deep branch of the ulnar nerve supplies the hypothenar muscles and the adductor and abductor muscles of digits 2 to 5, but it does not innervate the abductor pollicis brevis.

3. **B.** The deep fibular nerve is a branch of the common fibular nerve. It is primarily a motor nerve that innervates the anterior compartment of the leg. Its only cutaneous innervation is to the skin of the first web space. The saphenous nerve innervates the medial side of the leg and foot. The cutaneous branch of the superficial fibular nerve innervates the anterior part of the lower leg and dorsum of the foot. The sural nerve innervates the lateral side of the leg and foot.

CHAPTER 24. Dental Nerve Blocks

1. **C.** The lingual nerve was most likely damaged because there is a loss of both taste and general sensation in the anterior two-thirds of the tongue, which is innervated by the lingual nerve. The chorda tympani also carries taste from that area but does not mediate other sensations from the tongue. The auriculotemporal nerve is a posterior branch of the mandibular division of the trigeminal nerve and innervates skin near the ear and temporal region. The mental nerve is the terminal branch of the inferior alveolar nerve and innervates the skin of the chin.

2. **B.** The inferior alveolar branch of the mandibular division of the trigeminal nerve provides sensory innervation to the mandibular teeth and would require anesthesia to abolish pain. The lingual nerve provides taste and sensation innervation to the anterior two-thirds of the tongue and carries general sensory, taste, and parasympathetic fibers. It does not provide sensory innervation to the teeth. The buccal nerve provides sensory innervation to the inner surface of the cheek. The mental nerve is the distal continuation of the inferior alveolar nerve as it exits the mental foramen of the mandible, and it does not affect the teeth. The nerve to the mylohyoid is a motor branch of the inferior alveolar nerve that supplies the mylohyoid and the anterior belly of the digastric.

3. **E.** An infection of the submandibular space is usually the result of a dental infection in the mandibular molar area in the floor of the mouth (Ludwig angina). If the patient is not treated with antibiotics promptly, the pharyngeal and submandibular swelling can lead to asphyxiation. Quinsy, also known as peritonsillar abscess, is a pus-filled inflammation of the tonsils that can occur due to tonsillitis. Ankyloglossia, also known as tongue-tie, is a congenital defect that results in a shortened lingual frenulum, which can affect speech. Torus palatinus is a benign bony growth on the hard palate; a torus mandibularis is a similar growth on the inside of the mandible. Such growths are usually benign and do not typically cause pain. A ranula is a mucocele found on the floor of the mouth, often resulting from dehydration in older individuals, leading to the inspissation of salivary secretions. It can be caused by local trauma, but a ranula is usually asymptomatic.

4. **C.** A child's underlying permanent teeth can be damaged if there is an attempt to reinsert an avulsed primary tooth. There is also a risk of tooth fragment aspiration, especially in patients with altered mental status. The proper handling and prompt transportation of any avulsed teeth, except a primary tooth, are important for maintaining tooth viability.

CHAPTER 25. Abdominal Paracentesis

1. **E.** The inferior epigastric artery is a branch of the external iliac artery. It ascends deep to the rectus abdominis muscle to anastomose with the superior epigastric artery, a branch of the internal thoracic artery.

2. **A.** The inferior epigastric artery courses from a point lateral to the pubic tubercle and runs cranially beneath the rectus abdominis. This is important to remember because puncture of this artery can result in significant hemorrhage. The point for paracentesis needle insertion in the left lower quadrant is two fingerbreadths medial to and two fingerbreadths cranial to the left anterior su-

perior iliac spine. When the location or presence of ascitic fluid is in doubt, sonography can be used for clarification.

3. **A.** The potential for massive bleeding in patients with disseminated intravascular coagulation makes this a contraindication to abdominal paracentesis. Pregnancy, acute tubular necrosis, sepsis, and age are not contraindications.

CHAPTER 26. Auricular Hematoma Drainage

1. **C.** The auriculotemporal nerve, a branch of the mandibular division of the trigeminal nerve, passes posteriorly and deep to the ramus of the mandible and superior to the deep part of the parotid gland, emerging posterior to the temporomandibular joint to supply the skin anterior to the auricle and the posterior two-thirds of the temporal region. The nerve distributes to the skin of the tragus and adjacent helix of the auricle. The lesser occipital nerve, a branch of the cervical plexus, supplies the skin posterior to the auricle. The great auricular nerve, also a cervical plexus branch, supplies the skin overlying the mandible and the capsule of the parotid gland. The zygomaticotemporal nerve supplies the hairless patch of skin over the anterior part of the temporal fossa. The greater occipital nerve supplies the occipital part of the scalp.

2. **D.** A hematoma must be evacuated prior to packing or suturing.

CHAPTER 27. Cerumen Removal

1. **C.** The external surface of the tympanic membrane is primarily innervated by the auriculotemporal nerve, a branch of the mandibular division of the trigeminal nerve. Damage to this nerve would also result in painful temporomandibular joint movement, which receives innervation from the same nerve. Taste in the anterior two-thirds of the tongue is supplied by the facial nerve and would be unaffected in this injury. The sensory innervation of the nasal cavity is from the ophthalmic and maxillary divisions of the trigeminal nerve and would be unaffected by injury to the tympanic membrane. Sensory innervation to the larynx is provided by the vagus nerve, whereas the pharynx receives sensory fibers from the glossopharyngeal and vagus nerves. The palate is supplied by the maxillary division of the trigeminal nerve and would be unaffected by this injury.

2. **A.** The inner surface of the tympanic membrane is supplied by the glossopharyngeal nerve. The auricular branches of the facial and vagus nerves and the auriculotemporal branch of the trigeminal nerve innervate the external surface of the tympanic membrane. The great auricular nerve arises from C2 and C3 and supplies the posterior auricle and skin over the parotid gland. The lingual nerve does not have anything to do with the sensory supply of the tympanic membrane.

3. **B.** The vagus nerve is one of the major sensory nerves to the external auditory meatus and is the afferent limb of the cough reflex. The vestibulocochlear nerve mediates hearing and balance. Although the auriculotemporal branch of the trigeminal contributes to the innervation of the external acoustic meatus, it does not participate in the cough reflex. The facial nerve, which also contributes to the innervation of the external acoustic meatus, has no role in the cough reflex. The accessory nerve supplies motor innervation to the sternocleidomastoid and trapezius nerves.

CHAPTER 28. Ear and Nose Foreign Body Removal

1. **D.** The posterior inferior quadrant of the eardrum is the only portion of the tympanic membrane in which an incision risks minimal or no damage to important adjacent structures. Incision in the anterior and posterior superior quadrants of the eardrum would likely damage the malleus, situated immediately superior and medial to the tympanic membrane. The umbo is situated in close proximity to the handle of the malleus and might also be damaged. A vertical incision through the eardrum would almost certainly damage the malleus. Damage to the malleus from a surgical incision would interfere with auditory conduction through the middle ear cavity. This should be avoided to prevent conductive hearing loss.

2. **A.** The inner surface of the tympanic membrane is supplied by the glossopharyngeal nerve. The auricular branches of the facial and vagus nerves and the auriculotemporal branch of the trigeminal nerve innervate the external surface of the tympanic membrane. The great auricular nerve arises from C2 and C3 and supplies the posterior auricle and skin over the parotid gland. The lingual nerve has nothing to do with the sensory supply of the tympanic membrane.

3. **B.** The area of damage is in the external acoustic meatus, which is supplied by the facial, glossopharyngeal, and vagus nerves. The auriculotemporal and great auricular nerves supply the temporomandibular joint and external ear, respectively. The lesser occipital nerves supply the skin on the posterior aspect of the skull. The chorda tympani is responsible for taste from the anterior two-thirds of the tongue and sensation in the middle ear. The lesser petrosal nerve and tympanic plexus carry autonomic innervation to and through the middle ear and are not associated with the external ear canal.

CHAPTER 29. Burr Hole Craniotomy

1. **E.** The middle meningeal artery is a branch of the maxillary artery and courses between the dura mater and skull close to the area of the pterion. A fracture or blunt trauma to this location typically results in the laceration of the middle meningeal artery, resulting in an epidural hematoma. The external carotid artery ends behind the mandible by dividing into the maxillary and the superficial temporal arteries, and neither of these arteries directly supplies the meninges. The deep temporal arteries do not penetrate the bony skull and thus would not contribute to an epidural hematoma.

2. **D.** Subdural bleeding usually results from tears in veins that cross the subdural space between the dura and the arachnoid. This bleeding may cause a gradual increase in intracranial pressure and result in the leakage of venous blood over the right cerebral hemisphere, with a variable rate of progression. A subarachnoid bleed occurs due to the rupture of an artery into the subarachnoid space surrounding the brain, that is, between the arachnoid membrane and the pia mater. Hydrocephalus may result if the subarachnoid bleeding or subsequent fibrosis obstructs the flow of cerebrospinal fluid through the subarachnoid space or its reabsorption. In most cases, epidural bleeding results from tearing of the middle meningeal artery, and this rapidly expanding, space-occupying lesion can cause death within 12 hours. Intracerebral bleeding into the brain parenchyma involves focal bleeding from a blood vessel into the brain parenchyma, most often a result of hypertension or atherosclerosis. Typical symptoms include focal neurologic deficits, with an abrupt onset of headache, nausea, and impaired consciousness. Bleeding into the cerebral ventricular system may be due to trauma or the hemorrhage of blood from nearby arteries, especially those that supply the choroid plexus.

CHAPTER 30. Elbow Joint Aspiration

1. **D.** Fracture of the medial epicondyle often causes damage to the ulnar nerve, running in the groove behind the epicondyle. The ulnar nerve innervates the flexor carpi ulnaris muscle and the medial half of the flexor digitorum profundus muscle in the forearm. The nerve continues on to innervate the muscles of the hand. The flexor digitorum superficialis is innervated by the median nerve and the biceps brachii by the musculocutaneous nerve. The radial nerve innervates both the brachioradialis and supinator muscles.

2. **A.** The anular ligament is a fibrous band that encircles the head of the radius, forming a collar that fuses with the radial collateral ligament and articular capsule of the elbow. The annular ligament functions to prevent the displacement of the radial head from its socket. The joint capsule allows free rotation of the joint and does not function to stabilize it. The interosseous membrane is a fibrous layer between the radius and ulna, helping to hold these two bones together. The radial collateral ligament extends from the lateral epicondyle to the margins of the radial notch of the ulna and the annular ligament of the radius. The ulnar collateral ligament is a triangular ligament that extends from the medial epicondyle to the olecranon of the ulna.

3. **C.** The superior ulnar collateral branch of the brachial artery accompanies the ulnar nerve in its path posterior to the medial epicondyle and is important in the blood supply to the nerve. The profunda brachii artery passes down the arm with the radial nerve. The radial collateral artery arises from the profunda brachii artery and anastomoses with the recurrent branch of the radial artery proximal to the elbow laterally. The inferior ulnar collateral artery arises from the brachial artery and accompanies the median nerve into the forearm. The anterior ulnar recurrent artery arises from the ulnar artery and forms an anastomosis with the inferior ulnar collateral artery anterior to the elbow.

4. **C.** The common extensor tendon originates from the lateral epicondyle, and inflammation of this tendon is lateral epicondylitis, nicknamed "tennis elbow" because the tendon is often irritated during the backhand stroke in tennis. Because the extensors of the wrist originate as part of the common extensor tendon, extension of the wrist will exacerbate the pain of lateral epicondylitis.

5. **B.** Ginglymus is the technical term used to describe a hinge joint. It allows motion in one axis (flexion and extension in the case of the elbow) and is therefore a uniaxial joint. The other types of joints listed allow motion in more than one axis.

CHAPTER 31. Ingrown Toenail Removal

1. **E.** The deep fibular nerve supplies the skin of the first web space of the foot. The sural, superficial fibular, tibial, and saphenous nerves have a cutaneous distribution but not for the first web space.

2. **A.** The dorsalis pedis artery is accessible on the dorsum of the foot and can be palpated just lateral to the extensor hallucis longus tendon. The sural and fibular arteries do not supply the foot. The deep plantar artery is not palpable on physical examination. The anterior tibial artery becomes the dorsalis pedis artery at the ankle.

CHAPTER 32. Knee Joint Aspiration

1. **E.** The vastus lateralis muscle is located on the lateral aspect of the thigh. The distal portion of this muscle lies superficial to the proximal part of the lateral aspect of the knee joint capsule. When a needle is inserted superior and lateral to the patella, it penetrates the vastus lateralis muscle on its course to the capsule. The short head of the biceps femoris has its origin on the posterior aspect of the femur, merges with the long head of the biceps femoris, and inserts on the head of the fibula. The rectus femoris passes longitudinally on the medial aspect of the femur and inserts on the tibial tuberosity, via the patellar (or quadriceps) tendon. A needle inserted lateral to the patella would not penetrate this muscle. The sartorius originates on the anterior superior iliac spine and forms part of the pes anserine, which inserts on the medial aspect of the proximal part of the tibia. A needle inserted laterally to the patella would not penetrate this muscle.

2. **A.** Excessive compression of the prepatellar bursa, as occurs when working on bended knees, can result in pain and swelling of the prepatellar bursa, so-called "housemaid's knee." Prepatellar bursitis also affects plumbers, carpet layers, and other people who are often on their knees. The bursa normally enables the patella to move smoothly under the skin. The constant friction caused by these occupations irritates this small lubricating sac (bursa) located just in front of the patella, resulting in a tense, deformable cushion of fluid. Treatment usually involves simple drainage, but this may need to be repeated, and occasionally steroids are injected. Excessive irritation of the infrapatellar bursa when kneeling for frequent and long periods (as in prayer) can result in "parson's knee."

CHAPTER 33. Lumbar Puncture

1. **D.** A lumbar puncture is performed to obtain a sample of cerebrospinal fluid (CSF) from the lumbar cistern (the subarachnoid space below the conus medullaris) between L4 and L5 or L3 and L4. It is done in this region because the spinal cord ends at the level of L1 to L2 and the dural sac ends at the level of S2. Therefore, L4 to L5 is the safest place to perform the procedure because it minimizes the risk of injuring the spinal cord.

2. **B.** The highest points of the iliac crests are used as a landmark for locating the position of L4 to L5 for a lumbar puncture. They are identified by palpation and traced medially toward the vertebral column (Tuffier's line). The inferior angles of the scapulae lie at vertebral level T7 and the lowest ribs at T12. The sacral hiatus is located lower at the distal portion of the sacrum, and the posterior inferior iliac spines lie below S2.

3. **E.** CSF is found within the subarachnoid space, flowing to that space from the ventricles. The epidural space, positioned between the dura mater and periosteum, contains fat and the internal vertebral venous plexus (of Batson). The subdural space, between the arachnoid mater and dura mater, exists only as a potential space and does not contain CSF.

4. **A.** When a lumbar puncture is performed, the needle must penetrate the ligamentum flavum, the dura mater, and finally the arachnoid mater to reach the subarachnoid space where the CSF is located. The lumbar cistern is a continuation of the subarachnoid space below the conus medullaris. The pia mater is adherent to the spinal cord, and the posterior longitudinal ligament is attached to the posterior aspect of the vertebral bodies.

5. **C.** The subarachnoid space, containing cerebrospinal fluid (CSF), is located between the arachnoid and pia maters. The epidural, subdural, and pretracheal spaces do not contain CSF. Although the central canal, contained within the substance of the spinal cord, does contain CSF, puncture of this space would result in spinal cord injury. CSF circulates within the subarachnoid space and can be aspirated only from that location. The subdural space is only a potential space between the dura and

arachnoid mater. The epidural space contains epidural fat and Batson's venous plexus and is the site of injection for epidural anesthesia.

6. **C.** Lumbar puncture is generally performed at the level of L4 to L5. The spinal cord ends at L1 to L2 in adults, although it and can be as low as L2 to L3 in newborns.

CHAPTER 34. Nasogastric Tube Placement

1. **E.** The rima glottidis is the opening between the true vocal cords. The diameter of this opening is regulated by the laryngeal muscles to modulate the pitch of sound. The piriform fossa is a shallow space found on the lateral side of the laryngeal opening and is bounded laterally by the thyroid cartilage and medially by the aryepiglottic fold. Although a vestibule can mean any opening, in the head and neck, it refers to the anterior portion of the oral cavity. The vallecula is a depression behind the root of the tongue that holds saliva for lubrication and prevention of premature initiation of the deglutition reflex.

2. **A.** Patients with midface fractures have distorted anatomy. The sinus walls are thin and abut up against the brain. Attempts to place a nasogastric tube (NGT) in this situation may result in intracranial damage or infection. Distorted anatomy is also the reason NGT placement is contraindicated in patients who have undergone bariatric surgery. A bariatric surgeon should be consulted prior to placement of an NGT in these patients. Hematemesis in patients with cirrhosis may have a number of sources, including ulcers, Mallory-Weiss syndrome, and gastric or esophageal varices caused by portal hypertension. The placement of an NGT in such a patient is inadvisable because of the danger of rupturing varices, if present. A gastroenterologist should be consulted prior to attempting NGT placement in such cases. There are several ways bleeding varices are treated, such as by performing a banding procedure via endoscopy or by sclerotherapy.

CHAPTER 35. Paronychia Incision and Drainage

1. **C.** The common palmar digital branch comes off the superficial branch of the ulnar nerve and supplies the skin of the little finger and the medial side of the ring finger. The superficial branch of the radial nerve provides cutaneous innervation to the radial (lateral) dorsum of the hand and the thumb, index finger, and lateral middle finger over the proximal phalanx. The common palmar digital branch of the median nerve innervates most of the lateral aspect of the palmar hand and the dorsal aspect of the second and third fingers as well as the lateral part of the fourth digit. The deep radial nerve supplies the extensor carpi radialis brevis and supinator muscles and continues as the posterior interosseous nerve. The recurrent branch of the median nerve supplies the abductor pollicis brevis, flexor pollicis brevis, and opponens pollicis muscles.

2. **A.** The matrix of the nail is the layer of the nail where the nerves and vessels run. The pain experienced by this patient would therefore be due to the irritation of these small digital nerves supplying the nail region.

CHAPTER 36. Skin Abscess Incision and Drainage

1. **C.** This is a typical presentation of *Staphylococcus aureus* infecting the skin and the soft tissue, producing bullous impetigo. Areas of erythema develop into bullae filled with cloudy fluid.

These bullae often rupture, producing a characteristic honey-colored crust.

2. **C.** As noted above, this is a case of bullous impetigo and the drug of choice is a cephalosporin.

3. **A.** A fluctuant mass in the neck requires surgical evaluation because it may not be a simple abscess. Incising it without prior imaging (eg, ultrasound or computed tomography) risks major bleeding if it is a hemangioma or any other vascular tumor.

CHAPTER 37. Shoulder Joint Aspiration

1. **C.** The tendon of the long head of the biceps brachii muscle passes through the glenohumeral joint surrounded by the synovial membrane. The glenohumeral ligament attaches to the glenoid labrum. The long head of the triceps brachii arises from the infraglenoid tubercle beneath the glenoid cavity. The infraspinatus tendon passes posterior to the head of the humerus to insert on the greater tubercle. The coracobrachialis arises from the coracoid process and inserts on the humerus.

2. **D.** The patient is suffering from subacromial (or subdeltoid) bursitis. If pain on palpation is less when the arm has been elevated to the horizontal, the bursitis may be thought of as being more subacromial, that is, associated more with the supraspinatus tendon, because such a bursa may be drawn back under the acromion when the limb is abducted. The subscapular bursa, beneath the subscapularis muscle, would not present with superficial pain. It can communicate with the glenohumeral joint cavity. Inflammation or arthritic changes within the glenohumeral joint present as more generalized shoulder pain than this patient has. The teres minor muscle and tendon are located inferior to the point of marked discomfort.

3. **A.** The supraspinatus initiates abduction of the arm during the first 15 degrees of motion. Palpation of the tendon during this phase would result in pain from a supraspinatus tendinopathy.

CHAPTER 38. Transurethral (Foley Catheter) and Suprapubic Urinary Bladder Catheterization

1. **B.** If the membranous portion of the urethra is injured, urine and blood can leak upward into the retropubic space (of Retzius). It is limited inferiorly by the urogenital diaphragm and the muscle within (compressor urethrae), which would also be injured. The bulbospongiosus muscle and other perineal muscles, the corpus cavernosum, and the openings of the bulbourethral ducts are inferior and anterior to the region of injury.

2. **C.** The retropubic space (of Retzius) is the extraperitoneal space between the pubic symphysis and the bladder. A needle inserted above the pubic bone through the abdominal wall and into the space of Retzius will enter the full bladder but not the peritoneum. There is little risk of damaging major organs or vessels. Entry through the ischioanal fossa would not provide a direct route to the bladder. Entering through the superficial perineal cleft, perineal body, and deep perineal pouch carries a high risk of damaging important structures.

3. **C.** The superficial perineal space or cleft lies between the external perineal fascia of Gallaudet (fascia of the inferior perineal muscles in the superficial perineal compartment) and the membranous layer of Colles' fascia. Camper's fascia is the superficial fatty layer of the anterior abdominal wall and the perineum. Scarpa's fascia is the deep membranous layer of the abdominal wall. The perineal membrane is the inferior fascia of the urogenital diaphragm that forms the inferior boundary of the deep perineal

compartment. The superior fascia of the urogenital diaphragm bounds the inferior border of the anterior recess of the ischioanal fossa. There is no space between the urogenital diaphragm and the apex of the prostate gland.

4. **A.** Rupture of the spongy urethra leads to the accumulation of fluid (edema) in the superficial perineal cleft. The continuity of Colles' fascia (superficial membranous layer of the superficial perineal fascia) with Scarpa's fascia on the abdominal wall allows fluid to spread upward along the wall. Rupture of the pre-prostatic urethra, prostatic urethra, or urinary bladder would lead to fluid accumulation within the pelvis because these are not located in the perineum. Damage to the ureter would manifest in the abdomen or pelvis, depending upon the level of rupture.

Index

NOTE: Page numbers followed by f or t indicate figures or tables, respectively.